Postpartum Depression For Dummies®

P9-CKL-591

Ten Ways to Get Through the Day

Use these ideas to help you simplify your day and ease the overwhelming feelings you're probably having.

- **Make a short list of three tasks to accomplish each day.** For instance, set out to feed the baby, take a shower, and eat lunch.
- **Lower your expectations to a realistic level.** For example, use paper plates, order dinner out, and forget about sending baby announcements.
- **Repeat the positive statements on this Cheat Sheet** (or create and repeat your own).
- **Ask for help.** Odds are that people around you are politely waiting for you to call on them for help and would be delighted to, for example, pick something up at the store, babysit, make lunch, or fold your laundry for you.
- **Accept help that's offered.** When your neighbor, friend, relative, or other kind soul asks if he or she can do anything for you, practice saying, "yes!" and give them a specific task that would help you.
- **Gather the clutter (toys, baby blankets, and so on) into laundry baskets** instead of putting it all away, since it will all be on the floor again tomorrow.
- **Take breaks from tasks** (including taking care of your baby) when someone else is in charge.
- **Take your baby for a 15-minute walk** outside during the day (more than once if you're up to it) to help clear your head. Be sure to focus on breathing in lots of fresh air.
- **Set your alarm to go off with your favorite music** 15 minutes before your baby usually wakes up (it's worth it, trust me) so you can stretch your muscles, shower, and start your day in a peaceful way.
- **Drink lots of water and nibble high-quality protein** such as turkey, chicken, fish, or eggs (see Chapter 11 for more ideas) throughout the day.

Ten Truths to Remind Yourself Of Often

Carry this list around until these statements come naturally to you (then you know you don't need the list anymore!). Feel free to replace the underlined part of each statement with your own words. If you have difficulty truly believing any of these statements, review them and add your own spin on them with the help of a therapist.

- I'm a good mom because <u>I'm trying to get well and I care about my family</u>.
- I'm a good mom because <u>I'm getting help for myself and my child(ren) will benefit</u>.
- It's important to be kind to myself because <u>it will speed up my recovery</u>.
- I will take care of myself because <u>I need my strength to take care of my family</u>.
- I'm taking care of myself by <u>reading this book, seeing a therapist, and asking for help from others</u>.
- I have support people who <u>care about me and who are cheering me on</u>.
- I will ask for help and accept it because <u>that's what healthy people do</u>.
- This is only temporary — I'm looking forward to <u>enjoying my life</u>.
- I will follow the plan for recovery in this book because <u>I look forward to enjoying my life</u>.
- I know I'll get well because <u>I'm following an excellent recovery plan</u>.
- I know I'm not alone because <u>almost one in five mothers around the world has it too</u>.

Foods to Boost Your Mood

- Avocados
- Bananas
- Barley
- Chicken
- Dark chocolate
- Dried apricots
- Lentils
- Ocean fish (cold water)
- Rye crackers
- Turkey

BESTSELLING
BOOK SERIES

Postpartum Depression
For Dummies®

Cheat
Sheet

My Support Team

Although it's important to list the contact info of your professional support, it's just as important to list the everyday members of your team, even though you probably know them by heart. For each of the following members, list both a name and number.

Therapist

_____   _____

Doctors

_____   _____

_____   _____

Child care (babysitter/nanny/doula)

_____   _____

_____   _____

Support lines

Postpartum Stressline: 888-678-2669

Postpartum Support International: 800-944-4773   _____

National Hopeline Network: 800-773-6667   _____

Partner

_____   _____
              Work   Mobile

Close family members

_____   _____

_____   _____

Friends

_____   _____

_____   _____

Neighbors

_____   _____

_____   _____

Other important support people

_____   _____

_____   _____

Copyright © 2007 Wiley Publishing, Inc. All rights reserved. Item 7335-3.

For more information about Wiley Publishing, call 1-800-762-2974.

For Dummies: Bestselling Book Series for Beginners

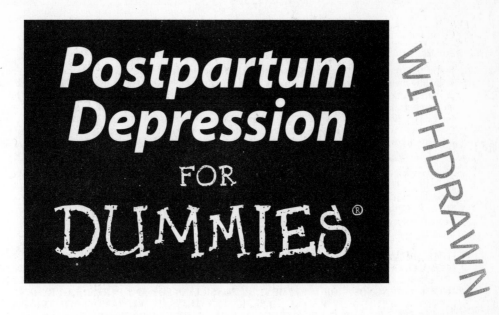

Postpartum Depression FOR DUMMIES®

by Shoshana S. Bennett, PhD

Foreword by Mary Jo Codey
Former First Lady of New Jersey

1807
WILEY
2007

Wiley Publishing, Inc.

Postpartum Depression For Dummies®

Published by
Wiley Publishing, Inc.
111 River St.
Hoboken, NJ 07030-5774
www.wiley.com

For general information on our other products and services, please contact our Customer Care Department within the U.S. at 800-762-2974, outside the U.S. at 317-572-3993, or fax 317-572-4002.

For technical support, please visit www.wiley.com/techsupport.

Wiley also publishes its books in a variety of electronic formats. Some content that appears in print may not be available in electronic books.

Library of Congress Control Number: 2006936818

ISBN-13: 978-0-470-07335-3

Manufactured in the United States of America

10 9 8 7 6 5 4 3 2 1

1O/RY/RS/QW/IN

WILEY

About the Author

Shoshana S. Bennett, PhD, is a licensed psychologist who founded Postpartum Assistance for Mothers in 1987 after her second undiagnosed postpartum illness. Dr. Bennett is the immediate past president of Postpartum Support International and the past president of California's state organization, Postpartum Health Alliance. She is a noted guest lecturer and keynote speaker, and her work has been the subject of numerous newspaper articles around the country.

Dr. Bennett has been a featured guest on national radio and television shows, including ABC's *20/20*. For years, her popular talk radio show *Mom's Health Matters* was heard worldwide, and, like her current tele-classes, focused mainly on subjects pertaining to pregnancy, postpartum, and parenting. She's also the coauthor of *Beyond the Blues: A Guide to Understanding and Treating Prenatal and Postpartum Depression* (Moodswings Press).

For 15 years prior to her current profession, Dr. Shoshana was a college instructor in the fields of special education, early childhood development, rehabilitation therapies, and psychology. In addition to three teaching credentials, she holds her second masters degree in psychology and a doctorate in clinical counseling.

Dr. Shoshana is available for speaking engagements, workshops, and telephone consultations. You can contact her through her Web site at www.postpartumdepressionhelp.com.

Dedication

To my daughter, Elana, whose beautiful and persevering spirit not only survived, but is thriving despite my emotional absence for so many years. And to my son, Aaron, whose love of learning and passion for self-growth propels me to demand the best from myself.

Author's Acknowledgments

I am especially grateful to the following people:

My children, who continue to be my best teachers — about being a mother and about remembering what is important.

My wonderful clients, who, by allowing me the gift of helping them recover, give my own suffering with postpartum depression a purpose and meaning.

My husband, who was the smiling, upbeat parent for our babies when I was ill and who has always supported me in pursuing my mission to pioneer in the field of postpartum depression.

My sisters, who encouraged me throughout the process of writing *Postpartum Depression For Dummies* by frequently checking in with love and care.

My dad, who has been an inspiration and role model, for expecting excellence in all my pursuits. And my mom (I miss her dearly), who showed me what unconditional love is all about.

My research assistant Laura Strathman Hulka, who checked facts and produced whatever obscure pieces of information I needed with lightning speed and thoroughness. And the enlightened editors at Wiley for understanding how important it is to add this topic into the *For Dummies* series and for helping me to bring the book to fruition: Jacky Sach, Tracy Boggier, Kristin DeMint, and Jessica Smith. Also, a big thank-you to Marlene P. Freeman, MD, who served as the technical reviewer of this book and lent her expertise to make sure I covered everything important for you to know.

Publisher's Acknowledgments

We're proud of this book; please send us your comments through our Dummies online registration form located at www.dummies.com/register/.

Some of the people who helped bring this book to market include the following:

Acquisitions, Editorial, and Media Development

Project Editor: Kristin DeMint

Acquisitions Editor: Tracy Boggier

Copy Editor: Jessica Smith

Technical Editor: Marlene P. Freeman, MD

Senior Editorial Manager: Jennifer Ehrlich

Editorial Assistants: Erin Calligan, Joe Niesen, Leeann Harney

Cover Photos: © Digital Vision/Getty Images

Cartoons: Rich Tennant (www.the5thwave.com)

Composition Services

Project Coordinator: Jennifer Theriot

Layout and Graphics: Lavonne Cook, Joyce Haughey, Barry Offringa, Laura Pence

Anniversary Logo Design: Richard Pacifico

Proofreaders: Charles Spencer, Techbooks

Indexer: Techbooks

Publishing and Editorial for Consumer Dummies

    Diane Graves Steele, Vice President and Publisher, Consumer Dummies

    Joyce Pepple, Acquisitions Director, Consumer Dummies

    Kristin A. Cocks, Product Development Director, Consumer Dummies

    Michael Spring, Vice President and Publisher, Travel

    Kelly Regan, Editorial Director, Travel

Publishing for Technology Dummies

    Andy Cummings, Vice President and Publisher, Dummies Technology/General User

Composition Services

    Gerry Fahey, Vice President of Production Services

    Debbie Stailey, Director of Composition Services

Contents at a Glance

Table of Contents

Foreword

*P*ostpartum depression — possibly more than any other mental illness — is a very private pain. Private because you can't believe you feel so empty and depressed at a time when you're supposed to feel so happy and fulfilled. You're afraid of appearing to be ungrateful, selfish, immature, or worse: A bad mother. So, you don't want to confide in anyone.

I thought I was all these things and more. I wasted a lot of time and energy on self-blame, believing my depression was caused by a personal failure or weakness — or both.

Don't do this to yourself. No one should have to go through that kind of anguish and humiliation. Accept the reality of PPD as an illness and recovery will be easier. Trust me. PPD is a mental illness, and mental illnesses have *nothing* to do with blame.

PPD doesn't care how ready and willing you are to have a baby. It strikes without regard for age, race, education, or economic background. And it robs you — and your family — of what should be a joyful time. As a mother, you deserve to fully enjoy your new baby. Your baby deserves a healthy mother who can provide the love and care he or she needs.

Back in 1984, when I experienced the first of my two bouts with PPD, I had no idea what it was. It wasn't something people talked about. I frantically searched every book about pregnancy and childbirth I could get my hands on for information about depression after giving birth. All I could find on the subject was a single paragraph that basically said "If your wife has postpartum depression, watch out! She's likely to accuse you of having an affair!"

Thankfully, the dark ages are over. *Postpartum Depression For Dummies* does the groundwork to help you get through this insidious illness. Think of it as a survival guide that arms you with practical, easy-to-understand information so you can avoid being trapped in your private pain the way I was.

Mary Jo Codey
Former First Lady of New Jersey

Introduction

. . . .

My family and I are survivors of my two life-threatening encounters with postpartum depression (PPD). After realizing that what I had been suffering from had a name and that it was unnecessary for my family and I to suffer for years, I vowed to myself that I would never let another woman go through this devastation if I could help it. It became my life's mission to educate women, their families, and health professionals about this affliction. When I started coming out of my second round of PPD in 1987, I began running PPD support groups out of my Northern California living room. (Up until that point, I taught special education and early child-hood development at local community colleges.)

After making my vow to help other women and their families, I went back to school and earned a second master's degree and a PhD. Then, fueled by my passion, I went on to become licensed as a clinical psychologist. Not counting the telephone classes I have led, since 1987 I have assisted over 15,000 women in dealing with and recovering from PPD.

My guiding star for two decades now has been identifying and treating women with PPD as quickly as possible so they could begin to once again enjoy their lives and families. So, when the wise and competent folks behind the *For Dummies* series approached me to write this book, I jumped at the chance. I knew that such a book would reach many more women than I could personally assist. And with this book, I hoped that women and their families wouldn't have to unnecessarily suffer for years — like I and my family did — from undiagnosed and untreated PPD.

About This Book

This book is intended for anyone who has PPD or thinks that he or she knows someone who has it. This includes women who have recently given birth, as well as their partners, family members, and friends. It's also a great resource for pregnant women, couples, and family members of pregnant women. In short, this book is meant for any women (and their friends and families) who may be at risk for PPD, which can be as many as one out of every five women who give birth.

However, this book isn't meant to be a medical textbook. Instead, like all *For Dummies* books, this one's meant to be an easily accessible and digestible guide that, no matter what page you turn to, can be immediately put to practical use. Even though this book isn't meant to be a textbook, my hope is that medical and mental health professionals will pick it up and benefit from what's inside (especially those who don't really believe in PPD).

The primary goal behind this book, then, is to enable you to understand the nature of PPD, and to help those suffering from it to recover as quickly and effectively as possible. I want you to know what to expect from PPD, including how this illness tends to behave, what the general treatments look like, and how to proceed through the recovery process. Although recovery can happen quickly, it won't be overnight, so I want you to have reasonable expectations about what's likely and what's possible.

Conventions Used in This Book

To help you navigate easily through this book (because I know how scrambled your mind can feel when you have PPD), I set up a few conventions that I use consistently throughout the book:

- Anytime I want to highlight new words or terms that I define in the text, I *italicize* them.
- **Boldfaced** text is used to indicate the action part of numbered steps and the keywords of a bulleted list.
- I use `monofont` for Web sites and e-mail addresses.

When this book was printed, some Web addresses may have needed to break across two lines of text. If you come across these instances, rest assured that I haven't put in any extra characters (such as hyphens) to indicate the break. So, when using one of these Web addresses, just type in exactly what you see in this book, pretending as if the line break doesn't exist.

You'll also notice that I refer to a mom's partner quite often throughout the book. As much as possible, I used the gender-neutral reference because I fully understand the fact that nowadays many couples are same-sex parents (and a good number of the couples I've counseled are same-sex parents). Sometimes, though, being politically correct is extremely tedious in writing, so in those cases, I used the masculine form — please note that this usage was only a technicality, though, and I in no way am leaving anyone out of the picture.

Finally, if I tell you that a client or some other person told me something, you can be sure that it's exactly what he or she told me. Unlike some books discussing mental health issues, I don't use composites of clients — pulling a little bit from Client A's history, a little bit from what Client B told me, and a little bit from what I read in a journal — to illustrate a point. If I tell you that something happened to a client, it really happened.

What You're Not to Read

Everything in this book has value — otherwise, I wouldn't have written it or included it. However, you may want to skip over some parts of the book, especially if you're pressed for time or don't have a need for certain types of technical or detailed information. Helpful but unnecessary information is usually denoted by a Technical Stuff icon or is highlighted in its own separate sidebar, which will be shaded gray.

Similarly, keep an eye out for my personal experiences, which I highlight with the Anecdote icon. This icon flags information that's extremely helpful and useful, but nonessential to your understanding of PPD.

Finally, if you're the one going through PPD, you may want to skip Chapter 16, which is intended for friends, family members, and partners of new moms suffering from PPD. On the other hand, you may actually find it useful to read about things from the perspective of those who love and know you best.

Foolish Assumptions

As any author does, I had some assumptions in my mind about you, the likely reader of this book, as I was writing it. By putting forth the following assumptions, I hope you'll feel liberated to make the best possible use of the material in this book:

- ✔ A lot of you have either been diagnosed with PPD or think that you may have PPD (or you're a family member or friend of someone who has it or who may have it).

- ✔ If you're pretty sure you have PPD, you're willing to talk to a qualified medical or mental health practitioner as soon as you can, and in any case, you won't make any kinds of major life changes or start with any kinds of medications (especially illegally obtained ones) without consulting a practitioner.

- ✔ You want to understand more about PPD, and you want an inside look at this all-too-common disorder from a trained psychology professional and from someone who intimately knows what you or your loved one is going through.

- ✔ You want to know that there's hope and light at the end of the tunnel. But, having said that, I also assume that you're ready to do what it takes to reach that light.

How This Book Is Organized

This book is divided into six parts to help you find information quickly and easily — whether you need general info on PPD or specific info on a certain treatment. The following sections give you a brief overview of the six parts.

Part 1: Bringing Postpartum Depression into the Light: What It's All About

Motherhood is challenging even without a mood disorder. So, in this part, I help you out by discussing the normal transitions of motherhood and then move into the basics of postpartum depression — who gets it and why and how you can tell the difference between the baby blues and PPD. I also describe the other five postpartum mood disorders so you can identify where you're at in the mix.

Part II: The Three Little Letters: PPD and You

After you've identified what you're experiencing, you can use this part to tune in to your thoughts and start turning the negative into the positive. Here in this part, I discuss the importance of seeing a competent professional, how and where to find one, the different types of therapists to pick from, and what to expect when you go to see one. Because hearing a diagnosis of PPD can provoke a wide variety of reactions, I mention many of them so that you can be prepared (or have something to identify with if you've already been there and done that).

Part III: Diagnosis Confirmed: Looking at the Treatment Options for PPD

In this part, I answer all your questions regarding treatment — whether you want to know about psychological, medical, or alternative treatments. For example, because there are four different types of groups that you might join for support, it's helpful knowing what to expect from each so you can choose well. Then I take you on a tour of medical and alternative treatments, including medications and herbs that are considered safe with breastfeeding. Finally, I round out the part with a chapter that shows you how to create a comprehensive plan for recovery.

Part IV: Traveling the Road to Recovery

Hopefully by the time you reach this part you're seeing a wonderful therapist. Here, I show you how to maximize your treatment to speed things along. I include a number of self-help tips as well — for example, eating specific foods, understanding the good and bad ways to exercise, and knowing how to let go of unrealistic expectations. Because emotional and physical support is so important to a new mom who's suffering from PPD, I also give you ideas about who to lean on, and I outline how to help your partner (if you have one) help you. The last chapter in this part is specifically written for the family and friends of the woman suffering with PPD.

Part V: Moving Beyond PPD

When all of your hard work has paid off and you've made it to the other side of the dark PPD tunnel, you're ready for specific suggestions on how to adjust back into your life — your new life. If you're contemplating having another baby in the future, I give you healthy ways to approach this important decision, including all the pros and cons. Plus, I show you the best way to develop a plan that will ensure a positive outcome (if you decide to go forward).

Part VI: The Part of Tens

In this part, which is great for quick and practical pieces of information, you can check out the most common fantasies of motherhood (see which ones you believed in before becoming a mom!). I also include a list of my favorite empowering thoughts to help you get through your day.

Icons Used In This Book

Throughout this book, I use icons in the margins to quickly relay certain types of information to you. Here are the icons you'll see and a short description of each.

When you see this icon, you'll know that I'm disclosing personal information regarding my own journey (or my patients' journeys) through this devastating illness to illustrate a particular point.

These reminders highlight the information that's good to jot down on your pad of notes (or that's just good to keep in mind as you go down the road to recovery).

I use this icon to flag a piece of interesting, but nonessential, information, such as the results of research or an experiment.

 This icon points out useful tidbits and practical advice.

 Because this icon alerts you when you need to be particularly careful about something, don't skip these icons!

Where to Go from Here

This book is written in a modular style, which means you can flip to any chapter and get a great deal of value from it without having read the chapters before it. However, for some of you — especially those in the medical or mental health professions, or those who have a friend or family member who may have PPD but who isn't in crisis — reading this book from start to finish will provide the most value. Otherwise, if you know what topic you're looking for, take a glance at the index or table of contents to find out where to find it.

If you're a new mom or a soon-to-be mom, you'll probably want to start with Chapter 1 because here new mom issues are truthfully stated, myths are busted, and the facts about PPD being a real illness are presented. If you have PPD, or think that you might, and you're feeling desperate for information, skip to Chapter 2, where I give you the lowdown on PPD.

Here's your first tip: If you're reading this book because you think you have PPD, before reading on, you may want to grab a pad of paper and a special pen or highlighter so that you can take notes and do the various exercises suggested throughout the book. Use this pad and pen as often as you like — and as often as you can — and refer to your notes frequently to see just how far you've progressed. If at any time you find the book overwhelming, just put it down. And only pick it up when you're ready to start reading again. Or, when you're ready, you can have someone else read it to you.

In some cases, *Postpartum Depression For Dummies* may be all that you need to recover from PPD. For most women, however, psychotherapy and perhaps medical treatment will enable a much faster and more effective recovery. What's most important for you to know, however, is that if you follow the suggestions in this book and get proper help, you'll indeed recover fully and completely from your postpartum crisis. Keep the faith, and read on!

Part I
Bringing Postpartum Depression into the Light: What It's All About

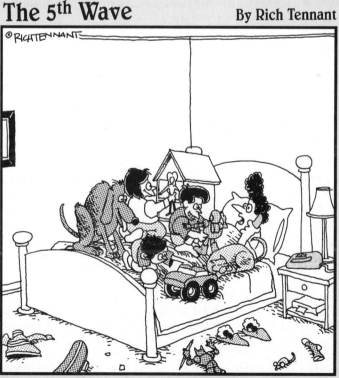

The 5th Wave   By Rich Tennant

"Normally things don't get me down. But lately, just getting out of bed has been difficult."

In this part . . .

Motherhood is an adjustment for any new mom, whether or not she has a postpartum mood disorder. So, this part gives you the lowdown on what to expect (consider this a friendly reminder if you've already been through the experience). I also discuss the difference between the baby blues and postpartum depression (PPD). Finally, I give you an overview of the six different kinds of postpartum disorders that can afflict a new mom.

Chapter 1

The Big Adjustment: Welcome to Motherhood

*E*ven if you're not hearing the "sound of music" as you read these words, it makes sense to start at the very beginning. And the very beginning, for purposes of this book — and for human life as we know it —is none other than motherhood. Yes, motherhood, that mythic time of life when everything goes according to plan, everyone is always happy, and things just couldn't be better.

Or, at least, that's what popular culture repeatedly implies. (Just last night I saw a commercial with a smiling, drop-dead gorgeous new mom bathing her infant and saying, "I never thought the love of my life would be bald and short.") But as anyone who has ever given birth or grappled with the demands of that new human life can tell you, this Shangri-La version of motherhood is more of an ideal than a realistic view of what to expect. This isn't to say that you won't also occasionally experience incredible joy and have peak experiences that would make the Dalai Lama jealous. On top of the usual busting of unrealistic expectations of motherhood, postpartum depression (PPD) adds a heavy layer. To be assaulted with PPD is a huge disappointment, to say the least — more of a shock, devastation, and feeling of failure to most.

Plain and simple, knowledge is power. Although the medical world still has many unanswered questions about postpartum depression, there's a growing consensus about many of PPD's general parameters and characteristics. By understanding a bit of what's known about the illness, you can go a long way toward empowering yourself to face this ailment. If you happen to be a partner, family member, or friend of a new mom who you think may be suffering from PPD, you can use the information in this chapter (and throughout the rest of this book) to make an informed decision about how you can best support that new mom and what steps, if any, you should take.

The Reality of Motherhood: Let Bootie Camp Begin!

On one hand, a whole world of popular culture continually puts forth a Disneyland version of motherhood. On the other hand, there's reality, which brings with it a whole slew of things that the same culture conveniently neglects to tell the new mom or mom-to-be. It's almost as if there's a collective conspiracy of silence dedicated to keeping new moms and moms-to-be in the dark so that no one scares them or frightens them off from willingly reproducing!

It would be impossible to make a complete list of everything that society typically glosses over when briefing new moms on what to expect of their new lives, but take a look at just a handful of important points every mom (or soon-to-be-mom) needs to know:

- **Labor and delivery is unlike anything you've ever experienced.** For some women, labor and delivery go pretty smoothly, but for others it's a huge ordeal. In any case, it will be intense and only barely resemble the 30-second video you may have seen in your childbirth class where a woman seems to take a few deep breaths and then it's over and the room fills with laughter and hugs all around. Even if you've already given birth once, you're unlikely to remember just how intense, difficult, or painful it was until it's happening again.

- **Being a mom, especially a new one, is exceptionally difficult work on many levels.**

  - **Physically:** As you're probably well aware, even though you're sleep-deprived, you still have the primary responsibility for taking care of a brand new baby. And that completely helpless human life form (why is it that of all the animals on this planet, human beings are the most helpless at birth?) has lots and lots of needs, from feeding to comfort and cleaning. And those responsibilities don't even factor in everything you've been responsible for pre-children.

  - **Psychologically and emotionally:** Even without a postpartum mood disorder, given the biochemical changes you've been subjected to and are still experiencing, plus the huge life change, you're likely to experience intense ups and downs as you adjust to your new life.

- **You might love your baby but hate the job.** It's completely normal to feel bored with the mundane, unstimulating maintenance tasks you're managing. Your feelings aren't personal towards your baby, though, and have nothing to do with your relationship with her.

- **Your time is no longer your own.** You can't just go out to the movies, have lunch with your friends, or take a trip whenever you want to. Instead, you have to factor in your baby's needs and well-being every time you make a decision about how to spend your time. And if you think you can bring Baby with you on all your ventures without much hassle, think again.

- **You're likely to encounter additional simultaneous challenges and pressures that you never expected.** No matter how well you've planned, and how supportive and stable your home environment is, you can be almost certain that a variety of substantial and unexpected challenges will emerge— from the financial and logistical to the emotional and even the spiritual. These challenges will test you on multiple levels simultaneously.

- **Being a new mother is *not* supposed to be the happiest time in your life.** Contrary to the persistent myth, it's only fair to say that new motherhood will be one of the most *challenging* times in your life.

ANECDOTE

Let the unsolicited opinion-giving begin!

As a new mother, you'll be amazed at how others will feel completely justified as they thrust upon you endless unsolicited opinions (they may have even started during your pregnancy). Throughout this book, I give you practical tips for allowing these rude and ridiculous comments to roll off your back. You're probably highly sensitive right now, so it may be more challenging at first. Just start practicing what you'd say if you heard, "Can't you keep your baby quiet?" or "Don't breastfeed in public — that's disgusting!" or "When are you having your next one?" Trust me — you may as well get ready for 1,000 earsful.

After my daughter Elana was finally delivered — my six-and-a-half-day labor ended with a successful C-section — I called my friend Leslie to tell her the good news. The anesthesia was still wearing off, and as you can imagine, I felt as if my body and my mind had been blown apart. Holding back the tears, I choked out the words "Leslie, Elana was born. I have my daughter." But instead of any kind of congratulatory or joyful response, the first thing out of Leslie's mouth was "Did you have her naturally?" Taken off guard, I briefly told her what had happened, and she replied very solemnly, "It's okay, you can always try again next time." I quickly ended the call and had to orient myself: Had someone died, or had someone just been born? Was I supposed to be mourning because I didn't have the "right" experience the way my "friend" defined it? Had I failed, or should I be celebrating the birth of my daughter?

On some level you may think that you should be giving all your time and energy to your baby. But ultimately, this won't work. It will merely exhaust you and deprive you of your joie de vivre. You won't be doing anyone — your baby, your partner, your other family members, your friends, and yourself — any favors by taking yourself off of your own to do list. Say goodbye to the old, and hello to the new, but somewhere in the middle, you have to remember the necessity of supporting yourself. This book spells out how you can, in a very practical way, make sure that happens.

The Reality of Postpartum Depression (PPD)

Allow me to start off head-to-head with the Big Question of the day (at least in pop culture, anyway): Does PPD exist, or is it a hoax that a bunch of new moms made up in order to get a little sympathy and to shirk off the hard work that being a new mom requires? As the history of diagnosing PPD shows, there's a long (and dishonorable) tradition of pooh-poohing the whole thing, a tradition that has caused untold numbers of mothers and their families to suffer far beyond what was necessary.

On a more positive note, although it's estimated that up to 50 percent of all cases of PPD still go undetected and women suffer in silence, the good news is that the U.S. is going in the right direction. PPD is finally beginning to receive more of the attention it deserves both in research and in doctors' offices.

Approximately 4 million babies are born in the United States per year, and along with many of them comes a postpartum mood disorder (affecting Mom, of course, not Baby). PPD is the most common, and statistically speaking, it strikes about 15 percent (in the medical literature the range shown is between 10 and 20 percent) of all new mothers. This is true for women in all countries and all cultures, and seems to hold fairly steady regardless of ethnic group, religious affiliation, class or education level, or any other distinguishing factors except age and socioecomonic status. (The lack of social, partner, and financial support available to teenage and low income moms is a strong risk factor and raises the percentage of PPD in these populations.)

PPD can also happen to any mom regardless of her medical, emotional, and psychological history. Unfortunately, no woman is immune. I sometimes hear women say "I won't get PPD. I'm not the type." But, this is wishful thinking because even though some are more prone than others, there's no "type" of woman who ends up with PPD.

Believe it or not, PPD is more common than gestational diabetes, preterm delivery, and pre-eclampsia. Being the most common complication of pregnancy, PPD affects at least 400,000 mothers every year in the U.S. alone. (For a comparative glimpse at the most common pregnancy-related complications and their frequency, check out Figure 1-1.)

In addition to the psychological harm that PPD can cause, there are potential physiological costs to the human body that not even the biggest doubter of the reality of depression can deny. Depression either causes, or is, at least, linked to changes in blood pressure; increases in stress hormones, such as cortisol and adrenaline; and increased risk of heart disease, among others.

The point here isn't to worry about these things. Instead, the point is that even the most stubborn scientific types — those who embrace only hard, physical facts and who tend to downplay or deny the reality of things that can't be touched or measured by X-ray — would be hard-pressed to deny that depression doesn't potentially cause some negative effects to the human body. So whether or not your doctor (or you) believe in the life of the mind and the spirit, if, as you read through this book, you find that you have PPD or are at high risk for it, you'll have plenty of hardcore physical-level justification for why you should take action sooner rather than later.

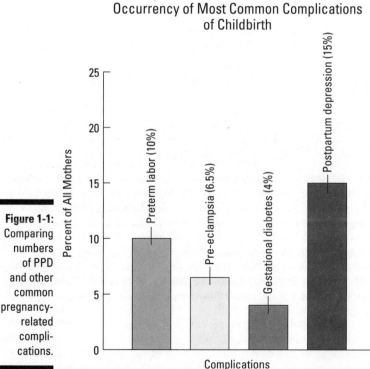

Figure 1-1: Comparing numbers of PPD and other common pregnancy-related complications.

Occurrency of Most Common Complications of Childbirth

The gender factor: A case for PPD

It's a known fact in the medical community that depression is twice as common in women as it is in men. The highest incidence occurs during the reproductive years (ages 25 to 45), and researchers don't think that's any coincidence.

Because there's a high frequency of depression before menstruation begins, before menopause, during pregnancy, and right after delivery, most researchers agree that there's a link between the reproductive hormones and depression.

Debunking Denial: A Glimpse from Yours Truly

Unfortunately a double-standard still exists between how society regards the physical health conditions that can be measured through a blood test or an X-ray and those that are considered to be mental illnesses. Researchers and practitioners in the field accept that PPD is quite physical (they can't yet measure it through a blood test, though). Nevertheless, many people still buy into that absurd stigma that because much of PPD manifests itself emotionally, somehow it's a sign of weakness and should be under the control of the person.

The real facts, however, are these:

✓ **PPD unquestionably exists, and it affects roughly one in every five new moms.** Ever since I began recovering in 1987 from my second life-threatening bout with PPD and all the way up to the present, I've been studying every piece of reliable research on the subject from all over the world. The articles I've written for different organizations and agencies in many countries contain the same basic information, because the women in their countries are experiencing the same symptoms.

✓ **PPD has physical (biochemical and hormonal) as well as psychological and emotional causes.** Although researchers devoting their professional careers to the field of PPD hold varying theories regarding the biochemical causes of PPD, no one disagrees that the brain chemistry of women who suffer with this illness has undergone powerful physiological changes. Although researchers believe that shifting hormone levels and changes in the hypothalamus and pituitary gland are involved, they still have much to discover regarding exactly what's happening and to whom — enter the annual conferences of international postpartum organizations, which are hopping with passionate folks eager to drink up the latest morsels of data from new research. Regarding the psychosocial causes, quite a bit of research shows specific risk factors, such as a personal or family history of depression, poor social support (especially poor partner support), and isolation. You find more about risk factors in detail in Chapter 2.

✔ **PPD isn't anybody's fault.** Contrary to what many suffering parents may think, PPD is entirely beyond their control, and they're in no way responsible for it. As with any other mood disorder, you didn't cause it, so if you're blaming yourself, stop. You wouldn't wish this on yourself or anybody else. You didn't ask for this or want it to happen — nor did anyone else want this to happen to you. And you're not responsible for your genes, either. If you have a family history of depression, you're no more responsible for being hard-wired for depression than you are responsible for your eye color. Now that you have PPD, however, that's not to say you can't do something about making it go away — hence the reason you picked up this book.

✔ **PPD is treatable.** In some cases PPD can be entirely prevented, and in other cases, a much faster recovery occurs with proper intervention and treatment. As with any other illness, the faster you get help, the better your prognosis for a quicker recovery. I have the best job on Earth, because I see women thoroughly recover from this illness every day.

Even though it's clear from my 20 years of professional experience in this field and over 5 years of personal experience battling the illness that all four of these general points are true, society as a whole doesn't always stick to them. The good news, though, is that modern-day society is definitely becoming more enlightened about the subject.

Denial's more than a river in Egypt

Even though society is making strides in coming to terms with PPD, many people still seem to think that it doesn't really exist. If you tell such people about a new mom who's suffering from PPD, they may show they're denial (and ignorance) by saying one of these things:

✔ "She's just feeling down."

✔ "She's just not mature enough to have a baby."

✔ "She's just being selfish and spoiled."

✔ "She just wants to call attention to herself now that the spotlight is on her new baby."

✔ "She'll get over it."

In part, these feelings come from a general societal belief, especially in America, that depression (whether postpartum or not) isn't real, and that almost anyone in any circumstance should be able to pull themselves out of it. For example, someone in this camp may say something like, "Well, I've been depressed too from time to time. So what? Just handle it. Just pull yourself up by your own bootstraps." (For a more detailed examination of that point of view, see Chapter 14.)

I'm a tough cookie, and a believer in taking responsibility and control of whatever you can to make things right. But I promise you that it's downright unhealthy and foolish to try this way of dealing with PPD. The implication with that effort is that it's shameful to ask for help. That idea isn't true at all, and I know you don't want your children growing up believing that. Use your strength to get proper help — you'll save yourself loads of unnecessary suffering, which is the smart and strong way to go about recovery.

Examining denial in other countries and cultures

Although most prevalent in America, these kinds of pick-yourself-up-and-dust-yourself-off perspectives are found in societies all over the world. On many occasions, I've heard partners and family members of depressed post-partum women say things like, "In my country, we don't have postpartum depression." But, rest assured, you haven't chosen the wrong country: Cross-cultural studies have shown that the U.S. isn't the only country that has PPD. Wherever there are women having babies — which is everywhere — a certain percentage of them will inevitably be hit with PPD.

Just as expectations about motherhood differ from culture to culture, attitudes about PPD — the causes, treatments, and the willingness of suffering women to come forward — also differ. PPD has been studied in almost every cultural environment in existence, including cities in North America and in the United Arab Emirates, rural African communities, Asian immigrants in the U.S., and many others.

Denying the reality of body chemical imbalances

For some people, not only is there a denial of depression generally, but there is a denial of the reality of biochemical and hormonal imbalances. These folks, like so many others, feel that a woman with PPD is just making up excuses, and that she just needs to buck up.

Similarly, you'll find those who, again, don't think the problem is biochemical, or they advocate naïve New Age or self-help medical beliefs. Parts of these alternative routes may indeed help the suffering woman, but the simplistic "just do this one thing" mindset isn't helpful at all. The woman's condition, in order to be fully treated, needs to be approached from all angles — biochemically, spiritually, psychologically, and emotionally.

You can align yourself with the universe and buck up all you want, but you simply can't "positive think" your way through PPD or any other kind of serious depression. If you have a mood disorder of some kind, you need to recognize that in all likelihood it has biochemical roots, and that your recovery will come much, much faster if you address it on multiple levels, including the biochemical level.

Celebrities raising awareness of PPD

What do Marie Osmond, Brooke Shields, former New Jersey First Lady Mary Jo Codey, Angelina Jolie, and Brittany Spears have in common? All of these famous moms have let the world know that they've suffered from PPD, and in doing so they have not only raised awareness generally, but have made it more "acceptable" to have PPD. By coming forward and candidly describing their personal experiences with this very real illness, all these women have helped erase the stigma further by illustrating that successful, intelligent, strong women can be hit with PPD — it's an illness, not a weakness.

Brooke Shields' 2005 book, *Down Came the Rain: My Journey Through Postpartum Depression,* was a useful wake-up call for many women who had been suffering in silence (and I highly recommend it). Marie Osmond also wrote a book called *Behind the Smile: My Journey out of Postpartum Depression.* Reading these books can prove useful for the new mom or mom-to-be, but remember that these brave and honest women are actresses and musicians, not medical or psychological experts or professionals.

In May 2005, actor Tom Cruise lambasted Brooke Shields for her use of medications to help her with her postpartum depression. Cruise, famous for being an advocate of his controversial Scientology religion, asserted that he knew the history of psychiatry, that Shields should not have been taking antidepressants, and that he could have helped her out of her depression through the use of vitamins.

The potential downside of these actors and actresses speaking out is that PPD seems to be in vogue now (it's the malady of the month!), and it may eventually end up being trivialized by its association with Hollywood stars. (Just because a new Hollywood mom is having an argument with her husband or separating from him doesn't mean she has PPD.) To emphasize how popular PPD is in the media, note that an interview with me in the "Ask the Expert" section in *Soap Opera Digest* appeared this year, because a character in one of the soaps had PPD. I was thrilled that the network wanted proper information so that the character could be portrayed more accurately.

The good news about these celebrity revelations — and even Tom Cruise's misguided attack on Brooke Shields and rant against psychiatry generally — is that PPD is being brought even further into the public eye. In the long run, all this attention is raising awareness, and hopefully helping more women get the kind of treatment they need in a timely fashion.

Allowing denial to cloud thinking

Denial is powerful and changes the way people think about things. And because many people (and unfortunately some doctors) deny that PPD is a real and serious illness, they have many inaccurate beliefs about PPD. At other times, the problem isn't denial, just lack of proper information. Without good information, lots of well-meaning people (including some professionals), may hold the following beliefs:

- Returning to work will cure it.
- Staying home will cure it.

✔ Breastfeeding will prevent it.

✔ Depressive types are the only ones who get it.

✔ Eventually it goes away by itself.

✔ It occurs only after you have your first baby.

Why some doctors may be hush-hush about PPD

Even if society as a whole tends to be in denial about depression and PPD, at least you can count on your doctor — the one who's making sure your pregnancy goes well, or the one who's following through with you after he helped deliver your baby — to give you the real scoop, right? Wrong. Many doctors are now gaining tools for warning their high-risk patients, but many are still in the dark as to how to handle these situations. Most are eager for the information, such as what to say and what to give their patients as resources — they just don't have it yet.

It's not that most doctors don't recognize the reality of PPD. And it's not that doctors don't understand the potentially harmful effects of depression on the human body. Instead, doctors have the following two major reasons why they tend to avoid the subject of PPD entirely (even if — sometimes *especially if* — the new mom in question seems to be at high risk of coming down with PPD):

✔ **To avoid putting moms or moms-to-be on the defensive:** Often, doctors are afraid that their new mom or mom-to-be patients may become defensive when they're told about PPD. For example, when the patient hears from her doctor about PPD, she may perceive that the doctor is saying that she's going to be a bad mother or that she won't be able to handle motherhood. And that, of course, can make just about anyone defensive.

✔ **To avoid causing unnecessary worry:** The majority of informed doctors tend to not bring up PPD with their patients because they don't want to worry their patients into actually coming down with PPD. This really makes little sense, and is a bit like thinking that pregnancy counseling may make a woman pregnant.

The point here is that information about PPD isn't what needs to be feared. Instead, it's the lack of proper information that can allow a bad situation to keep going or turn worse. If a woman is so obsessive or anxious that merely hearing about the possibility of PPD pushes her over the edge — "Uh-oh, what if I get this? Do I have this? How bad will it be? Do I have it yet? How about now?" — then she already needs professional treatment for her anxiety.

In spite of the reasons for not doing so, it's important for your doctor to clue you in. So, even though your doctor may have avoided the topic altogether, be wary if he's reluctant to talk about it or if he offers little information after you mention your concerns about how you've been feeling. Every doctor should make sure that all of his new mom or mom-to-be patients know about PPD as a matter of standard protocol, and you should expect your doctor to bring it up matter-of-factly, just as he'd bring up other common potential pregnancy disorders, such as gestational diabetes. Your doctor should also reassure you that PPD is nothing to be embarrassed about, nothing that you caused, and nothing that's indicative of a character weakness or deep-down flaw of some kind. If your doctor goes against the grain in any of these areas, you may want to find another healthcare provider. (Chapter 10 discusses all you need to know about your primary provider's role in your treatment if you're indeed experiencing PPD.)

In my own case, had I known in advance that there was something called PPD, that I was at high risk, and that treatment was available, my family and I would have been spared years of pain. So, take heed and make sure you understand where your doctor's coming from.

When Depression Begins in Pregnancy

Clients sometimes say to me, "Dr. Bennett, I think I'm having postpartum depression and my baby isn't even born yet! Is this possible?" My answer: You bet it is. The old belief that pregnancy protects women from depression and anxiety is long gone. Approximately the same percentage of women who suffer from PPD suffer from depression in pregnancy (around 15 percent). In fact, all of the mood disorders listed in Chapter 3 can also occur during pregnancy.

Each year (in the United States alone), about 400,000 women experience PPD, and many of these women had also been depressed in pregnancy. The two camps don't necessarily include the same women. However, some women who are depressed during pregnancy also suffer from PPD — in effect, they just stay depressed from pregnancy through delivery and afterwards. Other women are depressed during pregnancy but don't get PPD, and vice-versa. If a woman has experienced depression in her life before she becomes pregnant, she has a 50 percent risk of experiencing depression in pregnancy. In fact, about one-third of all postpartum mood disorders (PPD being the most prevalent) begin during pregnancy.

Distinguishing between pregnancy hormone changes and PPD

It's easy to dismiss warning signs of these mood problems as simply normal signs of pregnancy. For instance, a loss of appetite could be written off as being due to morning sickness. A big increase in appetite, on the other hand, including cravings for carbohydrates and sugar, could be overlooked as being an expected part of pregnancy. Tiredness, even though you've rested, can be a sign of depression, but too often practitioners quickly assume that this symptom is just normal for pregnancy. Likewise, poor sleep, mood swings, and worry are many times automatically passed off as usual and common.

Sometimes women who report depression are told that "Of course you're emotional. Your hormones are up and down." But, if a pregnant woman is unable to sleep or function or is considering suicide, something needs to be done. And she should be given help long before she feels that bad.

Although a more detailed description of therapeutic interventions for women who are depressed during pregnancy is beyond the scope of this book, as a beginning step, Table 1-1 can help you determine whether a pregnant woman has symptoms that would justify a deeper look and perhaps an immediate therapeutic intervention. You — or your friend, partner, or other family members — shouldn't wait until after the baby is born to seek and receive help.

Table 1-1	How to Tell Whether a Pregnant Woman Is Depressed	
Factor	*Normal During Pregnancy*	*With Depression During Pregnancy*
Tiredness, energy level	She gets tired easily, but if she takes a nap or a rest, it rejuvenates her and she gets her energy back.	It doesn't matter if she takes a nap or how much she rests, she still feels deeply fatigued.
Ability to experience pleasure	Some things may bother her, and her pleasure may be somewhat diminished, but she generally can feel pleasure and can enjoy a variety of things, and she looks forward to the birth of her child.	With depression, she has an almost complete lack of ability to feel or experience pleasure, and she may not look forward to the birth of her child.
Appetite	Her appetite increases.	She typically loses her appetite.

Factor	Normal During Pregnancy	With Depression During Pregnancy
Self-esteem	Her self-esteem remains about the same as it has always been.	Her self-esteem goes down and stays down as long as she's depressed.
Guilt	She experiences no unusual feelings of guilt.	She experiences ongoing feelings of guilt for no particular reason.
Insomnia	She may have some normal physical ailments or challenges, such as a full bladder or a backache, but she can fall asleep. And if she wakes up to go to the bathroom or for some other reason, she can fall back asleep.	She has trouble falling asleep and trouble falling back asleep if she wakes up to go to the bathroom or for some other reason. She may also tend to wake up very early and stay awake.
Self-destructive or suicidal thoughts or actions	She won't have any self-destructive or suicidal thoughts or take any self-destructive actions.	She may have self-destructive or suicidal thoughts or actions.

Understanding the urgency of getting help at this stage

When depression during pregnancy is overlooked, it can increase the risk of pregnancy complications. For example, consider the following facts:

✔ Depression is often associated with low birth weight (less than 2,500 grams) and up to twice the risk for pre-term delivery (less than 37 weeks, although with advances in medical science, this number, sometimes quite controversially, keeps getting lowered).

✔ Severe anxiety during pregnancy, which is obviously distressful for the pregnant mom, can also cause harm to the growing fetus due to a constriction of the placental blood supply and the presence of higher cortisol levels. Anxiety can also cause a heightened startle response in the newborn and can cause the newborn to be harder to soothe.

✔ When women are depressed during pregnancy, it increases the risk of many pregnancy complications. For instance, they often don't get proper prenatal care. Not only, then, do they tend to eat poorly and not properly gain weight (sometimes they even lose weight while pregnant), but they frequently self-medicate with alcohol or street drugs, which can be dangerous to the mom and the baby.

A Swedish study found depression and anxiety in pregnancy to be associated with the level of nausea and vomiting, prolonged sick leave during pregnancy, increased medical visits, more frequently planned C-sections, increased use of epidurals to control pain during labor, and longer labors.

A Brief Overview of Treating and Recovering from PPD

PPD is a mood disorder, and its cause is thought to be caused by many different factors. Some people consider PPD to be mainly of psychosocial or psychological origin, whereas others consider it to be mainly biochemical or even genetic (although the genetic link isn't yet proven, it's clear that women who have any history of depression in their family, including depressed male relatives, are at a higher risk of having PPD). As a result, treatment methods are a-plenty, and if what you're dealing with *is* PPD, you'll likely use a combination of treatments for the most effective healing process.

I talk all about each of the different treatments in Part III, along with a whole chapter devoted to creating a comprehensive plan (Chapter 10). But, for now, I give you the short-and-sweet version so you can get a taste of what to expect without having to swallow the whole cookie at once. (Feel free, by the way, to turn right to the section of the book that calls to you the most. If, for example, you need to know — right now — about how to deal with your family members and friends, that's where you should turn first.)

Timing is everything, so begin your treatment now

As a starting point, you need to know that although you'll definitely recover from your PPD crisis, and although a variety of treatments can be initiated right away, in most cases, you won't find a quick fix. Consider the following treatment scenarios and the expectations you should have of them in terms of Big Ben:

- ✔ **Taking medication:** If part of your healing path involves taking prescribed medication, start seeking help early because it may take a bit of time for you to find the right psychiatrist or medical doctor. Even after you find the right doc, it may take up to several weeks for the right medication in just the right dosage to be prescribed.

✔ **Changing communication habits:** To the degree that you have to learn how to communicate better with your partner, family members, and friends — for example, if you need to learn to ask for what you really need or if you need to learn how to become comfortable saying "no" to people's requests — treatment may take a while. Remember, like Rome, new relationship styles aren't built in a day.

✔ **Processing your emotions alongside a therapist:** If you're going to undergo a course of therapy with a psychologist or other mental health therapist, that too is not a one-shot deal or something that can be concluded in just a week or two.

If you've had long-term underlying psychological issues that have contributed to your PPD, you can expect that they'll take some time to thoroughly work their way out of your life. Similarly, if you've never really learned to face your feelings, and this is part of what's up with you, it's unrealistic to expect to get to the bottom of it in only one or two therapy sessions. The great news is that it takes far shorter a time to get rid of these old habits than it did to grow them, so you can accomplish this in far less time than you imagine.

Even though most of the treatments take time, you can still do several things right away that will help make a real difference and launch your recovery. Here are four suggestions that can be adopted immediately:

✔ **Carve out 15 minutes a day to read this book.** Some new moms or new moms-to-be will have no problem whatsoever reading through this book. Others, especially those who are feeling overwhelmed, may find it difficult to even pick the book up. If you're one of these people, remember this: The very act of carving out 15 minutes a day to read a few pages, which can prove tremendously helpful to you, amounts to a very courageous and intelligent act.

✔ **Take notes.** As you read this book, do it with pen, pencil, or highlighter in hand. Circle important points, take notes, and use asterisks. In other words, do whatever it takes to fully engage your mind with respect to how the information you're reading applies to you. If you were taught to not write in books, either break that rule or get a fresh notebook and write down notes next to the appropriate page numbers.

✔ **Keep a journal.** This suggestion is similar to taking notes, but here you're taking notes specifically about yourself. You don't have to write anything copious — just a paragraph or two a day can prove useful and therapeutic in the long-run.

If keeping a journal feels like that one extra duty that will put you over your limit, don't do it.

✔ **Take three sets of ten deep breaths a day.** Sounds simple, right? If you get tired easily, are anxious, or if you simply have an open moment during your day — maybe you're standing in line somewhere or waiting for the tea water to boil — go ahead and consciously, deliberately take ten deep breaths. These breaths will help relax your body and mind, and will take a little bit of the edge off of however you may be feeling. Most people space out at about breath number seven. So, be sure to stay conscious of the number of breaths you take. Even though deep breathing isn't a cure-all, it certainly helps if you can do it everyday.

Knowing your three main treatment options

The treatment options for PPD begin with a professional assessment. If you have, or think you have PPD, you need to see a professional who can help you determine whether you're actually suffering from this illness and whether you need additional treatment. (Flip to Chapter 5 for a discussion on seeking a professional assessment.)

If, after receiving your assessment, you're told that you do have PPD, your major treatment options include the following:

✔ **Psychological treatment:** Depending on your particular situation, you can almost certainly benefit from psychological treatment or therapy. As discussed in Chapter 6, you certainly shouldn't be afraid of being stigmatized by receiving therapy.

✔ **Medical treatment:** Medical treatment — which usually means taking prescription medication — can be enormously important and effective depending on your personal situation. For example, for some women, the road to as quick a recovery as possible requires taking prescription medication.

As discussed in great detail in Chapter 8, you have to consider many factors when deciding to use medications. This includes determining which of the many medications prescribed is best for you. Issues such as the impact of taking medication while breastfeeding are also considered in Chapter 8.

✔ **Holistic treatments (a hodgepodge):** In addition to conventional medical treatments, a variety of holistic or alternative treatments are available as well — from acupuncture to homeopathy (check out Chapter 9). Views differ on how effective these alternatives are. In most cases, however, they should be considered as an adjunct to, not a replacement for, standard medical treatment and psychological therapy.

Medical pros not excluded

Pediatricians, nurses, therapists, and other medical and mental health professionals with PPD are usually the last people to actually seek the help they need. When they finally make it to my office, they all tell me, "I'm the one who takes care of everyone else in crisis — I can't be in crisis myself." Or they say, "It's embarrassing — with my education I should be able to pull myself out of this and not need extra help." Nurses especially, take a long time to get the help they need. They're usually always putting others first and are used to waiting for their own needs. Often, by the time a nurse with PPD finds her way to my office, she's been suffering for quite a while. "Healer heal thyself" is what I remind all these professionals. But, with the bad comes the good: When these professionals experience PPD firsthand, their professions (and the mothers they help) benefit because they become richer professionally. As you can imagine, it's necessary for medical professionals, to walk the talk about taking care of themselves.

As Chapter 10 discusses, it's important that you receive a comprehensive treatment plan. You deserve to have a well-rounded recovery plan that focuses on all aspects of yourself — physical, emotional, psychological, and spiritual. Such a plan should be constructed with the help of a professional (ideally your doctor or therapist) and should integrate the various components from the treatment modalities that you intend to try. With such a comprehensive plan in hand, you know who you have to see and when, what you should be looking for, and what you have to do and when. It's rarely as easy as "one, two, three," but with such a good plan in hand, you have a valuable roadmap that systematically leads you on your path to complete recovery.

Fostering recovery on your own

In addition to the three major treatment modalities, there are a variety of other things that you can and should (and will!) learn to do to support yourself in your recovery from PPD. These include, but aren't limited to, the following:

- ✔ Obtaining a good understanding of what PPD is and isn't (see Chapter 2)

- ✔ Getting proper nutrition (see Chapter 12)

- ✔ Exercising sufficiently and appropriately (see Chapter 12)

- ✔ Taking a sufficient number of breaks and learning how to make sure you get whatever else you may need from the support people in your life (see Chapter 12)

- ✔ Creating an effective support team around you (see Chapter 14)

✔ Knowing how to communicate with those who aren't initially too helpful or understanding (see Chapter 13)

✔ Gaining an understanding of the risks of PPD and the steps you can take if you've already had PPD once and are thinking of having another baby (see Chapter 18)

Before You Begin, Take Some Hope for the Journey

If you happen to already have PPD, you may be feeling pretty bad, or even hopeless. I want you to take a deep breath —yes, right now — and acknowledge the possibility that even if you feel hopeless in this moment, you don't need to feel that way (and in all likelihood you won't be feeling that way for long). Here are seven reasons why you shouldn't feel hopeless:

✔ PPD, once acknowledged, can be effectively treated.

✔ As long as you're getting the proper treatment, you're going to be fine.

✔ Not only will you end up as good as new, but with the therapeutic work that you receive by reading this book, you may very well end up *better than new*.

✔ PPD wasn't your fault in any way, shape, or form, and you have no reason to feel guilty, ashamed, imperfect, or bad in any way.

✔ Not only will you be absolutely fine, but as long as you're getting the proper treatment, your baby will be absolutely fine as well.

✔ By reading this book, you've taken a giant step toward understanding PPD and toward getting proper treatment.

✔ You're not the only one who's ever had PPD. In fact, up to one in five women suffer from PPD. With proper help they make it through — and so will you.

Getting help when you need it is a strength, not a weakness! You prove your strength by pushing through the devastating feelings and getting the help you need in spite of how you feel. My clients first contact me feeling like crumpled heaps of exposed raw nerves, worn down and defeated. As I remind them of what they battled in order to get themselves to call me (babysitter, lack of motivation, hopelessness, fear, stigma of needing help), I reinforce to them how strong they are. Strength doesn't mean that you feel great — it means that you do what you have to do no matter what it takes.

Chapter 2

These Ain't No Baby Blues: PPD, Up Close and Personal

*H*ere's the way your mind works post-delivery: Any depression or anxiety that has been hanging around you in the past, however mild, typically becomes exaggerated. For instance, if you've dealt with low-grade depression before, after delivery it can go over the line and become postpartum depression (PPD). Or, if you've always had what you thought was a personality quirk of checking twice to make sure the stove burner is off, this "quirk" can become a full-blown obsessive-compulsive episode after delivery.

Research shows that the months both immediately before and after giving birth are the times when women are the most vulnerable for mood disorders. These disorders have various physical, emotional, and psychological causes, one of the primary causes being that dramatic hormone changes occur after delivery. The reproductive hormones estrogen and progesterone plummet even below pre-pregnancy levels, to just about zero. Cortisol also increases to high levels by the end of the pregnancy and drops significantly after delivery. These hormones are known to have a major effect on psychological functioning.

Many women, doctors, and postpartum depression researchers think that these dramatic hormonal changes, among others, contribute to postpartum depression, and many women who have postpartum depression seem to be very sensitive to hormonal changes. After delivery, about 80 percent of moms feel the baby blues, which is totally normal. But, if the brain chemistry of a woman is wired so that she already has a tendency toward mood imbalances, she's at high risk for PPD.

In this chapter, I start out by showing you the differences between PPD and its much milder "cousin," the baby blues. Then I delve into PPD itself so you can get an idea about its symptoms and timing. I also discuss the risk factors and causes of PPD (to the degree its causes are understood), as well as depression during pregnancy, a subject that's all too often overlooked.

Baby Blues: Cute Name for a Crummy Time

After pregnancy and birth, new moms often experience a general emotional letdown, along with a huge sense of responsibility for taking care of a newborn infant. They may think, "Why did I do this? Was I nuts?" It's also not uncommon for new moms to be disappointed by the amount of support they're receiving (or not receiving, as the case may be), especially when it comes to their partners. On top of all this emotional baggage, new moms face certain undeniable physical challenges too, including tiredness, lack of sleep, and the increased physiological requirements of healing from the birth itself. If she chooses to breastfeed or pump her breast milk for her baby, the mom has a greater requirement for sufficient nutrients, such as protein and iron, that she needs to provide for herself.

What the lighter side looks like

After giving birth, it's perfectly normal for a woman to have a bout of what has affectionately been labeled "the baby blues." Research shows that between 50 and 85 percent of all new moms experience the baby blues. It's interesting to note that the majority of women worldwide seem susceptible to them and, in fact, experience them to some degree. Feelings often include one or more of the following:

- Weepiness
- Stress
- Vulnerability
- Sadness
- Worry
- Lack of concentration

A case of the baby blues usually comes on within the first week after giving birth and typically peaks between the third and fifth days postpartum. The blues can persist for two or possibly even three weeks, but for the most part they dissipate by the end of the second week. Contrary to popular belief, the baby blues aren't more likely if a woman is giving birth for the first time, and the delivery method and use (or avoidance) of epidurals and other painkilling drugs don't seem to make any difference either.

To see how often the baby blues surfaces compared to PPD and a healthy postpartum experience, see Figure 2-1.

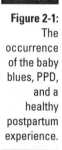

Figure 2-1: The occurrence of the baby blues, PPD, and a healthy postpartum experience.

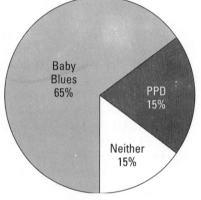

Baby Blues 65%

PPD 15%

Neither 15%

Some researchers write about the exact opposite of PPD happening to some new moms. An elevated mood where the mom is so cheerful she's giddy, which I call "the baby pinks," has been identified as something to watch out for. In this situation, even though the occasion is happy, the degree of the woman's elation is illogical. Many of these women experience a big drop in mood after a few days, which can lead to PPD or another postpartum mood disorder.

Getting support

Even though no research proves whether a highly supportive partner and social network help a new mom shake off baby blues more quickly than without them, it certainly makes sense that when a woman faces biochemical and emotional challenges, having a supportive partner and family environment makes life a lot easier for her.

Along with family support, all new moms need to have some basic education and information about the baby blues, if only to know that the condition isn't likely to last long and to help her distinguish them from PPD (see the upcoming section "Distinguishing between baby blues and PPD").

One way to get this information is to attend a support group for brand new moms. These groups, which are often arranged by hospitals or community healthcare centers, can prove to be useful because they not only dole out great info, but they also reassure the new mom that a bout of baby blues is normal and that many other women around her are feeling the same way. After chatting with other brand new moms for just a couple of minutes, the new mom can see that she's in good company and that her feelings are relatively mild.

When the Misty Blues Turn to Darker Hues

If you've been waiting for a few weeks for your baby blues to go away and they're still hanging around, or if you're unable to identify with other women in your support group because your blues just seem to feel worse than theirs, you may be dealing with something other than the mild baby blues. More than likely you're suffering from the more severe, but completely treatable, PPD. If you're not sure, don't worry, you've come to the right place. In this section, I help you determine what you're suffering from.

Distinguishing between baby blues and PPD

PPD and the baby blues look similar in some ways: They both involve some kind of low mood, worry, and feelings of sadness and irritability, and they both affect new moms. But, PPD is a more serious condition that requires a whole different level of intervention than the baby blues. Because of the seriousness of PPD, you need to know how to tell the difference between the two so you can get help as soon as possible.

Here are two basic ways to differentiate the baby blues from PPD:

- **Duration of the symptoms:** The first way to tell the difference is by noting how long your symptoms last — regardless of how mild they seem to be. Anything past two (or at the most, three) weeks, even if you feel only mildly blue, is now considered to be PPD.

Often a woman will feel down, stressed, and emotional for months and tell herself (and her partner, family, and friends) that she just has a case of the baby blues and that her feelings aren't bad enough to get help. Don't wait and assume that your feelings will eventually go away. Ignoring your symptoms for such an extended period only prolongs your condition and makes recovery more difficult. In fact, sometimes the baby blues hang on for the long haul and spiral down into more serious PPD symptoms.

✔ **Severity of the symptoms:** If, as a new mom, your symptoms interfere with your daily life in a big way, you may be suffering from PPD or another postpartum mood disorder (see Chapter 3 for details on the other disorders).

If your symptoms are in fact strong enough to affect your daily life, you need to contact a professional, even if it happens to overlap the baby blues timing of the first two weeks (or so) after pregnancy. The sooner you get help, the better.

In my own case, after the placenta was delivered and my internal hormones radically shifted, I immediately plummeted into a severe case of depression. In other words, as soon as the pregnancy hormones left my body, I found myself at the bottom of a deep psychological well and knew that something was terribly wrong.

Also helpful in distinguishing between PPD and baby blues is perspective. For example, whereas a mom with the normal baby blues typically has a perspective about becoming herself again, a woman with PPD usually loses that perspective. PPD is a thief — it steals away the woman's perspective and her feelings of competence and confidence. Generally, women with PPD feel as if they've lost themselves.

The question to ask yourself is this: "Do I generally feel like myself?" If the answer is "Well, I'm tired because I'm up with the baby a lot, and sometimes I cry for no reason, but yes, I'm still me," you have a case of the baby blues. If you answer the question with something like, "No, I don't know who this is, but it's not me," you're probably looking at PPD.

If you do feel as if you may be facing PPD, no matter what anyone tells you, don't wait to get help. If you're feeling that bad (or if you know a new mom who is feeling that bad), by golly, it may be PPD and help is needed now. If it turns out not to be PPD, no harm is done. The worst that happens is that help is sought, the new mom finds out it's the baby blues, and she leaves the therapist's office with a plan of action. And usually she starts feeling better right away.

Seek professional help when the baby blues persists past two weeks, or before that if

✔ You're unable to function normally

✔ You're feeling sad, angry, anxious, or scared for much of the day

✔ You can't cope with everyday life

✔ You have scary thoughts (refer to Chapter 3 for much more on scary thoughts)

Identifying the symptoms of PPD

The symptoms of PPD, and the severity of those symptoms, differ greatly from woman to woman. But even one of the following symptoms, no matter what the magnitude, may signal that you're suffering from PPD.

The following list comprises just some of the most common feelings, symptoms, and emotions related to PPD:

✔ Sleeping too much or inability to sleep at night, even when you're not up with your baby

✔ Irritability, anger, or rage

✔ Worrying much of the time

✔ Feeling overwhelmed or anxious

✔ Difficulty making even minor decisions

✔ Problems concentrating and lack of focus

✔ Change in appetite (usually loss of, but sometimes the opposite)

✔ Overeating or binging on carbs and sugar

✔ Loss of sex drive

✔ Sad a majority of the time

✔ Guilty feelings

✔ Low self-esteem or feelings of **worthlessness**

✔ Hopelessness

✔ Inability to experience pleasure

✔ Discomfort with the baby (uncomfortable holding or interacting with the baby)

✔ Physical problems without apparent cause (backaches or other pains that the doctor can't figure out)

I've often heard women lament that they've never really felt like themselves since the birth of a previous child. Sometimes this fact isn't clear to them until they begin to get help for their current bout of PPD. It usually turns out that they suffered PPD after the birth of another child, but they never received adequate help. Even though it can be a bit tougher to get rid of this depression that's been hanging on for years, the good news is that these women can still return to their old selves.

Given this general lack of confusion, it's extremely important to conduct individual assessments of new moms who may be suffering from PPD so that those women who are indeed afflicted can receive treatment and intervention as early as possible. If PPD goes untreated, it can become chronic depression — 25 percent of moms are still depressed after one year.

Understanding the risk factors

PPD can occur after the birth of any child, regardless of the baby's gender or place in the birth order. A popular misconception about PPD is that if it's going to happen, it will happen after the first baby. But, this belief isn't necessarily true. Many women who show up in my support groups or in my office are flabbergasted that they, in fact, didn't have any depression after their first child but they did with a later baby. Doctors don't know why this happens, but be aware that it does.

Even though PPD can happen to anyone (think roulette wheel), certain factors put a woman at higher risk than others. For example, the reasons for PPD can be biochemical, emotional, and psychosocial, and the factors may combine in such a way that makes a mom more susceptible after a particular birth. And, after a woman suffers from one bout of PPD, she's at an even higher risk after subsequent pregnancies (50 percent higher).

Your OB (or another professional that you're in contact with) should have already given you proper PPD information and should have alerted you if you're at high risk. The strongest predictors of PPD are depression and anxiety during pregnancy (about one third of all postpartum mood disorders start during pregnancy). And, whether you're at high risk or not, someone in your OB's office (or wherever you received prenatal care) should have screened you for PPD during and after pregnancy. If you haven't been screened, you can use the information in this chapter to self-screen. But, also remember to ask the OB (or other medical practitioner) to screen you in the office.

TECHNICAL STUFF

The thyroid factor

About 10 percent of new moms develop *postpartum thyroiditis,* which means that the thyroid gland is inflamed. This condition can result in temporary hyperthyroidism (overactive thyroid) or hypothyroidism (underactive thyroid). Some of the symptoms of hyperthyroidism are weight loss, anxiety, panic attacks, and insomnia. Symptoms of hypothyroidism are tiredness, depression, weight gain, and loss of memory. Sometimes postpartum thyroiditis goes away on its own, but for others it can turn into chronic thyroiditis.

Because this condition is so common, if I had my way, every new mother would be tested between two and three months postpartum just to rule it out. If she's depressed due to a thyroid imbalance, all the antidepressants and therapy in the world wouldn't fix it. The thyroid imbalance needs to be addressed directly — nutritionally, with alternative medicine, or with prescription medication (or a combination of all the options).

Especially if you have a family history of thyroid imbalance, ask your doctor (preferably an endocrinologist) to test your TSH, T4, anti-TPO, and antithyroglobulin. The last two test your antibodies, which may be too high (indicating an imbalance) even if the first two are within normal range.

A few factors make it more likely that you will suffer from, or are already suffering from, PPD. The more risk factors that apply to you, the more at risk you are. Ask yourself the following questions to assess your risk factors:

☐ Did you have PPD after the birth of another child?

☐ Were you anxious or depressed during your pregnancy, especially during the third trimester?

☐ Have you ever had PMS or PMDD (premenstrual dysphoric disorder)?

☐ Have you ever suffered from mood changes while taking birth control pills or fertility medication?

☐ Do you have a personal or family history of depression or anxiety?

☐ Have you ever had an eating disorder?

☐ Do you have good physical and emotional support?

If you answered yes to any of the preceding questions, you're at risk for experiencing PPD. Hormonal changes are a big factor. If you have ever had PMS or PMDD or have struggled with mood swings from hormone medication, you're more likely to react strongly to hormonal changes, which means that the changes due to childbirth may make the suffering more intense. Also, a woman's perceived support — both of the physical kind (someone doing chores, making her food, and so on) and the emotional kind (someone to talk to and lean on) is crucial for a healthy postpartum period. If she feels alone and unsupported, she's at high risk for PPD.

Traveling in time and place

As medical science becomes more enlightened, it doesn't embrace and promote as radical a split between mind and body as it used to. Now medicine is starting to put forth a more integral, useful, and usable definition of PPD. More and more medical doctors, healthcare providers, and caring professionals in all disciplines are now informed about PPD. Recent legislation in some states is increasing awareness of those working with pregnant and postpartum women so that many more doctors are conducting at least preliminary screenings for maternal depression. More than 60 percent of moms who get PPD have an onset of PPD within the first six weeks following delivery.

In other countries, the general level of knowledge about PPD is far ahead of what's found in the United States. In France, England, Australia, and Canada, for instance, the detection and assessment of PPD is considered a priority. In Canada, at the very first well-baby check, the doctor notes any sign of depression on the part of the mom and sends her to a clinic for help.

When you're well and have the strength to participate in this important and growing movement, as a member of Postpartum Support International, you can join hundreds of other passionate individuals to help promote legislation, education, and resources for postpartum women and their families. Check out the following Web site for details: www.postpartum.net.

The rates of depression during and after pregnancy are also higher among women with eating disorders, especially bulimia and binge-eating. Perfectionism, which is the fear of making mistakes, seems to be a factor linking eating disorders to PPD. Interestingly, women with eating disorders are at just as high a risk for developing PPD as women who have a history of depression. (A personal history of depression raises the new mom's risk of PPD to 30 percent.)

What will further increase your risk for PPD is the presence of any stressor in your life that occurs around the time of your baby's birth. In other words, moving to a new location, selling a house, or adding on to the old house right before delivery isn't a good idea. In fact, this is the absolute worst time for your mental health to do any of these things. Before you make any big changes, wait until things have settled a bit in your life — usually a few months postpartum is sufficient.

Considering Special Situations Where PPD May Be on the Horizon

No one is immune to PPD. It can happen to anyone — even dads and women who didn't give birth. And in addition to the high risk factors already discussed earlier in this chapter, there are specific situations that make parents especially vulnerable. These specific situations are highlighted in this section.

If Baby is seriously ill

Having a baby with serious health challenges is no picnic, and unfortunately, these challenges can cause moms to spiral into PPD. These moms are often tending to their ailing infants so much that they pretty much ignore their own needs — eating, sleeping, and taking breaks, for starters. Moms with babies in the Neonatal Intensive Care Unit (NICU) are prime examples. Often these moms, no matter how strongly they're urged to contact me, choose not to until they're literally falling over and unable to function. They practically live at the hospital and they're constantly wracked with guilt. They're thinking, "If I would have done things differently, my baby would be fine. It's my fault that he's suffering." Nurses practically have to kick these moms out of the NICU to go home.

When a mom of a child born with disabilities sees other babies leave the hospital thriving, she's left with the sinking feeling of knowing that her child's health issues may always be a factor in her and her child's life. When the baby is well enough to come home, no matter what the health challenge was or still is, it's often then that mom crashes. She's filled with anxiety about taking care of her fragile child and continues to put her needs last (if she even recognizes them at all).

If you're in this situation, I understand intimately how scary and anxiety-producing this can be (my daughter spent time in the NICU). It's heart-wrenching to see your little one lying there hooked up to monitors and IVs. As tough as it is to see your baby having to deal with all of this, you have to keep the following in mind:

- ✔ It's harder for you than it is for her.
- ✔ Your baby needs you to have the strength to care for her when she comes home (finally). So, make time to eat and sleep.
- ✔ Take breaks away from the hospital.
- ✔ If you have other children, spend time with them — they need you, too.
- ✔ Remember that it's not your fault.
- ✔ Lean on your partner or a therapist, friend, or other support person.

Many of my clients throughout the years are mothers of children with various disabilities (it has helped tremendously that my first career was in the field of special education). Counseling and support groups for them and their partners can be extremely helpful so they meet other moms and parents in similar situations and receive tools to help with their grief and plans for the future.

If Baby passes on

It's a cruel fact that even when a pregnancy ends without a live baby to show for it, PPD can still rear its ugly head. All the body "knows" is that it's no longer pregnant. No matter why or how the pregnancy was terminated — by nature or by human choice — the symptoms of PPD are often present. The mom usually has some level of grief due to the loss of her baby, but she can also experience a biochemical reaction of her pregnancy hormones dropping, which can cause PPD.

A significant percentage of women experience high levels of anxiety after a miscarriage for about six months, and they're also at increased risk for obsessive-compulsive disorder and post-traumatic stress disorder. Men, even though they grieve differently than women, can also experience depression and anxiety following a termination. Resolve is an organization that specifically helps with the painful subject of infertility — whether it's the inability to get pregnant or the inability to stay pregnant. Check out this helpful resource at www.resolve.org.

With her next pregnancy and postpartum period, a woman needs to be monitored for anxiety and depression because it's normal for her feelings to surface at this time (she may be depressed about her last loss, anxious about losing this one too, guilty about being happy, and so on).

In the case of a stillbirth or death of a newborn, professional help for the couple is most definitely recommended. Several organizations are dedicated to helping women and couples through these devastating experiences. For example, visit Helping After Neonatal Death (HAND) on the Web at www.handonline.org and The Compassionate Friends at www.thecompassionatefriends.com.

Different types of support groups are also available, and these professional organizations can often point you in the direction of an appropriate group that specifically fits the type of loss you've experienced — miscarriage, stillbirth, neonatal death including SIDS (Sudden Infant Death Syndrome), or any other situation where the death of a baby occurs.

If babies come in pairs (or more)

More than 25 percent of mothers of multiples have depression and anxiety disorders during pregnancy and after delivery. Some of the reasons for this high percentage of depression and anxiety include the following:

- ✔ **The high rate of preterm deliveries:** Mothers of preterm infants experience a higher level of depression than mothers of full-term infants, and multiples are notorious for being born preterm.

- ✔ **Sleep deprivation:** It's difficult enough getting the sleep you need with a single screaming baby, let alone with many mouths crying and eating throughout the night.

- ✔ **Social isolation:** Because organizing yourself, the babies, and all of the baby stuff takes so much work, it's challenging to meet anyone out of the house. Many moms of multiples feel that it's just not worth it.

- ✔ **The never-ending demands of the babies:** When one's napping, the other one's screaming, and at least for a while, sleeping and feeding schedules are close to impossible (and maybe not your style or choice). And if you're breastfeeding or pumping, you'll feel like a continuous milk machine.

If you're a teenage mom

Young mothers — under the age of 19 — have an extremely high risk (as much as 48 percent) of becoming depressed postpartum. Two of the main reasons are isolation and lack of support. Think of it this way: Their parents often kick them out of the house, the fathers of their babies take off, and their friends are busy living regular teenage lives. As you can see, PPD affects the teenage mom's ability to have relationships, which, in turn, lowers her self-esteem even more.

Like their adult counterparts, these moms often cry, are lonely and sad, have difficulty sleeping, and experience mood swings. But some symptoms are more unique to teenage moms. For example, many teen moms with PPD are scared and feel unprepared for motherhood. They also feel torn between the responsibilities of motherhood and being a teenager, and they may fear being abandoned or rejected by friends and family. Because their world is different from the adult reality and because they often can't identify with adult moms with PPD, teen moms desperately need their own support groups to help their isolation — whether they're in-school groups or community groups.

Extending beyond Biological Moms: PPD in Dads and Adoptive Moms

Just as PPD in moms that deliver their babies is becoming well-accepted and much more understood, news is suddenly cropping up about PPD in people who didn't actually birth their babies. This is confusing and odd for many people to grasp. Even though it isn't really a funny fact, many folks are surprised and sometimes humored that postpartum dads get depressed too. And women who adopt babies are also at risk. This section explains.

Letting go of preconceptions: Dads with PPD

Men, too, have PPD after their babies are born, and it's at the rate of at least 10 percent. Their symptoms are different from the fluctuating moods and emotions that moms with PPD exhibit. Fathers seem to have more tension and short-temperedness as the main symptoms of their PPD. Other feelings are confusion, fear, anger, frustration, and helplessness. Fathers with PPD are concerned about their partners, their disrupted family life, and their financial problems. They also have increased expectations for themselves, decreased sleep, confusion over their new role, and increased responsibilities (if the mother has PPD or is otherwise ill). It's assumed, for obvious reasons, that a dad's depression isn't hormonally induced.

The strongest predictor of whether a father will become depressed postpartum is the presence of PPD in the mother. The father whose partner has PPD has between a 24 to 50 percent chance of developing PPD symptoms. The other factors that put dads in the high-risk category are previous bouts of depression and instability in the relationships with their partners. It's interesting to note that the onset of a father's depression occurs later in the postpartum period than the onset of PPD in moms. In Chapter 16, I discuss why partners, if the partners weren't receiving adequate help themselves, sometimes become depressed as the moms recover.

When fathers suffer from PPD, their baby boys are especially affected. These boys have been found to have twice as many behavioral problems in their first few years as other children without depressed fathers. So, if you think your partner may be depressed, be sure to encourage him to find help as soon as possible — if not for his own sake, for the sake of his kids. Your therapist may be able to refer him to an excellent counselor who has expertise with daddy depression.

While working with moms, I often suggest that their partners accompany them to a therapy session. During that session I check in with the partners to make sure they're receiving the support that they need. I can tell if a dad is depressed, no matter how he tries to cover it up with statements such as "I'm just here for her — I'm fine." Sometimes (but more rarely) a dad has the awareness to know he's suffering and will call me directly to ask for an appointment.

Even though this is changing for the better, men often avoid going to support groups. But, they're usually willing to talk on the phone with another dad who's "been there." Even if that's all he does, it will be helpful. Your therapist may have a reference — person or Web site — for him, so be sure to ask. Two of the many good Web sites for postpartum dads are `www.postpartumdads.org` and `www.postpartum.net/fathers.html`.

Feeling the weight without the labor: Adoptive moms

Even though they aren't going through loads of hormonal changes from pregnancy and delivery, women who adopt babies are also candidates for PPD. As with any other mom, PPD in adoptive moms can begin within the first year after the baby enters the home. Many moms who adopt have a history of infertility, and because of this infertility, some have taken a variety of medications to help them conceive (some of these meds themselves can cause depression). Then, despite the medication, these women face the despair of not conceiving. Others have no problem conceiving, but they end up experiencing many miscarriages. This inability to carry and birth a baby isn't only difficult on these women emotionally, but also physically and hormonally.

These moms have a difficult time when they're hit with PPD because they usually aren't given permission (by themselves or by others) to feel depressed after finally having a baby. They feel and hear things such as, "Isn't having a baby what you've wanted all these years? How can you complain about anything now?" Or, "You've spent all your savings, energy, and time on this project, so you should just be happy."

Because these moms typically aren't screened in OB offices, other professionals, such as pediatricians, family practice doctors, and adoption agencies need to be on the lookout for symptoms of depression. These professionals also need to understand that it's difficult enough for a mom with PPD who delivered her baby to acknowledge that she's in distress because she's afraid that her baby will be taken away. So, they need to take into consideration the fear of adoptive moms who, for good reason, often have that worry to begin with.

The sudden impact of becoming a mother — often the primary caretaker — may also be a factor in PPD, as well as the sleep deprivation that accompanies having an infant in the home.

Chapter 3

You Mean There's More? Five Related Postpartum Disorders

. . . .

In This Chapter

▶ Identifying the categories you fit in

▶ Knowing how to handle the postpartum disorders

▶ Allowing others to support you

. . . .

*W*ouldn't understanding PPD be relatively simple if it were the only postpartum mood disorder out there? Perhaps, but no such luck — there are five more! No need for you to become any more overwhelmed than you may already be, though. After you know a bit about the other five, you may find that some of the other feelings you've been experiencing are demystified. And you also may be greatly relieved to know what PPD is and what it isn't — for example, how it differs from some of the scary reports you've heard on the news.

Penciling in Some Lines: A Quick Comparison of Mood Disorders

No matter how many times a doctor waves the diagnostic manual (as if it's a magic wand), a woman will rarely fit neatly into the six postpartum disorder categories (counting PPD itself). These disorders are separated into these categories simply for the purposes of research and treatment. So, as you read this chapter, you may realize that you identify with the feelings of more than one of the postpartum disorders. Don't worry though, this variety is very common. For instance, I was an absolute smorgasbord of these disorders. I had a few symptoms of some and a lot of the others. Whatever you do, don't be distressed or confused if you aren't sure where you fit, because it doesn't matter what combination of symptoms you're living with: They're all treatable.

With any of the postpartum disorders, you can expect to find a wide range of severity — from mild to moderate to severe. Regardless of which level you're at, one thing is for sure: When you suffer from a postpartum disorder, it always feels bad. In this chapter and throughout this book, though, I provide tons of information to get your wheels turning on the road to recovery.

Because the scientific community isn't in complete agreement (rarely does that exist in any field!) regarding the number of women who are affected by each of these postpartum disorders, I present the most commonly accepted statistics throughout this chapter. And I start with the numbers in Figure 3-1 — which shows the relative occurrence of each of the six disorders in postpartum moms who are suffering from a mood disorder. Postpartum bipolar disorder isn't included in the chart because the occurrence rate isn't clear yet.

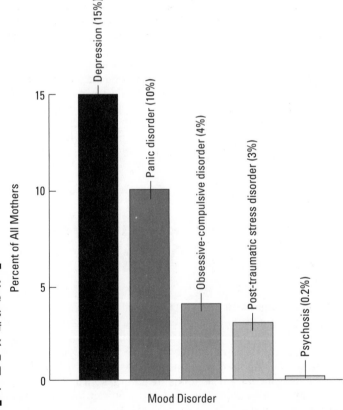

Occurrence of Postpartum Mood Disorders

Figure 3-1:
The relative occurrences of each of the six postpartum mood disorders.

When Fear Strikes: Panic Disorder

A panic attack is much more than just a feeling of high anxiety — it's a temporary feeling (though duration varies) that comes and goes in waves, and it feels as if you're enveloped (smothered, really) in absolute, irrational, and uncontrollable fear. About 10 percent of new mothers experience them. Often moms with panic say they feel like they're losing it. Others say they feel like they're going crazy. With panic attacks, many women often report a sensation of claustrophobia and feel the need to run outside to breathe. Also, to show you just how strong these feelings can be, consider this: If a mom is fortunate enough to fall asleep in the first place, an episode can awaken her straight out of her deep sleep.

I remember bolting upright in bed numerous times, having difficulty catching my breath, and thinking I was having a heart attack. It's terrifying. Sometimes the panic is made worse by thinking about particular subjects or going to specific places. For example, every time I'd get close to my OB's office, I'd become so dizzy, lightheaded, and nauseous that I'd have to pull over onto the shoulder of the road. It took three tries before I actually made it into the office for my postpartum checkup.

Here's a list of common feelings associated with panic attacks:

- ✔ Claustrophobia
- ✔ Dizziness
- ✔ Fear of going crazy
- ✔ Fear of losing control or dying
- ✔ Fear of more panic attacks
- ✔ Hot or cold flashes
- ✔ Numbness or tingling
- ✔ Sensation of skin "crawling"
- ✔ Shortness of breath
- ✔ Tightness in the chest
- ✔ Trembling

Searching for the root of an attack

Unfortunately, you usually won't be able to identify particular triggers for your panic attacks. For example, you may be serenely sitting on the couch with your preschooler reading him a story, when, wham, a panic attack comes over you. Because of this unpredictability, moms with panic disorder are often afraid to go out with their babies because they're worried a panic attack may strike at the store, park, or worst of all, in the car. They think, "What if I get a panic attack and I lose control of the car?" Making the situation even worse is the fact that moms with panic are usually big "what-iffers" who are worried about every possible negative scenario.

Even though postpartum panic is unpredictable, doctors have found that most often, moms who have postpartum panic attacks have a personal or family history of panic or anxiety. This history may either be on mom's side or dad's side of the family (blood relatives). It isn't necessary to ask your parents, grandparents, aunts, or uncles if they've had anxiety or panic attacks before, but if you happen to know they have, it can help fit the puzzle pieces together during your professional assessment. Hyperthyroidism (overactive thyroid) can also cause panic attacks, so get your thyroid checked if you haven't already.

Calming your panic

Psychotherapy and medication (including thyroid medication, if necessary) are the most well-known treatments for relieving panic. If you're using an antianxiety medication to help, sometimes your doctor will advise you to take it regularly even if you're not feeling panicky. The reason: Preventing a panic attack from hitting in the first place can actually calm your system down a few notches so it won't be as vulnerable to automatically reacting with more panic. As with any other habit, you can train your body to react differently — in this case, without panic. So, if your MD has prescribed an antianxiety medication to help treat your anxiety or panic attacks, don't try to be "strong" and not take it. It's understandable that you're trying not to become dependent on the pills, but by avoiding taking the medication, you may be doing yourself a disservice.

Specific nutrients (see Chapter 12) have demonstrated success in relieving these symptoms as well. Alternative treatments are also starting to emerge. Acupuncture, for instance, has been showing promise for increasing melatonin, a brain chemical that relieves anxiety and insomnia.

Sometimes you can't avoid a panic attack, even when you use all your tools — both psychological and biochemical — but you can train yourself to ride out the panic when it hits. Whatever you do, don't fight it — you'll just make it worse. When you start to feel that sensation of a wave washing over you, your job is to get control of the fear before the fear gets control of you. To control the fear, try out the following techniques:

- ✔ **Talk to yourself.** Tell yourself, "This is only a panic attack. No one has ever died from a panic attack. It's just adrenaline shooting through my system and it will go away soon."

  It's immensely helpful (and it'll become easier as you practice) to hold on to what you rationally know (for example, that panic attacks aren't deadly) because fear takes you to the irrational (and scary) in a split second. You'll find pretty soon that you can keep your perspective even in the middle of the worst of it.

- ✔ **Wiggle or tap your feet on the floor.** Moving around can help you stay grounded. Panic focuses your energy on your chest and everything above, which is why your breathing becomes so shallow. And when your breathing is shallow, you begin feeling dizzy and lightheaded.

  Because it's impossible to be grounded and have a panic attack at the same time, my clients report that the panic stops more quickly when they use this technique. Concentrating on your feet, which are rooted to the earth, serves as an additional purpose of distracting you from your fear.

- ✔ **Go outside if you can.** Look up at the sky and breathe as deeply as possible. Getting out into the big wide-open can help you avoid that closed-in feeling that often accompanies panic.

- ✔ **Avoid cruising the Internet and news of any form.** Most news that's reported is negative and anxiety-producing. So, unless you're specifically visiting a known and trusted Web site, the Internet will probably end up increasing your anxiety, not relieving it. It's understandable that you may feel desperate to find help, but searching when you're anxious is highly unadvisable because much of the information on the Web is unscreened and often untrue — and will get you riled up for no reason at all.

  If you can avoid local, national, and international news for a while, do it. (By the way, when I say "news" I mean all kinds of news, including TV, Internet, radio, and newspaper news.) The news heightens anxiety even without postpartum panic! If your partner is watching the news in the living room, for instance, I suggest you go into another room or ask your partner to wear a headset until the news is over. And if you're reading a magazine or book that starts to raise your anxiety, put it down and do something else. When the postpartum crisis has passed, you'll probably be fine picking up that scary mystery novel again.

If nothing else works, carrying an antianxiety medicine in your diaper bag or purse can be helpful — these medicines work very quickly to relax you. My clients say that they get peace of mind just knowing that the medicine is always available. They remind themselves that the worst that can happen is that they have to take the medicine and they'll be fine. If something else helps you relax, such as a homeopathic remedy or a special quote from a book, then by all means, use what works.

When left untreated, panic disorder can lead to agoraphobia, which is a fear that causes a mom to not want to leave her home at all. I don't bring up this idea to scare you — I just want to nudge you to get help the help you need before you reach that point.

Helping others help you

If you're experiencing panic attacks, I'm sure you've run into those people who say, "Just calm down and relax." Even though they probably have the best of intentions, you know that someone telling you to "just relax" when you're in the middle of a panic attack, is hardly helpful. Usually this response just upsets you more because you can't relax — that's the whole problem. So, tell those around you what helps and what doesn't. For example, you can ask them to say the following things (or others like them):

✔ "It's fine if you don't want to go tonight. If going out feels like too much to handle, stay home and take care of yourself."

✔ "It must be scary for you when you're having panic attacks. If you need a hug, let me know. I'm here."

Facing the Aftermath: Post-Traumatic Stress Disorder

Post-traumatic stress disorder, a condition that dredges up past experiences and causes a person to become anxious and depressed, can often strike postpartum women. In fact, approximately 1 to 6 percent of postpartum women are suffering from it right now. When a woman experiences post-traumatic stress, a traumatic event or period of time from her past may come back to haunt her.

For example, one of my clients, around two weeks postpartum, suddenly began having disturbing memories of her father chasing her around the house when she was very small. Her father had been physically abusive, hitting her and her older brother with belts, metal spatulas, brushes, and whatever hard instruments he could grab while in a rage (which was a few times a week). Her nightmares, which began around the same time as her daytime memories, were bad enough to awaken her throughout the night. And, much to her horror, she felt so fiercely protective over her baby daughter that she even kept the baby from her loving husband (who was a doting new daddy). Rationally she knew this made no sense, but she felt powerless on an emotional level to stop the feelings and behaviors. With some energy psychology techniques and cognitive behavioral therapy, my client fully recovered.

The most frequent symptoms of postpartum post-traumatic stress are

- ✔ Intense anxiety
- ✔ Fear
- ✔ Extreme sensitivity and awareness of surrounding stimuli such as noise
- ✔ Startling easily
- ✔ Flashbacks of the past trauma(s)
- ✔ Recurring nightmares

If you've experienced any type of abuse — sexual, emotional, or physical — you're at high risk of suffering from post-traumatic stress disorder. Traumatic labors, deliveries, or health issues with yourself or your baby can also cause a postpartum post-traumatic stress reaction.

This isn't to say that you'll definitely have a reaction, but it's better to be prepared just in case. Do everything possible to help protect yourself from this unpleasant experience. For example, if you're aware of any traumatic past experiences, tell your OB/GYN so that he or she can do the following:

- ✔ Be prepared to be especially tuned in to you during the birth and postpartum periods and to put this information in your chart for hospital staff.
- ✔ Give you a referral to an excellent therapist specializing in trauma who can start helping you before the baby comes, if possible.
- ✔ Give you a referral of a doula who's trained to take care of you emotionally during labor and delivery and also during the postpartum period.

Post-traumatic stress in the delivery room

Traumatic memories may begin to surface during labor and delivery, which is when a woman is at her most vulnerable. So, midwives and birthing doulas try to elicit information about past trauma from their clients before the birth. By doing this, they can prepare themselves to provide the extra support, nurturing, and modifications needed for the woman's comfort. For example, one of my clients who had experienced sexual abuse at the hands of her father and other male relatives anticipated that just being naked, feeling out of control, and being examined during labor and delivery would be terrifying. Her OB and doula reassured her that they would accommodate any and all preferences she had if at all possible. One of my client's wishes was that she would be draped with a sheet whenever possible, so she'd hopefully feel less vulnerable and less exposed. Just knowing that she had such support from the professional team helped make the outcome quite positive and much easier for her than expected.

Reducing post-traumatic stress

Psychotherapy and medication are still the most common treatments for post-traumatic stress disorder. However, even though talk therapy is useful with PPD, many professionals believe that it has little value in post-traumatic situations. These professionals feel as if talking about the traumatic events has the opposite effect and can continue to traumatize the person.

Alternative methods, such as powerful energy psychology techniques, are also becoming more recognized as treatment. Some of these techniques include Eye Movement Desensitization and Reprocessing (EMDR) and Emotional Freedom Technique (EFT). General holistic and alternative techniques are discussed in Chapter 9.

Also helpful for reducing your post-traumatic stress is giving yourself lots of compassion. Obviously, you've already been through some bad experiences, so don't beat yourself up on top of it — that's just mean. It's all too easy, for example, to put yourself down for acting "silly" about having nightmares regarding things that happened so long ago, or to feel frustrated with yourself if you've already dealt with this issue in therapy and thought you were done with it. Remember that even the most intelligent, organized, spiritual, and grounded women are still human. No one is immune to this reaction or any other.

If you're having trouble being kind to yourself, imagine that you're speaking to your best girlfriend who's going through the same thing, and say to yourself what you'd say to her:

✔ "You've been through so much."

✔ "This is a common reaction to scary experiences."

✔ "I love you and I'm so glad you're taking healthy steps to feel whole again."

If you've had therapy before for a particular traumatic experience, and you're wondering why it has popped up again to haunt you, remember that you're vulnerable right now. You're not weak, just vulnerable. As a matter of fact, women are at their very most vulnerable during pregnancy and postpartum. If a mood disorder or memories of traumatic events are going to surface, they typically surface now. And if they have shown themselves prior, they resurface at this time. This is due to a number of factors that are still being researched, but in part because of the hormonal upheavals affecting brain chemistry. Just remember that the more stressful experiences you've had in your life up to this point, the more at risk you are to have a post-traumatic stress reaction.

Helping others help you

If your closest support people don't have a clue what's happening inside you, they may jump to false conclusions and therefore, be unable to support you like you need. So, if you're suffering from post-traumatic stress disorder, explain to those around you that your startle reactions, nightmares, and anxiety are due to one or more traumatic experiences that you've lived through. You don't necessarily need to spell out the specifics to all of your support people, but you can if you think it would be beneficial to you. Feel free to let your support people know that you'll talk when you're ready and that in the meantime, they shouldn't ask. Finally, tell them that you may need a lot of reassurance that the scary memories will eventually stop.

Sometimes a family member will call me, alarmed at the behavior of the new mom, my client. I urge the new mom to communicate to the family member the same way I'm suggesting to you, and it helps the situation considerably. Usually my clients are bugged less from worried support people when the supports have the information and don't need to guess anymore. Often my clients need to release some embarrassment about their "scared" behavior and give themselves some compassion before they're able to share some of the necessary information with those around them.

Spell out as clearly as possible to your support people what it is that you need from them, whatever that may be (hugs, reassurance, space to be alone to journal, companionship, and so forth).

ANECDOTE

Post-traumatic stress: The experiences of yours truly

The first time I was ever in a hospital was when I was 3½ years old. My appendix was about to rupture. No one told me where I was going or what was about to happen. All I knew was that my tummy hurt. At the hospital, I was whisked away from my mother and put in what I thought was a laundry basket or garbage bin and wheeled down a corridor. I was placed on a table and saw a huge needle coming at me. Right before a horrible-smelling wet cloth was placed over my nose and mouth (what I now know was ether), I asked timidly what they were going to do to me. I was told not to bother myself with that.

My mother wasn't permitted in my room after the surgery (it was 1958, and parents weren't even allowed in the hospital room after a child's surgery), but she fought hard enough and was finally let in. In recovery, I thought my arm with the IV was dead because I was told not to move it. So for weeks after the IV was removed, my arm just hung at my side like a useless appendage. I actually had nightmares about my arms falling off.

The next time I needed to go to a hospital was to have my baby (I've always been very healthy).

Instantly during labor I felt like a little girl completely at the mercy of the adult medical staff around me. I felt helpless and frightened. I never dilated past six centimeters and I thought I was going to die from pain. I was having front and back labor because my baby was transverse and posterior (sideways and "sunny-side up"). At that time, I had what I now know was an out of body experience due to the pain and fear. I visualized a crystal ball exploding into a billion pieces, which I now believe signified my Self being destroyed. I was finally given a C-section and my baby had to go to the intensive care unit because of a collapsed lung and an infection. When I returned home, I was tortured with nightmares about losing my baby in a big hospital with evil people and trying desperately to find her. Sometimes I was the baby, and sometimes she was. All the feelings from my trauma at 3½ mixed together with the traumatic six-and-a-half-day labor and delivery. Because I never received the help that I needed — the help I'm determined to give you now — my post-traumatic stress disorder lasted for years.

Breaking the Cycle: Handling Obsessive-Compulsive Disorder (OCD)

Obsessions, as you can probably guess, are unpleasant, intrusive thoughts that repeat over and over in your mind for no apparent reason. Approximately 3 to 5 percent of new moms develop these obsessive thoughts. Even when there isn't a problem to solve, the mind may hold on to a particular worry or thought and spin it around hundreds of times a day (annoying at the least, and anxiety-producing and scary at the worst).

On the other hand, *compulsions,* which are different from obsessions, are particular behaviors that the mind "tricks" you into thinking you must do repeatedly. The compulsive behavior may be in response to an obsession (for instance, you're obsessed with a thought of accidentally hurting your baby, so the compulsive behavior may be to hide the kitchen knives). Or, you may feel a powerful urge to check something, count, wash, clean, or do some other behavior. Sometimes these behaviors are rituals, such as a series of behaviors that you think you need to do in a particular order. And other times the compulsions are behaviors such as repeatedly checking the baby's breathing no matter how many times you've checked it that hour and boiling the pacifiers and lining them up in the dish drainer in the exact same way every time. Unfortunately, there are no percents yet in the literature associated with the number of moms who wrestle with compulsive behaviors.

Some women just have the obsessive thoughts, others only have the compulsive behaviors, and still others have both. Remember that occasionally having the same worry pop into your head or having a preference to eat your cereal from the same bowl is normal. But, if you have a lot of obsessions and/or compulsions that distress you and get in the way of you enjoying your day, you may have *obsessive-compulsive disorder* (OCD).

A personal or family history of OCD puts you in the high-risk category for suffering from postpartum OCD. Fortunately, most women are aware that they've had some degree of obsessive thinking or compulsive behavior (or both) since before they became pregnant. On the other hand, some women have noticed these behaviors in themselves since childhood, but they never had a name for what they were suffering from until after the postpartum evaluation. In these cases, the OCD usually didn't get in the way of the woman's life before now, so she never felt the need to get help for it. If these behaviors are mild before pregnancy and delivery, they'll typically become huge afterward, and go over the line into an actual disorder.

Before these behaviors go over the line, however, women with obsessive or compulsive tendencies don't always consider these tendencies to be a problem. In fact, those traits, such as having a strict attention to detail or great follow-through can be considered assets. For example, one of my clients who's a surgeon had prided herself on receiving many accolades from her higher-ups in the hospital for her insistence on sterilizing all her surgical instruments twice and lining them up perfectly before each operation. During therapy with me she became worried that she would lose this edge when treated for her postpartum OCD. I assured her that she would always be able to keep the behaviors that she wished to keep, but let go of the rest that she was feeling postpartum. And that's exactly what happened.

If you have a tendency toward OCD, the conditions you experience after birth, such as sleep deprivation, stress, and hormonal changes, can make your obsessive thoughts and compulsive behaviors worse. If you haven't already, make a plan for yourself as soon as possible regarding sleep, specific nutrition changes which may help with anxiety and depression (see Chapter 12), and breaks.

The obsessive side of OCD

Having had postpartum obsessive-compulsive disorder myself (complete with the horrifying images it often produces), I was convinced that I had to make this particular disorder a subspecialty of mine. Mothers who suffer from the obsessive side of OCD unfortunately never obsess about anything positive. Instead, they always obsess about the scariest topics that their overactive, buzzing minds can land on. The thoughts constantly flip through their minds until they begin focusing on the most upsetting scenario possible. Each woman's worst-case scenario may be different, but common themes involve sharp objects stabbing the baby or the baby being dropped from a high place.

Discovering the irony behind the scary kind of postpartum obsessions

Not all moms with postpartum OCD have the symptom of scary thoughts about their babies being harmed (and I hope you are spared this), but it's common enough to warrant writing this section.

The irony of OCD is that a mom who has it is the most careful, protective mother of all. Her protective instincts are constantly working overtime. This mom can walk into a room and instantly anticipate every possible danger to her child — a sharp corner on the coffee table, a wobbly chair, a glass knick-knack by the phone, and so on. She's so tuned in to these remote dangers that her obsessions can become absurd. The scenarios she creates in her mind are so unlikely that they could make another person want to chuckle in disbelief.

For example, one of my clients started obsessing about her baby catching HIV. One thought led to another until she couldn't even take her baby to the local store. She would envision an HIV-infected person using the public restroom at the store and then touching the shopping cart, which would somehow infect her baby.

Every object a mom with OCD sees can suddenly turn into a potentially dangerous item. For example, she envisions a vacuum cleaner cord wrapped around her choking baby's neck. Or, maybe, she "sees" a kitchen knife that she had always used to prepare dinner stabbing her baby. Does she want to hurt her child? Absolutely not! She has the exact opposite intent: She's so obsessed with safety that she envisions her worst fear of not being able to keep her baby safe. And what's the most horrifying thought of all? That she herself would be the one to accidentally do the harm.

Even though a mom with OCD understands logically that the chances of horrible things happening to her baby are almost impossible, she justifies her worry by saying, "But it *could* happen." So, the theory regarding why a mom with postpartum OCD has thoughts about harming her baby is this: She obsesses on the most horrible thoughts possible, and the absolute worst thought is that she herself may be the cause of that harm. Her obsessive, anxious mind lands on these self-incriminating thoughts, often in a barrage of nonstop horror. Her brain is like a dial that's set to "worry mode," and if one obsession stops, it's simply replaced with another.

Overreacting to OCD

Professionals who haven't received specialized training on postpartum obsessive-compulsive disorder sometimes wrongly mistake it for postpartum psychosis. This misdiagnosis is particularly damaging to the mom because the mom is already worried that she's psychotic, or about to become so, and a danger to her baby. The mom's worst fears are confirmed, ironically, by the people who are supposed to be helping her. Even worse, sometimes well-meaning professionals whisk the mom into the hospital or has her baby taken away, which further convinces the mom that she's a danger to her child. The unnecessary damage and suffering that happens in this situation can take quite a while to undo.

Along the same lines, and even without the misdiagnosis of the ill-trained professionals, many moms with OCD think that they're going crazy and that they're always on the verge of hurting their children. That's why they doubt themselves, and don't trust themselves to be alone with their babies. They say, "If I'm capable of *thinking* such a horrible thought, what would stop me from actually *doing* it?"

For example, when a scary piece of news is released about a mom hurting or killing her baby, obsessive moms worry that they may be capable of snapping and becoming that mom (which is why I continually recommend that depressed and obsessive new moms avoid the Internet and other sources of local or national news). I get flooded with calls from women with postpartum OCD when there's a news report of this kind. I reassure them that they're obsessing about becoming psychotic because they have OCD, not psychosis. I tell them that the fact that their thoughts and behaviors are distressing to them and don't feel like thoughts they would normally have indicates that they don't have psychosis. I say, "If you were psychotic, you wouldn't be calling me right now. Because you'd be having a break with reality, you wouldn't be able to recognize that you're having bizarre thoughts that don't make sense. Let the fact that you're distressed be reassurance to you that this is just OCD." I also emphasize that OCD doesn't turn into psychosis. The two conditions are distinct entities (see the section, "Immediate Attention Needed: Psychosis" later in this chapter for details on psychosis).

Moms who are suffering from OCD aren't a danger to their babies. They're simply overprotective. There isn't one report to date of any mother with postpartum OCD, ever following through on any of her scary thoughts. She's just afraid she will, which is a huge difference from actually going through with the thoughts. In fact, most moms with OCD will do away with themselves before they would ever hurt their children. When these moms don't trust themselves, they can go into another room and leave their babies safe in the crib for a few minutes as a precaution.

The compulsive side of OCD

Sometimes the anxiety from compulsions is tied to superstitious or obsessive thinking. If, for instance, the mom has an obsession about her baby dying, she may worry to herself, "If I don't fix that blanket on the baby in that exact way ten times, the baby will be smothered and it will be all my fault."

Often the fear is that something bad will happen if the behavior isn't indulged. Safety is always the theme — a mom has compulsive behaviors as an attempt to keep herself or others (or both) safe. Here are the top obsessions (thoughts) and compulsions (behaviors) that result for postpartum obsessive-compulsive disorder:

- A need to count things repetitively, such as bottles
- A need to check things repetitively, such as doors to ensure that they're locked, and the baby's breathing
- A need to constantly clean and tidy up
- Germ phobia
- A need to have things "just so"
- Terrifying images or thoughts of harming the baby or watching the baby be harmed
- Intense shame and disgust about these thoughts
- Behaving in ways that reduce the anxiety about the thoughts they're having (for example, hiding sharp objects)
- Distrust of herself, especially when alone with her baby

Putting OCD to bed

Psychotherapy and medication can be useful in treating postpartum OCD because it's associated with low serotonin (the brain chemical that's most responsible for moods). So, doctors usually first try to treat OCD patients with medications that help increase serotonin. You can also use several non-medical tactics to get rid of your compulsive behaviors and thoughts.

Delaying your compulsive behaviors

If you're cleaning, checking, or doing other activities compulsively, no matter how challenging, try your best not to indulge in those behaviors when you're feeling the strong urges. No one knows how difficult this direction is more than I (as someone who had severe postpartum OCD), but I also know how therapeutic it will be for you when you're able to resist the compulsions. Your first step may be delaying the compulsive behavior for five minutes (if you can't do that, just try one minute to start with). That way, you'll be able to see for yourself that nothing terrible happens when the behavior isn't immediately carried out (like your mind says it ought to). During the delay period, distract yourself the best you can with some other positive behavior. Make sure these positive behaviors are

- ✔ Carried out in a different area of your home than the one you're currently in (or outside the home, if necessary)
- ✔ Incompatible with the compulsive behavior (in other words, one that you can't do at the same time as the one you're trying to avoid)

After you've mastered five minutes, try to increase the time period. When you've reached a 15 minute delay, often the need to carry out the behavior, which intellectually you know isn't necessary in the first place, will have lessened to the point where you're able to avoid it entirely. This will help raise your self-esteem substantially because you'll feel so much more in control of your behavior.

The rule of thumb my clients try to follow is this: When they get that "I must do that task now" compulsive feeling in their bodies (it's always accompanied with at least some anxiety), they simply aren't allowed to succumb. Only when that feeling is *not* present, do they give themselves permission to, say, clean their kitchen. In other words, if they feel the compulsive sensation, they need to wait until the feeling subsides and they're "grounded" again. Then, if they still want to, they can accomplish the task in a calm way — not in a frenetic one.

When you indulge in the compulsive behavior, it actually makes the OCD worse, much like a tire going around in the mud, digging deeper and getting more stuck in the rut. Keep in mind, though, when you try to refrain from these activities, you may notice that your anxiety temporarily increases. But, I assure you that it will eventually drop back down and you'll feel better than ever. Also remember that I didn't tell you all this so that you'd start obsessing about it and add it to your worry list! Instead, I'm only trying to encourage you to get help from someone who truly understands postpartum OCD.

Letting go of negative obsessive thoughts

Women suffering from OCD can have terrifying thoughts or images of their babies being harmed. If you get a scary thought, try not to dwell on it. These thoughts have nothing to do with the real you, or say anything about you as a person or as a mom. Instead, say to yourself:

- ✔ "This is just the OCD making me think that I'm dangerous. It's only a thought and it has no power over me."

- ✔ "I'm an excellent mom who's trying to protect her baby. My baby is safe with me."

When you're trying to ward off your compulsive, scary thoughts, be sure to stay away from the Internet and any other sources of news — newspapers, magazines, radio, and TV. Moms suffering from OCD are often drawn to information that's scary and anxiety-producing. Here's why: When you're trying desperately to keep your baby safe and the magazine by the checkout counter reads, "Protect your baby from this horrible illness! Read page 42," guess who buys the magazine? That's right: You! You think, "If I resist and don't buy this magazine, I may miss some essential piece of information that may save my baby from a horrible fate. And then my baby's suffering will be all my fault."

If you have OCD and it tries to suck you in to all of the negativity of the world through the use of fear tactics, get mad instead of anxious. Say to yourself something like, "How dare those publishers try to make us mothers feel like we're not good enough if we don't buy their silly magazines! I'm not buying into that nonsense!" By choosing to get angry, you'll feel more in control and less afraid. And remember that the magazines conveniently placed at the checkout counter are only there to sucker you into feeling anxious so that the publisher can sell more copies. Eventually you won't need to feel angry in order to feel in control. Instead, you'll be able to recognize what's going on and laugh about it. Anger, for the time being, is just a helpful stepping stone.

Helping others help you

As with every other postpartum disorder, you don't have to suffer through it alone. Clue in your support people as much as possible. For instance, if you're having scary thoughts or other irrational obsessions, let your support people know that you need lots of reassurance that the OCD is the only reason you're having these thoughts. Have your support people help you hang on to what you rationally know is true by telling you the following things (or things that are similar):

- ✔ "These thoughts are just the OCD speaking."

- ✔ "These are only thoughts — they have no power over you.

- ✔ "You're a good mom and a good person."

Even though getting reassurance from your support people is important, the most powerful way to get reassurance is to give it to yourself. As soon as you can, start relying more on giving yourself these same messages. As uncomfortable as this may be at first (you'll probably trust others more than you trust yourself), it really is the cornerstone of your success. You see, as great as it is to receive reassurance about yourself and all the things going on in your life from those around you, relying on them too often will eventually undermine your confidence in yourself and in your own knowledge. I understand this may be confusing, because on one hand I'm suggesting letting others help you and on another I'm saying lean on yourself, but my point is to find a balance between relying on others and trusting yourself.

If you're getting therapy, which I hope you are, it's often helpful to bring your partner or another close support person with you to an appointment so he or she can learn how to best support you (and about the disorder in general). Because your urge to indulge the compulsive behaviors can sometimes spill over onto the people you're closest to, your therapist may make sure that your partner or support person is only checking, counting, or cleaning things once (even if you ask that person to do it several times). After that one check, if you think that it needs done again, you'll have to do it yourself. At first, your support person's unwillingness to check things more than once will probably be annoying to you. But don't get mad at the other person! He or she is just following your therapist's directions. In the long run, remember that cutting down on the compulsive behaviors will help you recover faster.

Riding the Emotional See-Saw: Bipolar Disorder

Bipolar disorder (previously known as manic depressive disorder) is identified by its huge mood swings. One week the person may feel like she's on top of the world, and then suddenly she may drop into the pit of depression and be curled up in bed and unable to function. The huge upswing is called mania and the downswing is major depression. A woman's first episodes of bipolar illness sometimes surface postpartum. Because the symptoms of depression are listed in the section on PPD, I speak more about the manic episodes here.

Here are the some of the most common experiences associated with mania:

- ✔ Perceived need for less sleep
- ✔ Sudden bursts of energy that make you want to get many things done quickly
- ✔ Extreme happiness
- ✔ Inappropriate humor

✔ Shopping sprees

✔ Poor judgment

✔ Anger

✔ Sexually overactive and inappropriate

✔ Obsessing about religious topics

If you have a personal history of bipolar disorder, you're at a 20 to 50 percent risk for a postpartum bipolar episode. If you had a postpartum bipolar episode after a previous delivery, now you're at a more than 50 percent risk.

As with any other mood disorder, pregnancy and giving birth greatly increase your chances of suffering from bipolar disorder, especially if you've been diagnosed with it before. In fact, as with any other mood disorder, there's no other time in your life when the chance of having a bipolar episode will be greater than right now. If you have a blood relative who has been diagnosed with bipolar disorder (even if *you* haven't) you're also at a higher risk than others. So, if you have any personal or family history of bipolar disorder, make sure your doctor knows.

Often a client may not know if she has a family history — no one ever received the diagnosis or mentioned the diagnosis. But, if I ask her about specific behaviors she may have seen in relatives, such as dramatic mood swings, everything often clicks into place. For example, one of my clients, who I suspected had bipolar disorder, replied this way when I asked her about big ups and downs in her relatives: "Oh, yes. My Aunt Margie would be in great moods some weeks. One time I went to visit her and she baked every recipe from this one cookbook, which took her all night! The next time I visited her, I was looking forward to all this fun and she barely wanted to do anything. I was really bored, because she just lay around on the sofa until my mom picked me up."

So, if your doctor or therapist asks you about your family history, don't forget to mention any strange behaviors that you remember in your relatives because this can help you (and the professional) identify what may be hanging around in your genes.

Balancing the scales of bipolar disorder

If you have PPD and you have a family history of bipolar disorder, your psychiatrist may put you on a mood stabilizer along with your antidepressant. Your psychiatrist does this because if a person with a tendency toward bipolar disorder is given particular antidepressants, or an antidepressant without a mood stabilizer, it can cause mania.

Natural treatments, such as minerals, to keep bipolar disorder under control have become more popular. It's fine to use these natural treatments as long as your medical practitioner knows what you're taking and has given you the green light to move forward. Some medical folks know more than others about alternative methods of treatment, though, so feel free to shop around until you feel comfortable with the level of expertise. (Check out Chapter 9 for more general info about natural or alternative treatments.)

In the end, it doesn't matter which path you decide to take to control your symptoms. The key is to give yourself permission to use whatever works. The best thing you can do for yourself and your family is to take whatever steps necessary to feel happy (but not happy like that nun in *Sister Act* — you know who I'm talking about).

Whatever treatment plan you and your doctor choose, make sure you're faithful to it and your normal health regimen, which includes nutrition, nighttime sleep, and exercise. It's imperative that you give the plan some time to work. It's easy to become impatient and quit the medication right before it may start working. Or, when the medication is already working, it may be tempting to stop taking it because you think you don't need it anymore. That's a mistake. You're feeling better because of the medication, so don't stop — at least not yet. You want to be feeling fully yourself for at least a few months before you and your doctor discuss weaning you from it.

Besides medications and treatment plans, knowing how to self-monitor so that you can tell when your mind is beginning to spin out of control is also important. Doing so may take practice, but it's worth the practice because catching a manic episode before it happens can save you a lot of energy and heartache. Know your warning signs so you'll be prepared to call in your professional support team if necessary.

If, for example, one of your warning signs is shopping too much, and you find that you just bought the same sweater in all nine colors, call your doctor or therapist. You can also run down your checklist of nighttime sleep, good nutrition, and so on, to make sure you're on track and are taking care of yourself. If you feel you don't need sleep at night or are sleeping too much during the day, those may be warning signs. Mastering how to put on the reigns when you start to spin will be of great help to you.

Helping others help you

Sometimes it's easier for a close support person to notice if you're not acting like yourself than it would be for you to notice. Often it's the partners who recognize the signs first. So, let your closest support people know that you're counting on them for reality checks every now and then. But, make sure you actually listen to those who know you the best. Sometimes you may not agree with them, but at least pay attention to the behaviors they find worrisome and get checked out just in case.

Immediate Attention Needed: Psychosis

Postpartum psychosis is *not* a severe case of PPD — it's altogether a different beast. So, you can imagine why the general public becomes tremendously confused when, for instance, a psychotic mother kills her baby and the media calls it postpartum depression.

A mother with postpartum psychosis is in her own reality, which is why this is a particularly dangerous and scary mood disorder. The mom often floats in and out of being in a normal person's reality, but it's impossible to count on her being rational from minute to minute. Sometimes she'll seem to be talking to herself or others and not making sense, and then suddenly she'll be totally lucid and carrying on a normal conversation.

The main reactions associated with postpartum psychosis are

- ✔ Auditory hallucinations (hearing things others don't, such as "special messages" meant only for her from the TV, radio, computer, or newspaper)
- ✔ Bizarre thoughts about needing to kill her baby
- ✔ Confusion
- ✔ Disorientation
- ✔ Extreme agitation
- ✔ Insomnia
- ✔ Paranoia (false beliefs that others are trying to harm her)
- ✔ Tactile hallucinations (feeling things that aren't there, for instance spiders crawling up her arm)
- ✔ Visual hallucinations (seeing things others don't)

Postpartum psychosis typically begins within the first few days following delivery, which overlaps the baby blues period. More than half of all cases of postpartum psychosis begin the first week, and more than 75 percent begin within the first 2 weeks. So, if the new mom is still in the hospital at this time, the day nurses in the postpartum ward should pay close attention to the night nurses' notes because the new mom may be acting bizarrely at night, but may seem normal during the day (or vice-versa).

Luckily, only one or two new mothers in a thousand experience psychosis. But, when it happens, it's always considered to be a medical emergency because with it comes a five percent suicide rate and a four percent infanticide (mom killing her baby) rate.

Similarly, only a handful of times in the 20 years that I've been practicing has a psychotic mom contacted me directly. It's usually a family member or a doctor who contacts me after the woman has been hospitalized. One of the most bizarre parts of psychosis is that the mom usually doesn't know that she's ill. She may know that others aren't thinking the same way she is, but she typically believes she's correct. And even though she'll float in and out of the psychotic state, she's in another reality most of the time. So, in other words, if you're worried that you may be psychotic, chances are that you probably aren't.

Although this area needs more study, here's what professionals know so far regarding rates of recurrence: If a woman has had psychosis or bipolar disorder before in her life, or if she has a family history of either, she has between a 20 and 50 percent chance of experiencing postpartum psychosis. And if she has had a previous postpartum psychosis, she zooms up to a 70 percent risk after she delivers another baby.

Don't get anxious or scared about any of this information, especially if the personal or family history part applies to you. Instead, just make sure you see a specialized professional who can guide you with a plan of action.

Combating psychosis

If you're experiencing any of the symptoms listed for psychosis, please see a medical professional immediately because postpartum psychosis is always considered to be a medical emergency. Like any other postpartum disorder, psychosis is also treatable, but you need to be in the hospital until you're more stable. In the hospital you'll be safe and will be assigned to a doctor who will oversee your medication and make sure you're recovering.

If you're unable to be hospitalized due to a lack of insurance or another financial difficulty, you need a support person by your side at all times — I mean literally in the same room — until you're more stable. With psychosis, you never know what thought will float into your mind at any moment. Even though your thoughts may be quite irrational and even delusional, psychosis will make you believe they're true. That's why you aren't safe to be alone or by yourself with your baby at this time.

Even though it may be difficult, be sure that when you use the bathroom you keep the door open so your support person can be close if necessary. And, when you're spending time with your baby (which you should most definitely do if you're up to it), make sure you always have another adult with you until you're completely stable.

Warning your loved ones

If I've said it once, I've said it a thousand times: Don't try to deal with a post-partum disorder on your own, especially if it happens to be postpartum psychosis. So, as you're on your road to recovery, make sure your closest support people understand that you're in the middle of a scary crisis and that they shouldn't leave you alone for even one minute until you're stable.

As you begin to feel better, it's typical to have strong feelings about what just happened (or may be still happening) to you. And hearing that you "lost your mind" or "went crazy" can be embarrassing and hurtful. So, make sure to tell your support people not to use those demeaning terms. Tell them to use the clinical word — psychotic.

Also after recovery, you may feel fear. It can be scary to hear stories about the things that you did and said, and the ways you behaved when you were in a psychotic state. To know that you were that out of control can be alarming and scary to many women. Your therapist, doctor, and informed support people can reassure you that the worst is over, and that there are ways of helping to prevent other occurrences.

Well-meaning relatives may suggest that you find a postpartum depression support group. But, be sure to tell them that it's not the right thing to do quite yet. Your experience may be different from anyone else's there, and you may not relate to others (or they to you). Individual therapy is recommended before you pop into the group. After a postpartum psychosis, you'll usually have some depression to deal with, so at that point, attending a support group may be helpful.

Part II
The Three Little Letters: PPD and You

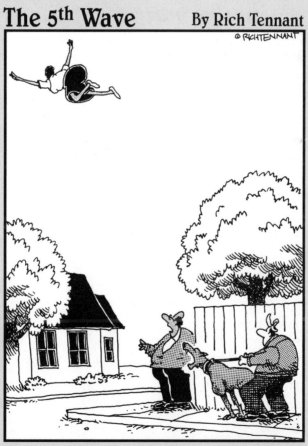

The 5th Wave   By Rich Tennant

"Dora's anxiety has always manifested itself in the 'flight response.'"

In this part . . .

Making an initial realistic assessment of whether or not you have postpartum depression (PPD) is probably high on your priority list right now. These chapters help you by providing the tools to do exactly that. I also discuss the advantages of seeking a professional assessment, and I give you an idea of what a diagnosis of PPD really means. Finally, this part ends with a description of how to find a good therapist to help you recover as quickly and effectively as possible.

Chapter 4

Looking Within: Is PPD Your Big Bad Wolf?

*O*bviously, if you're feeling depressed, you want to feel like yourself again as quickly as possible. The first step is to be clear about what you're dealing with. The quicker you're able to identify how you're feeling both emotionally and physically, the easier it will be to outline a plan of recovery.

Postpartum depression (PPD) fogs your thinking and makes it difficult to find clarity in anything, especially these new emotions you're feeling. So, I've written this chapter to help you pinpoint what you're experiencing. When you understand what you're experiencing, you're then able to clue in your support people as to what help you need. Because you'll be able to put words to and describe your thoughts and feelings, the professionals on your treatment team will also have more of the necessary information to best help you psychologically and physically.

Facing the Beast Head-On: Tuning In to Your Emotions

Some women are crystal (and painfully) clear about what they're thinking when they have PPD. If you're one of these women, great. If you're already aware and honest about what's filling your mind, then you're one step closer to being able to change those disempowering thoughts to empowering ones.

If, on the other hand, your thoughts and feelings are all jumbled together in what feels like one big mess, you've joined the majority of women with PPD. A good therapist can help you disentangle the mass of put-downs, guilt, and other negativity so that you can finally tune in to the thoughts behind the emotions and change them (see Chapter 6 for more on finding a good therapist).

To help yourself tap into your emotions, say what you're thinking or feeling out loud. If you're more than mildly depressed, though, wait until you're with a therapist. Don't worry about sounding coherent, just start talking and trying to express your emotions. Pretty soon you'll start hearing your own voice articulating some difficult and complicated feelings, which may surprise you. The reactions of my clients when they start voicing their pain range greatly. Some women cry from relief that, finally, even though the act was uncomfortable, they not only acknowledged their feelings to themselves but also expressed them to someone else (me). Other women cry with despair because they're not sure they'll ever get out of the deep hole they feel they're in. And still others find themselves giggling at the absurdity of their depressed or anxious thoughts.

As you begin to tap into your emotions, assess whether you're having any of the following feelings (if you do, consider them signs of a possible bout with PPD):

- ✔ **You feel guilty a lot, have low self-esteem, and are self-critical.** New moms in general tend to doubt themselves, but if you're feeling bad about yourself, are quick to feel guilty, and tend to put yourself down, you've crossed the line.

- ✔ **You feel sad a lot of the time.** If you're generally not feeling like yourself and you're sad more often than not, this behavior is a signal that you need to make an appointment with a professional. However, if you're just mildly sad off and on, but it doesn't get in the way of your day and the sadness is gone by the third week postpartum, this behavior is normal.

- ✔ **You have scary thoughts.** Scary thoughts can entail anything that's disturbing to you, and they therefore vary quite a bit. Many women with PPD report that their scary thoughts focus on the subject of not getting well and needing to be hospitalized forever. However, the most obvious thoughts that need attention are thoughts of harming yourself or your children. Having scary thoughts about harm coming to you or your children doesn't necessarily mean anyone is in danger. For example, the thoughts that often accompany postpartum OCD are frightening but not dangerous (see Chapter 3 for the details on that disorder), but you definitely need a thorough evaluation. The important differences between the kind of thoughts that are emergencies and the kind that aren't are also discussed in Chapter 3.

✔ **You lose your temper frequently and easily and feel anger or rage.** Sometimes PPD shows up more as anger than classic sadness. If you're snapping a lot at little or big people, or if you fill with rage for any reason, consider this a warning sign.

✔ **You feel easily overwhelmed.** If even the smallest tasks, such as washing dishes, paying bills, or making phone calls, are too much for you to bear, your blues are probably more serious than the average downer days. When the brain chemical serotonin is low, which is most often the case with PPD, overwhelm occurs. Overwhelm can feel puzzling and frustrating when the same tasks that used to be no big deal suddenly feel too complicated and difficult to handle.

✔ **You feel hopeless.** Hopelessness comes when a person is very depressed. If you're having thoughts that you'll never recover, that life's not worth it, or anything that comes close to those, get help immediately.

✔ **You worry excessively.** New mothers are an anxious bunch, but typically the worry doesn't take over the day. If you're having trouble turning off your mind, if the littlest things bother you more than you think they should, or if you start obsessing over anything and everything, please seek help. (I'm not listing typical worries, such as health problems of the baby, because you might add them to your "worry list" if they're not already there.)

✔ **You have difficulty making decisions.** If the normal myriad of daily no-big-deal decisions seems to have become more complicated, pay attention what's going on with you. What to wear, whether to drive or walk, which item to buy — all of these can be debilitating with PPD.

If I was able to get to the grocery store at all during the worst of my PPD, it would take me at least four hours to mobilize — organizing my thoughts and putting them into actions seemed close to impossible. I remember one time catching myself standing in front of the produce section staring at the fruit. I was just standing there staring. I literally couldn't make up my mind on what to buy. It was a surreal experience. I was standing outside myself watching this woman, me, who I used to know, and was thinking, "What's my problem? I have a master's degree and two teaching credentials and I can't decide whether to buy apples or pears?!" This situation for me was simultaneously ridiculous and tragic. At that time, I was unable to find any humor in the situation. You can access humor only when you're clear that the condition is just temporary. At that time, I knew no such thing. I thought that this was the new me and that I had lost myself forever. Now, looking back, I can see the funny parts because I have the perspective. I know now that I would be able to live through it.

Because PPD clouds your judgment while you're trying to make even the tiniest of decisions, now isn't the time to try and make major life decisions if you can avoid it, such as moving, divorcing, or changing jobs.

If you notice that you're being more forgetful and that you're having a difficult time processing information, don't fret. This PPD symptom is definitely annoying, but I promise you'll get your get your brain back as you recover from the illness. Although frustrating, you won't experience the severe kind of memory loss like you'd find with Alzheimer's (but many a mom has voiced her concern to me before being reassured). You won't forget where you live or what your name is. However, if you walk back into your house repeatedly, just to forget the same item time and time again, rest assured that this forgetfulness is typical. At this stage, you may be concerned that you'll forget the baby and leave without her, but you won't. You may feel like you're in the middle of a silly sitcom and want to change the channel. Try your best to keep your sense of humor — this nuisance, like all the other symptoms I list in the previous bulleted list, is temporary.

I remember wondering whether I also delivered 50 IQ points from my brain when I birthed my baby. Suddenly I couldn't remember easy vocabulary, and I would immediately forget what my husband had said to me a minute before. I couldn't read, since by the end of the sentence I had forgotten what the beginning said. If you have a similar problem, don't worry — it's only temporary. I suggest that you not try to read right now — it will only frustrate you. If your normal self (before the PPD) liked to read, your reading and understanding the printed page again will probably be an indication of your old self coming back.

Minding Your Mentality: A Look at Self-Talk and Dark Thoughts

It may be obvious to you when your mood is low, but you may not be able to tell how low it really is. For example, often all you know is that you feel awful, but you may not be able to gauge your mood with any precision or be able to tell if what you're feeling is normal or over-the-line depressed. It's even a bit trickier becoming aware of what you're actually thinking. But, when you are, that awareness can provide you (and your support people) essential information to help figure out how serious your condition is and where you fall on the continuum. This section gives you some guidance on paying close attention to your thoughts and assessing them.

Hearing what you say to yourself

Self-talk is extremely important, so I mention it in different ways throughout this book. Your energy is probably scarce, so why waste it by using self-talk that serves only to beat yourself up? Battling PPD takes a lot out of you, so pummeling yourself with put-downs is like standing in the middle of a boxing ring and kicking yourself when you're down.

The vicious cycle goes like this: The more depressed you are, the more you tend to beat yourself up, which, in turn, makes you more depressed. If it's unusual for you to put yourself down and if your self-esteem and confidence are usually high, it'll be more obvious if your self-talk is suddenly negative — and this is a warning sign that you may have PPD. If, on the other hand, you've had a longstanding habit of self-deprecation but it's worse now, this change is also a warning sign.

After you take a good, hard look at all the things you say to yourself, you're likely to be in for a big surprise. Take one of my clients, for example: After listening to what she was telling herself throughout the day, she was astounded. "Dr. Bennett," she said, "I'm so mean!" My client considered herself a compassionate person, so what amazed her most about this assignment was that she wouldn't have dreamed of saying those nasty things to anyone else she cared about — so why should she say them to herself?

The rule for self-talk is this: If you wouldn't say it to anyone else you love, don't say it to yourself. This rule isn't just a recovering-from-PPD thing either — it's a rest-of-your-life thing. Don't be kinder to yourself because you're suffering. Be good to yourself always because it's the right thing to do.

Whenever I tell my clients that I knew as soon as they contacted me that they were good mothers, they usually respond quizzically, yet intrigued. These women are desperate for any evidence that proves their own negative thoughts about themselves wrong. I hardly ever know these women when they first call, but I know they're good moms because bad mothers don't try to get help. Bad mothers don't care how their behavior is affecting their child or children. Only good moms try to improve the quality of their family's life by getting some help for themselves.

Some of the most common statements that I hear from women who are struggling with PPD and who in turn become paralyzed by the thoughts are

- ✔ **"I'm weak and incompetent."** The shame underlying this statement may keep a woman from calling a support group where she'll see that she's not alone and that others will accept her and work with her toward healing.

- ✔ **"What kind of mother will others think I am if I'm out and about all the time?"** If a mother's feeling guilty and shameful about wanting to leave the house a lot, she may not be willing to come forward and tell anyone because she assumes that other people will judge her the same way she's judging herself.

✔ **"I admit that . . ."** Whenever I hear the word "admit," I know the mom is feeling shame about her PPD. If she says, "I admit that I'm not enjoying my baby" or "I admit that I can't do everything myself," what she's really saying is that she thinks poorly of herself and thinks that she must be a weak person or bad mother.

If you're identifying with these types of statements, try eliminating the word "admit." For example, instead of saying, "I admit that I can't wait to go back to work outside the home," say, "I can't wait to go back to work outside the home." "Admit" implies shame, but just being honest acknowledges your feeling without judgment and is simply matter-of-fact. You have nothing to be ashamed about, so make your speech reflect that truth.

✔ **"I'll always . . ."** or **"I'll never . . ."** Loss of perspective is another common symptom of PPD. So, if you find yourself frequently using absolute terms, such as in "I'll always feel like this" or "I'll never get my old self back," I urge you to revise your wording. Say instead, "I'm worried that I'll always feel like this, but I know that's just the PPD talking — it's not the truth."

Remember that by revising your wording, you reinforce the positive truth and serve your mental health well. Affirmations work, so if you're going to use them, please say truths, not lies.

Recognizing the difference between fantasies and reality: A word about suicide

You need to know that with PPD, as with depression in general, comes a risk of suicide. PPD tragically takes lives every year, and this suffering of families is totally needless. As you see throughout this book, severe PPD can make you feel worthless, perhaps even like a burden to your family. However, there's an enormous difference between feeling the huge weight and working to remove it, as opposed to actually acting on it in a way that harms you and leaves your family forever agonizing.

So, moms with PPD (and moms without PPD who are burned out) often have what I call *escapist fantasies,* which are fantasies of getting away and leaving the pain behind. When I was going through PPD, I daydreamed about getting on a bus and riding as far away as I could. Even though these daydreams weren't pleasurable, they did provide a sense of temporary relief.

These thoughts occur most frequently with PPD because overwhelm is always present with the illness (technically speaking, overwhelm develops when *serotonin,* a brain chemical, is low). When you have PPD, the escapist fantasies can be frequent, occurring several times each day. A woman with PPD tends to feel guilty when she thinks about what these fantasies may imply about her as a mother. A normal but stressed-out mom may also face similar thoughts periodically, but she typically doesn't obsess about what a terrible mom she must be. She doesn't take herself on guilt trips as a depressed mother does. As a matter of fact, when I drop in to new moms' groups to speak with them, most of the moms seem to have a healthy perspective and even laugh about these thoughts. Remember, though: These fantasies aren't suicidal thoughts — they don't show any intent to harm and show no actual plan to end anyone's life.

Some of the time, women with PPD have darker escapist fantasies or thoughts that follow this train: "If I were to walk out into the street and a bus were to come and run me over, that would be okay." Or these women may think, "If I just didn't wake up tomorrow morning that would be fine." These moms don't really want to die — they just want the pain to stop. They also don't want to take the responsibility of making that terrible decision to kill themselves.

Occasionally, escapist fantasies escalate into the circumstance where a woman *purposely* puts herself in dangerous situations so that some disaster might befall her. When a mom feels worthless, it's easy for her to think she won't be missed and people around her will get over her death easily. (This couldn't be further from the truth! Your family needs you!) If her fantasies take this course, they now need to be treated more as a death wish and as a potential precursor to suicide — not simply as an escapist fantasy. And in case you're skeptical about how much of an issue suicide really is with PPD, consider this fact: It's estimated that at least 400 mothers in the U.S. alone commit suicide due to PPD each year.

If you're intending to hurt yourself, and have an actual plan by which to do so, I urge you to *get help immediately.* This is an emergency. Let at least one support person know so he or she can stay with you *at all times.* Call your therapist if you have one, or your doctor, and tell him or her what you're thinking. If you need to drive yourself to a hospital or call 911 (or an alternate emergency number if you don't have 911) so that a healthcare professional can pick you up and drive you to the hospital, do it. *Suicide isn't an option!* Do whatever it takes to keep yourself safe. No need to worry about being in a hospital — recovery is often quick and you'll be home, feeling much better, soon. You should have a follow-up healthcare plan with a therapist (and probably an MD) when you're released. People devote their lives to helping others in your situation, and you will get well. Take it from me — I've been there.

Here are two suicide hotline numbers in case you're not sure whom to call:

1-800-273-TALK

1-800-SUICIDE

I have worked with many young and grown-up children whose mothers have ended their own lives. Believe me, if you could see the pain and devastation I've seen in these children, you would never in a million years consider putting yours through this.

Watching for Warning Signs of the Physical Kind

Physical signs of depression and anxiety in new mothers are easy to overlook. For instance, many new moms aren't sleeping a lot at night. But the key question is why aren't they sleeping? Are they able to sleep but they're awakened every hour by their babies, or are they waking up even when their babies are sleeping? The same goes for eating. Is the new mom not eating because she's not setting aside the time to feed herself, or is she not eating because her anxiety level is shooting through the top of her head, which is causing a knot in her stomach? The same question should be asked for any kind of self care — showering, getting dressed, calling your friends back, and so on. PPD can make any of these daily activities challenging, due to low self worth, low energy, and an overwhelming desire to avoid social contact (mostly to avoid the "How's motherhood" question).

Your closest support people know you the best, and so they can provide a good reality check for you. These people are the ones who can tell you if you're not acting like your normal self. They can help you identify possible PPD if they notice some of the common signs.

Later in this chapter, I give you a more in-depth self-screening test. For now though, keep an eye out for the following red flags. Make note if you

✓ **Have trouble sleeping:** Often the inability to sleep is the initial sign of PPD. If you have a difficult time falling asleep at night when your baby is sleeping, or if you fall asleep easily only to wake up a couple of hours later for no apparent reason, you may be experiencing PPD.

✓ **Cry frequently and easily:** Crying for no apparent reason — for example, every time you see the cat food commercial — is very normal during the first two weeks following delivery (this is called the baby blues). After a couple of weeks, if you're still often bursting into tears (even if you're not sad), get checked out.

✔ **Lose your appetite:** What you need to notice in the appetite category is whether or not you actually feel hungry. If you feel hungry but aren't setting aside time to eat, that's a different issue entirely — in that case you just need to take a closer look at your schedule and re-prioritize.

On the other hand, if food is no longer interesting to you, this factor is warning sign. A loss of appetite is quite common with PPD. At the beginning of your recovery, it may feel like you basically need to force-feed yourself to get some good nutrition in your body (hop over to Chapter 12 for some simple ideas).

✔ **Want to eat everything in sight:** Contrary to the previous point, some women have the opposite reaction to their brain chemicals shifting. If you're always hungry (and often crave sweets and carbs) and rarely, if ever, feel satisfied — as if the mechanism that typically alerts the brain that the stomach is full is out of commission — consider this factor a heads up.

Had my OB been trained to identify PPD, he may have noticed that, even though I left the hospital down to my pre-pregnancy weight, two months later I was 40 pounds overweight. I felt like a human vacuum cleaner, consuming everything in the refrigerator on a daily basis. The voluminous amounts of food I was consuming was shocking to both me and my husband, but the hunger was always present.

Evaluating Your Postpartum Slump

You may be wondering how you can tell for sure if what you're experiencing is regular new-mom behavior or PPD. Some of your friends who recently became mothers may also feel worried and guilty sometimes. So, should you dismiss yours as normal and try to forget it or should you pursue it further? The rule of thumb is, if you feel that something is "off" and you aren't yourself, chances are good that you have PPD.

It never hurts to find out more information. Educating yourself is never the problem — it's the lack of education that can be harmful. By finding out more about what you have (or don't have, as the case may be), you'll be able to normalize what is expected for all new moms, or you'll see what needs more attention.

So, any way you look at it, you have nothing to lose (and everything to gain, really) by digging deep and assessing your inner self and getting a professional evaluation, if your own assessment leads you to concern. You may be wondering why I recommend having two separate assessments. The main reason is that informal, do-it-yourself tests can be valuable for giving you information and helping you think about your condition, whereas formal tests, which you'll find in doctor's offices and clinics, have been researched and evaluated as tools to measure PPD. I discuss getting a formal professional evaluation in Chapter 5. But, for now, in this section I provide a self-test that I recommend for anyone who thinks she may be struggling with PPD. This test can help you begin to identify what's going on inside and where to go from there.

In the following self-test, check any of the boxes next to the statements that apply to you. If you or a support person has noticed something about you that isn't indicated on this self-test, I suggest you add it on the side, so you can refer to it later, if you make an appointment with a doctor or therapist. Here are the statements to consider:

- ☐ I have missed appointments lately.
- ☐ I don't enjoy the things I used to.
- ☐ I worry a lot about my health.
- ☐ I worry a lot about my baby's health.
- ☐ I don't want to be with the baby.
- ☐ I'm not interested in sex.
- ☐ The thought of being alone makes me feel panicky.
- ☐ Parts of my body hurt but the doctor can't find a reason.
- ☐ I don't feel hungry.
- ☐ I'm angry a lot.
- ☐ I'm not making enough milk for my baby.
- ☐ I cry a lot.
- ☐ I feel like my life is over.
- ☐ I'm not bonding with my baby.
- ☐ I'm tired all the time, even when I rest a lot.
- ☐ I don't feel comfortable around my baby.
- ☐ I crave sweets and carbs and eat all the time.
- ☐ I don't want anyone else to hold my baby.
- ☐ My family would be better off without me.
- ☐ I can't sleep at night, even when my baby is sleeping.
- ☐ I feel sad a better part of the day.
- ☐ My baby doesn't like me.
- ☐ I have a difficult time focusing.
- ☐ I'm not a good mother.
- ☐ I don't have support, and I feel like I'm all alone.

If at least five items on this list describe you, you may have PPD. I suggest that you make an appointment with a therapist who has specialized training in PPD (see Chapter 6) so you can receive a full assessment. And if you're feeling hopeless, feeling like your life is over, or feeling like your family would be better off without you, please get help immediately.

It's easy to downplay your PPD and therefore delay in getting help. You may be thinking, "I'm not that bad. It's not like I want to kill myself or hurt my baby or anything. I can tough it out." Don't wait. Lots of women think that in order to justify getting help they need to be severely depressed. Actually, though, the faster you catch the PPD (if it's mild to begin with), the easier your life can be as you recover because you can spare yourself the typical spiral downward.

Chapter 5

A Professional Assessment: What's Huffing and Puffing at Your Mind's Door?

· ·

In This Chapter

▶ Unraveling the confusion about the PPD diagnosis

▶ Preparing yourself for an evaluation

▶ Being screened professionally for PPD

▶ Handling the news of your diagnosis

· ·

*I*f you have postpartum depression (PPD), or if you think that you may have it, you should most definitely not shy away from seeking professional evaluation and treatment, because the faster you get help, the faster you'll begin to feel better. The ideal professionals to give you an initial assessment include an informed, experienced, and sympathetic psychiatrist (a medical doctor with special training in mental and emotional disorders) or a clinical therapist, such as a psychologist (PhD). Knowledgeable psychologists can assess and evaluate you plus give you information regarding medications (if necessary). A psychiatrist, on the other hand, can assess and evaluate you and can also actually prescribe the medication if necessary and appropriate.

Having sought an assessment, you may receive a diagnosis of PPD, and for some people this can be confusing, scary, and even overwhelming. In order to help set your mind at ease — and to prevent a diagnosis of PPD from, ironically, making you feel more depressed — this chapter briefly explains the history (and difficulties) of diagnosing PPD and then focuses on what a modern PPD diagnosis looks like, what it means, and how you can best deal with it.

The Difficulties of the Diagnosis

Besides the fact that it ignores the reality that PPD has been known as its own unique disorder since at least the 1830s (to save you a headache, I won't digress into the details here), the present terminology used by the *Diagnostic and Statistical Manual of Mental Disorders,* 4th Edition (DSM-IV) is quite confusing. The DSM-IV, which is the thick manual that doctors and therapists use to diagnose mental health disorders, is confusing for the following reasons:

✔ It contains no actual diagnosis called *postpartum depression.*

✔ The same woman may be described and diagnosed differently on different occasions (because of the all-over-the-place, up-and-down nature of PPD).

✔ The medical records of patients hospitalized for PPD or other psychiatric illness after childbirth often use different terms to describe and diagnose.

✔ The present terminology confuses not only those responsible for medical care, but the criminal justice system and insurance systems as well.

As a result, a woman with PPD often has her rights sacrificed or compromised. For example, when members of the criminal justice system hear "postpartum something or other," they tend to overreact.

Although my colleagues and I are taking steps in the right direction by educating medical and mental health practitioners as well as the sufferers themselves, it remains to be seen if substantial progress will actually occur by the time the next edition of the DSM arrives. Luckily, excellent professionals are also working on clarifying and standardizing the official medical terminology.

Taking a Pre-Assessment: The Edinburgh Postnatal Depression Scale

I have two favorite formal PPD assessments, both of which may be used by the diagnostician as part of the evaluation. One is the Postpartum Depression Screening Scale (PDSS), and the other is the Edinburgh (pronounced "edin-burrow") Postnatal Depression Scale (EPDS). The PDSS is excellent, but only available for professionals to purchase and administer. It can't be printed here for copyright reasons.

Pediatricians paying attention

Pediatricians are in an excellent position to catch PPD in parents. In increasing numbers, pediatricians are doing a great job of tuning in to the mental health of their patients' caregivers. Doctors speak so much about the impact of a baby's environment on his or her health and growth — what could possibly be more important than the primary caregiver's psychological wellbeing?

Many pediatricians are now routinely conducting brief screenings of the moms during well-baby visits, and moms with depression are being identified. Sometimes the Edinburgh Postnatal Depression Scale is administered, and other times the screening may be just a couple of simple questions. For instance, asking the mom whether she has lost interest and pleasure in doing things and whether she's been feeling down or worried, can, by themselves, start identifying moms with PPD. In about five to ten minutes, the results of the screening are explained to the mom, as well as the impact of the depression on her child, and then a referral is made. Some pediatrician offices now have a staff person who's designated to make a follow-up call to the mom. Even though pediatricians rarely see fathers, these docs are also beginning to pay attention to dads' mental health.

Pediatricians are getting the message that children of depressed parents are about three times more likely than their peers to suffer from depression, anxiety, or addiction. Thankfully, when a mother's PPD is treated, her kids show improvement in their own symptoms within three months.

The EPDS is available only for researchers and clinicians for their private use, but I obtained permission to reproduce it here for you (thank you to J.L. Cox, J.M. Holden, and R. Sagovsky, who published the EPDS in the *British Journal of Psychiatry,* Volume 150 in June 1987). Note that the EPDS shouldn't be used by itself to diagnose, but you can take the quiz now to help you see where you stand. And if you'll be consulting a doctor or therapist, bring the results with you to discuss your score as part of the entire assessment. The diagnostician should have an EPDS manual that thoroughly explains how to interpret the various scores.

Answering a handful of questions

If you're curious to see where you may fall on the continuum of PPD, take this quick test — the EPDS. Taking it isn't a requirement, so feel free to skip it if you want to.

For the following questions, please circle the answer that comes closest to how you've felt in the past seven days:

A. I have been able to laugh and see the funny side of things:

0 - As much as I always could

1 - Not quite so much now

2 - Definitely not quite so much now

3 - Not at all

B. I have looked forward with enjoyment to things:

0 - As much as I ever did

1 - Rather less than I used to

2 - Definitely less than I used to

3 - Hardly at all

C. I have blamed myself unnecessarily when things went wrong:

3 - Yes, most of the time

2 - Yes, some of the time

1 - Not very often

0 - No, never

D. I have been anxious or worried for no good reason:

0 – No, not at all

1 - Hardly ever

2 - Yes, sometimes

3 - Yes, very often

E. I have felt scared or panicky for no very good reason:

3 - Yes, quite a lot

2 - Yes, sometimes

1- No, not much

0 - No, not at all

F. Things have been getting on top of me (translated from British English to American English, this means, "I've been feeling overwhelmed."):

3 - Yes, most of the time I haven't been able to cope at all

2 - Yes, sometimes I haven't been coping as well as usual

1 - No, most of the time I have coped quite well

0 - No, I have been coping as well as ever

G. I have been so unhappy that I have had difficulty sleeping:

3 - Yes, most of the time

2 - Yes, sometimes

1 - Not very often

0 - No, not at all

H. I have felt sad or miserable:

3 - Yes, most of the time

2 - Yes, quite often

1 - Not very often

0 - No, not at all

I. I have been so unhappy that I have been crying:

3 - Yes, most of the time

2 - Yes, quite often

1 - Only occasionally

0 - No, not at all

J. The thought of harming myself has occurred to me:

3 - Yes, quite often

2 - Sometimes

1 - Hardly ever

0 - Never

Total Score:

Add your circled scores for each question. If your score is 14 or greater you may have postpartum depression or anxiety. But no matter what your score is, if you're not feeling like "you," speak with your healthcare provider. The next section explains how you can go about discussing your results.

ANECDOTE

Assessing a mom after going the whole nine yards (months, rather, and ten of them)

From Thomas M. McNeilis, D.O., F.A.C.O.G., Professor at Dixie State College

The postpartum period in a mom's life gets very little attention because most of the time and preparation during pregnancy are focused on the delivery. Moms are left to cope on their own as they return home from the hospital (which is usually in less than 48 hours). If they happen to have complications such as a C-section, medical problems, or a traumatic birth, attention is focused on the infant and not so much on mom's well being. Compounded with those facts is the point that there's an overlap of symptoms of depression with symptoms of pregnancy that tends to obscure a diagnosis of PPD, so it often gets overlooked. Add to that mix the ignorance everywhere, even in parts of the medical community, about PPD, and you can see that getting a diagnosis right away is sometimes a fat chance.

Some commonly held but false beliefs are still prevalent in society, and my colleagues are no exception in their belief of them. For example, consider these:

- Pregnancy protects against mental illness.

- Depression is very obvious in pregnant women.

- Most women have symptoms of depression only after birth.

The symptoms I look for in a new mom after she delivers are feelings of sadness, guilt, hopelessness, and worthlessness; difficulty concentrating; sleeping too little or too much; loss of interest in activities that she usually enjoys; recurring thoughts of death or suicide; and a change in eating habits. I keep a close eye on the mom if she experiences complications in the birthing process, such as C-sections and traumatic births, and if her baby has physical challenges, such as cleft lip and palate, RDS, jaundice, and so on.

From my experience, it's important to diagnose these symptoms during pregnancy and the postpartum period for the following reasons:

- PPD interferes with infant bonding.

- Women that have these symptoms are less likely to seek physician help and tend to have poor prenatal self-care.

- PPD can lead to substance abuse and self-medication.

- PPD can cause medical or obstetrical complications.

- PPD can lead to suicidal thoughts.

- If women exhibit symptoms of depression during pregnancy with the marked change of fluids, electrolytes, and hormones, they're more prone to a relapse or worsening of symptoms postpartum.

Discussing your pre-assessment with a professional

Your EPDS score isn't a diagnosis — it just gives you and your healthcare professional good information and a place to start. Sometimes pediatricians' or OB/GYNs' offices have a pile of EPDS forms on waiting room tables with instructions to complete the form and hand it to the doctor or nurse on your way in to the appointment. If the designated person in the office sees from your score that you need a complete assessment, he or she will (hopefully) refer you to a competent mental health professional.

If you aren't offered this information, make sure you ask for a referral. And, even if your score is low, feel free to request the name of a specialist in PPD anyway. The test is exactly that — only a test. It may not touch on the particular symptoms that are plaguing you.

Receiving a Competent Professional Assessment

When OB/GYNs and family practice doctors use the EPDS or another simple screening method, it's usually part of a very quick screening (usually five minutes or less), and from the results of that screening he or she may recommend that you see a mental health professional for a more complete evaluation. Anyone — including a nurse, doctor, technician, or another staff person in the office — can give the initial screening as long as he or she is trained to ask the right questions and to interpret the results accurately.

Making sure your doctor has proper PPD training

Not all those folks who are designated to screen you in the doctor's office for PPD have the proper training to do so. You may receive terribly insensitive questions such as, "Do you want to kill your child?" This happened to a few of my clients before they came to see me, and it was devastating for each woman. Often the woman, who may not have ever had that thought before and who may be obsessive, suddenly starts focusing on that worry. The thought "Am I capable of hurting my child?" may begin to plague her. Even if this question doesn't become a worry, it's still misleading and feeds into the misconception that PPD means you want to hurt your child.

There's no way to really know in advance if the person who's initially screening you has received proper training. You can ask, but I don't think you'll get helpful information. The most important point in this whole section is that if you want or think you need a full assessment by someone who specializes in PPD, then get one. If you need help, chances are you know that already. Sometimes, depending on your insurance, specialists require a screening first, which isn't anything to worry about. Just know that if you're asked questions that don't apply to you, they don't apply to you, end of story.

The mental health practitioner who gives you a complete evaluation, on the other hand, must have adequate training. You definitely need to speak to someone with specialized training in identifying and handling PPD. I outline exactly how to find a competent therapist in Chapter 6.

Going another round to establish a diagnosis

After you've been screened and are referred to a competent professional (or have found that person yourself), you'll go for a more thorough evaluation. It's usually at the end of this evaluation that you receive a diagnosis. Different therapists have their own methods of evaluation, but much of the appointment involves the therapist asking you general questions about your physical and emotional well-being, followed by more specific questions. The therapist may use your initial screening (the EPDS or another one) as a guide.

For example, I work in a very practical fashion. Sometimes one of my clients has already taken the EPDS or another screening test, but usually she hasn't. In a nutshell, I ask the mom about the following:

✔ Her hormonal history

✔ Her family and personal history of mood disorders

✔ The quantity and quality of her sleep

✔ Whether she has an appetite

✔ What she's eating and drinking

✔ The major stressors she's facing

✔ Whatever else she feels is important for me to know

After she and I feel that I have a good understanding of what she's experiencing, I outline a solid plan for her so she knows exactly and simply what she needs to do to start recovering.

A pediatrician's perspective

From Geoffrey R. Kotin, MD:

"As a pediatrician in a large HMO practice, I often meet new mothers for the first time at the two-week well-baby visit. This appointment provides an opportunity for me to assess not only the health, growth, and development of the newborn, but also the level of bonding between parents and infant and, to some degree, the emotional health of the mother. Most new mothers are very engaged with their babies. I see them cooing to the infant, cuddling him or her, and I sometimes need almost to pry the baby away to do my exam. So, mothers who distance themselves (physically or emotionally) from their baby or seem excessively tired, tearful, or anxious raise my level of concern about the possibility of postpartum depression.

Pediatricians are concerned about depression in mothers because intuitively, they think that a mother who's depressed would interact differently with her baby than a healthy mom, which can possibly lead to some adverse effects on the child. Current research does suggest that postpartum depression affects child development, behavior, and health. The following list shows these possible effects (though, remember that not all children of depressed mothers will suffer from these problems and if they do, many are able to overcome the effects and develop normally):

- Children, especially boys, of PPD mothers didn't perform as well as children of well mothers on cognitive tasks, such as language, at 18 months.

- Several behavioral effects have been documented. Infants of withdrawn mothers have been found to spend more time fussing and crying than others. Infants of intrusive depressed mothers cry less but have been shown to avoid looking at their mothers and engaging with them. Insecure attachment to the mother in late infancy can be a consequence of PPD and can have repercussions later in childhood. Increased problems at school entry have been noted, such as anxiety and, in boys, higher rates of conduct problems and hyperactive symptoms.

- There is concern that in some situations PPD may be a predisposing factor for child abuse.

- PPD can impact appropriate use of healthcare resources and consequently child health. Infants of mothers who reported having depressive symptoms were found to receive less consistent preventive healthcare, including immunizations, and to have more visits to emergency departments than infants of mothers who didn't report depressive symptoms.

In our clinic, mothers are asked to complete the Edinburgh Postnatal Depression Scale at each well-baby check in the first year. Women who score 12 or higher are encouraged to contact their primary care clinician or the mental health department for further evaluation (and we help with contact if necessary). They're also given a list of other resources, including literature recommendations and Web sites of organizations that provide help to mothers with PPD."

Reacting to Your Diagnosis

Not surprisingly, if the DSM-IV diagnosis of PPD is both misleading and confusing to professionals, it can be even more misleading and confusing for you, the layperson. To top it off, if you happen to have PPD, you're already subject to feeling overwhelmed, anxious, and confused by new information when it comes in.

The good news is that many competent psychiatrists, doctors, and clinical psychologists skip the confusing language after they've evaluated you and simply tell you that you have PPD.

When your doctor reveals your diagnosis, you may experience a number of emotions, including relief. This relief comes from the fact that you now at least know that what you've been experiencing actually has a name. Plus, your healthcare provider will probably sit down and talk with you, explaining to you the variety of treatments for PPD and the fact that the depression will go away over time.

If you hear negativity about your prognosis or sense worry on the part of the practitioner regarding your PPD, you should find another professional who understands PPD. A practitioner with specialized experience knows that this illness is treatable and will go away.

In addition to the relief of having a diagnosis, you may also react in several other different ways, the most common of which include the following:

✔ **Denial:** If you experience denial, you may say any number of the following things (or something like them) to yourself:

"No, depression of any kind, including postpartum depression, is something that happens to other people, but not to me."

"Because I'm not having scary thoughts about hurting myself or my baby, I don't really have whatever this "postpartum thing" is, and therefore, the professional who evaluated me must have made a mistake." (Unfortunately, there actually is a misconception that, in order to have PPD, you need to have feelings about hurting your baby or not caring about him or her.)

"I'm not that bad off. Everybody feels this way after they have a baby. This is just the blues."

Thankfully, you have this book and other resources available to you, which means that you'll be able to verify for yourself, based on your symptoms, whether the professional evaluation is correct (in the vast majority of cases, it will be).

✔ **Shame:** Usually when a woman feels shame, she has a preconceived, negative notion of what this illness is all about.

For example, if you think that having PPD means that you're "crazy," not ready to be a mother, inadequate, or weak, you may find yourself wanting to fight your diagnosis. After all, who wants to be a member of that club? If you believe that PPD means something negative about you as a person and a mother, *which it certainly does not,* then you'd feel unnecessarily ashamed.

✔ **Inadequacy or weakness:** Often, the disempowering question that goes along with this reaction is "Why can other mothers handle this and I can't?"

The incorrect assumption is that PPD is happening only to you. Almost one in five mothers experience PPD, so chances are you're meeting others with PPD every day (presuming you're outside and around other people). The very woman who you're convinced feels gloriously happy may have the therapy appointment right after you, so never assume. Just remember: PPD isn't a character weakness — it's an illness. Many strong, intelligent, good mothers are going through this right now with you — whether you've met them yet or not.

✔ **Guilt:** If you experience this emotion, you may say to yourself "Maybe I caused this. Maybe I did this to myself."

Often I'll hear what sound like confessions from new clients who have just received the news that they have PPD. They imply that the PPD is their doing. They say "I've always had low self-esteem. Now it's worse than ever. I should've been done with this problem before I became a mother."

You didn't bring the PPD on. This isn't your fault. You wouldn't wish this on yourself or anyone else. Even if you think that your personality or an unhealthy way of thinking may have fed into your depression, the PPD still isn't your fault.

✔ **Self-pity:** This is the "why me?" reaction. After all, it isn't fair that you have PPD and others don't. Your reaction is normal, so go easy on yourself. There's a time and a place to feel bad for yourself. That way you can move through this part of recovery and keep moving forward.

At this point, I suggest to women that they throw themselves a pity party (see Chapter 13 where I give you tips on doing this), which allows them to move on to accepting their diagnosis and receiving treatment.

Although it may not seem like it when you first hear it, your diagnosis is a step in the positive direction. This is because after you accept the frustrating reality, you suddenly have the capacity to take action, to mitigate the biochemical, psychological, and environmental effects it's having on you, and to get back on track with life the way you want it to be (which may be even better than before you had your baby). So if and when you hear the diagnosis, sit back, take a few deep breaths, open your heart and mind, and assume that on some level this is a very good thing you're being told.

This isn't to say that you should accept whatever the doctors or therapists tell you, and that you must agree to whatever therapeutic plan they recommend. If you feel extremely uncomfortable with what they recommend, you may want to seek out a second opinion with another expert in PPD (Chapter 6 has tips to help you find a knowledgeable therapist). After you find assistance that you feel good about, get on the therapeutic recovery track as soon as you can.

Chapter 6

Seeking Out a Therapist to Keep Your Proverbial House Standing

· ·

In This Chapter

▶ Realizing why you need to seek out a therapist

▶ Motivating yourself to attend therapy

▶ Selecting the right individual therapist

▶ Discovering the different types of therapists

▶ Paying for your therapeutic treatment

▶ Locating and interviewing your prospective doc

· ·

*A*lmost everyone who has postpartum depression (PPD) can benefit from working with some type of therapist. Even if you have excellent support at home from your partner and family, and even if a community of caring friends surrounds you, working with a mental health professional can prove tremendously helpful. For one thing, your social support network consists of people who are emotionally involved with you, and it may be difficult for them to remain objective (even if one or more is a therapist). Also, it can feel wonderful to be totally uncensored in the therapist's office and dump your feelings out without fear of hurting anyone else's. Even more importantly, a well-trained therapist, unlike your partner or family members, can bring to bear the depth of their overall therapeutic skills and experience, and if you hit the jackpot, they'll also have specific knowledge about, and experience with, PPD.

Many women who consult with me say that they waited for a while before making an appointment because "it wasn't that bad." They erroneously thought that seeing a therapist meant that they had to feel seriously ill and that only those in the "deep end" need that kind of assistance. Very soon after the appointment begins, these women realize that it was foolish to wait — they could have used the help a lot sooner. No matter if the depression is mild, moderate, or severe, it's best to get help as quickly as possible. Even if you aren't sure that you actually have PPD, go anyway and receive an assessment. Any decent therapist with expertise in this field can tell you if you're adjusting normally or if what you're experiencing is PPD. Even if you have the normal baby blues, getting some solid suggestions from a therapist can help you through it. Hearing that what you're experiencing is normal, by the way, is validating. I recommend it highly.

This chapter focuses on how to find the right therapist for you. Topics covered include choosing from among the many different types of therapists, understanding why therapist visits are so important, finding out about ways to pay for therapy, and knowing when you should stick with — or ditch — a particular therapist.

Understanding the Role and Importance of a Therapist

It goes without saying (but I'll say it anyway) that the main reason to see a therapist or counselor is so that you recover more quickly, more completely, and more easily than you would if you did it alone. Untreated PPD can turn into chronic depression and set you up for relapses throughout the rest of your life. For example, 25 percent of women with PPD will still have it after 12 months, if it goes untreated. So, it's imperative that you get treated as quickly as possible.

If you're in the hospital due to severe postpartum depression, bipolar disorder, or psychosis, therapy will be mandatory — and for good reason. You'll have a lot to process regarding what you've been through and what you're still experiencing. When you're discharged from the hospital, an outpatient plan with a therapist should be lined up for you. Make sure you follow through with the therapy until you're well and functioning as you want to be.

In case you need more motivation, there's one more reason to get therapy sooner rather than later: Untreated PPD may have a huge effect on your relationships and the individual members of your family. So, just in case you're feeling guilty (therapy will help you with this symptom of PPD too!) for spending the time and money on yourself for treatment, think of it this way: You're really investing the money in your whole family's health and future.

Untreated PPD can have the following effects on family members:

- Infants of depressed mothers sometimes have higher heart rates and have difficulty engaging socially. And, they weigh less, make fewer facial expressions and sounds, and are slower to walk. Finally, these same infants can be fussier, less active, and less responsive to other people. Infants of moms with PPD can also have signs and brain patterns of depression.

- Toddlers of depressed mothers are at higher risk for mood problems, have poor self-control, don't get along well with their peers, have neurological delays and trouble paying attention, and have behavior that looks like their mothers' depressive behavior.

- Preschoolers of depressed mothers can be less cooperative and more aggressive, can have less verbal understanding, can have more problem behaviors and less expressive language, and tend to perform poorly on school readiness tests. Spending one to two months with a severely depressed mother increases these kids' chances of becoming depressed by the age of 15.

- Marriages also can suffer if you don't receive proper help. Without solid professional help, the changes in your mood and behavior can be quite confusing and be misinterpreted by your partner, which can lead to hurtful arguments and yelling matches. You and your partner need guidance in order to adjust to the ups and downs of this illness. (For in-depth information on helping your marriage and getting partners their own help, see Chapter 15.)

A new study, which was conducted by researchers at the Cincinnati Children's Hospital Medical Center and featured in the August 2004 issue of the Archives of Pediatrics and Adolescent Medicine, determined that a mentally healthy father can dramatically help to correct the devastating impact that a depressed mother can have on the behavioral and emotional health of the child. The report is based on data that was collected from 822 children, ages 3 through 12, from two-parent families all over the country.

Don't be afraid if you've already waited a few months before finding help — even though you may have been depressed for a while, that doesn't automatically mean that your children are psychologically damaged. And if they have been affected, please know that children are remarkably resilient. The most important thing is that you get help so you can enjoy your life — and, in turn, your family will benefit. Simply congratulate yourself for finding help now and not waiting any longer.

Finding the Motivation to Go to Therapy: Demolishing Mental Blockades

This section isn't a discussion about finding the right therapist (that's discussed later in this chapter), or about arriving at your therapy sessions in a timely manner (something you may need to ask for support on, both in terms of having someone watch your new baby and in terms of driving or taking public transport if you really aren't up to getting yourself there safely). Instead, the focus here is on the kinds of mental and emotional blocks that people in general — and new moms in particular — often have about taking part in the therapeutic process. In other words, it's one thing to decide or agree to go to therapy, but it's another to actually go.

Very often my clients are aware that they had previous problems before their PPD, but they thought the problems were never bad enough to seek therapy, or they just never made the time to get those issues handled. Sometimes it takes a crisis to finally get the help that has been needed for years. That's part of the silver lining of going through PPD. You can emerge better put together than when you first fell into the pit. I've yet to meet a woman who regrets finally receiving the help — it's always such a relief for her. Let that be you!

In the beginning: Contemplating therapy

Most women who suffer from PPD will, at some point during their illness, consider whether they should seek psychological treatment from a professional therapist. Different women have different reactions when contemplating therapy. For example, in general, there are three different categories of women and reactions:

✔ Women who resist therapy from the very start and never seek or agree to receive professional help

✔ Women who decide right from the start to get support from a professional therapist

✔ Women who are on the fence, perhaps deciding or agreeing to go to therapy only after they find that things are clearly not going well for them

In large part, those women who resist even contemplating going to therapy do so because of the mainly negative images and stereotypes that society has with regard to therapy. From movies and books to the ideas that people throw around with each other in casual environments, therapy often gets a bad and undeserved rap. I could go on for hours listing all of the negativity that comes out of these sources, but the emphasis wouldn't help you heal. So, just know that the negativity you hear or read about is a bunch of hooey.

Just like with most services and products, those people who are satisfied usually don't have much to say about it (my clients have lots to say, of course!), whereas the much smaller number of people who have something go wrong make a great deal of negative noise and capture your attention. If you're a new mom who thinks that she may have PPD and that therapy just may help you, try to have an open mind and heart as you read through the rest of this chapter — the duration and severity of your illness could very well depend on it.

Confronting fear of the "therapy" label

It's true, many people are afraid of therapy. But, for the most part, they aren't afraid of what actually happens during or as a result of therapy. Instead, they're afraid of being stigmatized or labeled as someone who *needs* therapy. They may think "What if my friends or co-workers find out and think I'm nuts? What if it ends up on my permanent record?"

But the reality is that you do need support, that psychological treatment through therapy just might prove extremely valuable, and that whatever people think — or what you think other people might think — simply isn't relevant. Try to follow this thinking: What other people think about me is none of my business! It may also be useful for you to know that the therapist is bound by strict rules of confidentiality. Everything you say within the therapy session will stay between the two of you (with a couple extreme exceptions).

Thankfully, even in America, the notion of a negative lifelong branding or stigma for having gone to therapy has greatly diminished as many people from all walks of life — movie stars, politicians, sports figures, businesspeople — have readily acknowledged that not only have they gone to therapy, but it has proven immensely valuable to them. But still, you may find yourself afraid. If that's the case, as they say, "feel the fear and do it anyway."

Knowing that therapy doesn't mean you're weak

Closely related to the fear of therapy and the possibility of being stigmatized is the idea of appearing weak. Unfortunately, there's a myth, especially here in America, that everyone is supposed to be able to pull themselves up by their own bootstraps (see Chapter 14 for more on accepting the fact that you need a support circle). If you're resisting therapy, you may be thinking "Yes, maybe there is something called PPD, and maybe it's real, but a new mom with a baby should still be able to get through it on her own. After all, other women have babies, and they somehow manage to handle all their problems just fine."

Don't fall prey to this internally-voiced doubt or fear. The fact that you have (or may have) PPD is *not your fault.* You didn't cause it, you didn't ask for it, you didn't bring it on, and you aren't solely responsible for getting yourself through it. Rather than a sign of weakness, seeking appropriate support is a sign of strength and wisdom. If you care for yourself, your child, your partner, your family, your friends, your co-workers, and everyone else who's in your life, you do whatever it takes to get well as quickly and effectively as you know how. For the great majority of women, that plan includes therapeutic support of some kind, regardless of what anyone (including the doubting part of yourself) thinks about you for having sought such support.

Revisiting previous bad experiences with therapy

Some women with PPD who find themselves resisting psychological treatment have just had bad experiences with therapy. In other cases, they've merely heard about someone else having bad experiences. Obviously, if you know someone who had PPD and gave a particular therapist or counselor a very negative review, that's one professional you'd probably want to avoid. Otherwise, keep an open mind and give it another shot because, undoubtedly, as with any other service or professional, there are indeed bad — inexperienced, inadequately trained, ineffective, uncaring, — therapists out there. But sometimes, the therapist may be fine — it's just a bad fit for the two of them. In other words, that same counselor may be perfect for the next woman.

The bottom line is that you should most definitely not let the fact that there are a few bad apples out there prevent you from ever taking another therapeutic bite again, especially when you can really use the professional support that can be provided. (Imagine someone having a run-in with a bad auto mechanic and vowing to never fix his or her car again.)

Gracefully accepting your need for help

It's not uncommon for a woman who's suffering greatly from PPD to convince herself that she's actually doing just fine and that she certainly doesn't need any professional psychological treatment or assistance. Especially when she's right on the verge of making the decision to seek out or go ahead with therapy or counseling, she may tell herself that her PPD will go away on its own. (Note that even though PPD can eventually go away on its own, often it won't, and it can easily turn into long-term chronic depression.)

If you need therapy, then you need therapy. All the wishing, hoping, and praying that your PPD will just suddenly go away on its own is extremely unlikely to work. What's true, however, is that receiving psychological treatment from a qualified and caring professional is among the most important and effective things that you can possibly do to address your PPD. And just think: If it really wasn't that bad, you probably wouldn't even be reading this book!

Understanding your partner's reaction

If you're contemplating therapy, and you're married or otherwise share your life with another adult, you may have to deal with your partner's ideas about therapy in addition to your own. Partners often have strong emotions when it comes to therapy. That is, your partner's fears, doubts, anxieties, and so forth, both about therapy in general and your PPD in particular, may get stirred up by your decision to look into therapy.

Chapter 15 contains a general discussion about working with your partner, including how to work things through with your partner when you don't see eye to eye. Remember that your partner may be scared for you, your relationship, and your child. Even if you're feeling overwhelmed, in this situation, it's key for you to muster as much compassion toward your partner as possible. Not just compassion, however, but compassion coupled with strength and clarity. If psychological treatment is what you need, you have to be strong and clear with your partner that this is what you're going to do, even if he's uncomfortable with it. You're seeking therapy because it's one of the most effective treatments for PPD (and because it will help you, your relationships, and your child).

Talking yourself into, not out of, therapy

Henry Ford supposedly once said, "Whether you think you can or you can't, you're probably right." In other words, he was implying that the power of the mind shouldn't be underestimated. Based on the various fears and considerations described in this chapter, you can probably either talk yourself into or out of seeking and regularly attending therapy.

If you could have done what was necessary with respect to your mind and your emotions on your own, without any therapeutic intervention, you certainly would have already done so. Instead, the truth is that you probably need just the kind of help that a good therapist can provide. Talk yourself into therapy — do whatever it takes to face your fears and doubts and fully embrace the probability that therapy will make a huge positive difference to you — and you're well on the way to a full recovery.

Seeking Help When You Suspect You Have PPD

So you're pretty sure (or maybe certain) that you have PPD. So what now? First and foremost, don't get scared. Remember, it's not information that's your enemy — it's a lack of information that can be harmful. I don't mean you should jump up in glee because you now know you have PPD. I just mean that knowing your situation is a good thing, and it leads to finally finding real help. Here are the other things you don't want to do: Don't hide, don't go into denial, and don't just hope the PPD will go away on its own. Gather all the inner strength you can muster and go to war with the PPD demon — if you heed my advice, you'll win that war!

Your sources for finding professional guidance include the following folks:

- ✔ Your OB/GYN or primary care physician who may direct you to other community resources or medical professionals

- ✔ A postpartum depression organization (see the appendix for some organizations I recommend, along with their contact info)

- ✔ A therapist who has specialized training in PPD (which is discussed in the section "Finding the Right Therapist for You" later in this chapter)

- ✔ A support person who can find a resource for you

The last bullet is important because you may not feel capable of making the phone call yourself. Overwhelm and depression can make ordinarily simple tasks such as finding a number or an e-mail address feel like too much to handle, so don't feel bad if you need to ask someone else for help making the connection.

Recognizing the stumbling blocks: Why women don't get help

One of the most interesting (and unfair) parts of PPD is that the common emotions of guilt, shame, and embarrassment (which ironically get in the way of a woman reaching out and getting the help she needs) are actual symptoms of PPD. If your PPD is making you believe that you're a weak and incompetent person for not bucking up and handling your life, chances are you're embarrassed about coming forward to get support. After all, who wants to be associated with an inadequate bunch of people?

Try comparing PPD to other health situations. For example, can you imagine a person with diabetes or heart disease feeling too embarrassed to call the doctor's office? Of course not! So, the same concept should apply to postpartum depression.

The resource you first contact may or may not be the person or organization you stick with. But, it's the first step, and that contact can lead you to the resources that will help you recover.

Finding the Right Therapist for You

You've probably noticed that information about PPD is everywhere. The problem is that much of what you may be hearing is misleading or downright wrong. The key to receiving correct information is to listen to only reliable resources — those therapists, doctors, and counselors with specific training in PPD. If you're asked a worrisome question (even from a professional) or see an alarming article, you need to talk to a professional who specializes in this area to get some reassurance.

Consider the following example: Last year one of my clients was asked by the nurse in her obstetrician's office, "Are you thinking of drowning your children?" The well-meaning nurse was simply following the list of follow-up instructions for new mothers that the doctor had given her. Unfortunately, that one question had a negative effect on the woman. After that experience, my obsessive client, who had never had a drowning thought in her life, started doubting herself and the safety of her children when they were with her. Luckily, in therapy, she realized that the drowning question had nothing to do with her. It was simply evidence of a professional's lack of training.

So, now that you know it's important to be careful of whose advice you follow, you're probably wondering how you go about actually finding and choosing a therapist. Well, you've come to the right place. The following sections show you exactly what to look for in a therapist.

Knowing what to look for in a therapist

There are several characteristics that you should keep in mind when looking for a therapist. For example, you want to work with someone who is

- **Adequately trained and licensed:** All things being equal, you want to work with someone who has more, rather than less, training (refer to the upcoming section "Choosing a Licensed Therapist" where the various types of therapists are described).

- **Competent and generally effective at what she does:** You may be able to asses a therapist's competency through word of mouth, but often you'll have to make a judgment — relying on your gut instinct — upon meeting a potential therapist for the first time.

✔ **Open-minded and compassionate (especially if she isn't previously experienced with PPD):** If you have a first impression one way or another, you should trust that first impression.

When I first started working with other women with PPD, I couldn't find a psychiatrist who knew much about this specialized field. But, I did know one who was open-minded and willing to soak in as much information as he could. I started referring all my clients to him if they needed medication, and now this doctor has quite a popular reputation in this area.

✔ **Geographically close to you (if possible):** If you're choosing to see someone in person, you should probably be within a 30-minute drive to your therapist. But, if you have to spend longer traveling to someone's office in order to see a real expert in this specialty, it'll be well worth it. Because I give consultations for women and their families all over the country (and internationally), I work by phone or Webcam. It's convenient for everyone, and it works great.

✔ **Ideally, specifically knowledgeable in the field of PPD:** To find out a therapist's expertise in PPD, you can ask a potential candidate about her level of experience and you can ask what PPD-related organizations she belongs to.

If a therapist has little or no experience with PPD, you don't necessarily have to eliminate her, but do make sure that the therapist you choose is open-minded, willing to learn, and compassionate. For example, she should be willing to read up on PPD, go to conferences, receive training, and really get up to speed on the subject.

If you think a therapist is judging you, blaming the PPD on you, or thinking that PPD isn't "real", move on! There are many self-professed "experts" in PPD. Just by asking the right questions, you can usually avoid them (see "Assessing the Therapist You've Chosen" later in this chapter).

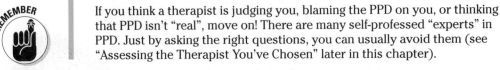

MIA: Formal training

Unfortunately, there's still no specific graduate training program anywhere in the United States that thoroughly addresses PPD — not for doctors, not for psychologists, not for social workers, not for anybody. If a therapist wants to be adequately trained in PPD, she or he has to attend a specialized in-service training or conference.

Postpartum Support International (PSI) offers such trainings on a regular basis. The great news is that professionals who work with pregnant and postpartum women are eager for this information, and are attending (by increasing numbers every year) these excellent in-service programs.

The gender bender: The equal weights of Mars and Venus

This may come as a surprise to many women — and men as well — but when considering a therapist or counselor, gender doesn't matter. Many women (and male partners and other family members and friends) automatically assume that a female therapist or counselor (or, for that matter, medical doctor) is better for a woman suffering from PPD, but this isn't necessarily the case.

Some of the very best therapists, counselors, and doctors that I've worked with over the years have been male, and some of the very worst have been female. Sometimes, because males know they're unlikely to ever experience PPD, they're more open to, and work much harder at, understanding just what the woman is going through. As a result, they end up being far more compassionate and effective. Conversely, some of the female therapists, counselors, and doctors (some who are mothers themselves but didn't have PPD), exude judgment and disdain, and can be quite cold.

Ultimately, it's the person — the individual practitioner — who you must evaluate, so don't let the gender of a possible candidate bend your mind toward an unfairly positive or negative evaluation and therefore a bad decision.

Choosing a Licensed Therapist

The process of choosing the right therapist may at first seem a bit daunting, especially if you're suffering from PPD and feel easily overwhelmed by new tasks. But, with a little bit of up-front knowledge about the different types of therapists (and other helpful professionals) who are out there, this process should be a great deal easier for you. Keep in mind that, ultimately, there's no wrong way to start. Getting help is what's most important, and if the first person you go to isn't the one you end up with, at least you'll have started and be that much closer to finding the right person.

Sorting through the assortment of therapists

A wide variety of therapists exist, and if you live in a major metropolitan area, you'll have many choices before you. If you live in a smaller town or in the country, however, you may have to work a bit harder to find the right type of therapist. But, remember, even if you find the right type of therapist, that person still may not be the right one for you. A person's credentials are far less important than who they are as a person, how open they are to learning about PPD (if they aren't already familiar with it), and how compassionate they are (see the section "Finding the Right Therapist for You" earlier in this chapter).

Nonetheless, knowing a little bit about the different types of therapists (and their credentials) can prove very useful as you initiate your search. Here's a short description of each of the different types of licensed therapists that could help you down the road to recovery:

- **Clinical psychologists:** *Clinical psychologists* focus on the diagnosis, treatment, study, and prevention of all types of mental and emotional disorders. A clinical psychologist has a PhD (doctorate level, which is the highest) or sometimes a PsyD in psychology. Even though they aren't able to prescribe medication, clinical psychologists will have received intensive clinical training in patient assessment, research, and the use of different types of psychological therapies.

- **Psychiatrists:** *Psychiatrist*s are medical doctors who receive four years of special training in addition to what's necessary to obtain their medical degree. In addition to training in psychotherapy, psychiatrists have received advanced instruction focusing on psychiatric diagnoses, psychopharmacology, and the management of mental health issues and disorders through medication. In short, these physicians are considered to have the greatest expertise with respect to prescribing medications for mood disorders, including PPD.

- **Social workers:** These professional therapists, who can't prescribe medication, either have a Masters in Social Work (MSW) or they're considered Licensed Clinical Social Workers (LCSWs). *Social workers* are trained to understand social and environmental factors and the impact of these on emotional and mental disorders.

- **Marriage and family therapists:** These professionals have an MFT (Marriage and Family Therapist) license, which, like the social worker, is a master's degree level license. *Marriage and family therapists* are trained in individual, couple, and family therapy, but they can't prescribe medication.

- **Counselors:** *Counselors* are master's level mental health professionals who have LCPC licenses, which means that they're Licensed Clinical Professional Counselors. These professionals can't prescribe medication.

- **Psychiatric nurse:** These professionals have an APRN (Advanced Practice Registered Nurse) license. *Psychiatric nurses* are registered nurses who have sought additional education and training and have obtained the equivalent of a master's or even a doctoral degree. They can generally provide a full range of psychiatric care and, depending on the state in which they practice, they may have the authority to prescribe medication.

Other potentially helpful professionals

Some individuals aren't licensed as therapists, and because they don't have licenses, they should never practice therapy. But, these individuals may still prove valuable to you in other ways — especially if you can't locate one of the many types of licensed therapists (or can't find one that you feel comfortable working with). I'm not referring to the local bartender or the woman who runs your hair salon, but rather individuals who are somehow in the helping professions and who may have either general therapeutic expertise or specific knowledge about PPD.

Certified midwife

A *certified midwife* is someone — almost always a woman — who's educated in the discipline of midwifery and who's certified by the American College of Nurse-Midwives. A certified midwife is able to provide primary healthcare to women, including prenatal care, gynecological exams, care during labor and delivery, and postpartum care for both moms and their babies.

If a midwife knows that you have a history of depression or have had a previous bout of PPD, she can do many things during your pregnancy, labor, delivery, and immediate postpartum period to either help you avoid, or at least reduce the intensity of any PPD you experience. However, after you've given birth and find that you're experiencing PPD, you typically wouldn't approach the midwife who assisted you because this kind of therapeutic intervention is beyond her primary competency. But, if you've developed a close relationship with the midwife, she may be able to offer you some initial therapeutic support and help until you find an appropriate therapist or counselor.

Pastoral counselor

Members of the clergy, such as priests, ministers, and rabbis, often have both training and experience in mental health issues. If you have a close relationship with a member of the clergy who is open-minded and well-informed, you may be able to receive help from him or her. For instance, this clergy member may provide an initial therapeutic way station for you and help you find a therapist with more experience and knowledge about PPD.

Be wary of clergy members who have outdated or backward views about PPD, such as it being "your fault" or "God's way" or anything else that tries to place blame on you. If you come across a backward-thinking clergy member, get out as soon as you can, and think about finding a new congregation for your religious worship.

Personal, life, business, success, or spiritual coach

In recent years there has been a dramatic rise of individuals offering services as coaches, including personal coach, life coach, business coach, success coach, or spiritual coach. Many of these individuals hold licenses in other fields, or are certified in hypnotherapy, neuro-linguistic programming (NLP), or specific types of coaching. Some coaches are skilled counselors and may be able to serve as a stopgap measure, or they may be able to help you find a qualified therapist. But, generally speaking, they won't be competent in helping you address something as specific and intense as your PPD.

Paying for Therapy: Don't Shortchange Yourself

Most people are willing to spend whatever it takes to attend to "real" ailments, such as something that can been seen on an X-ray or heard with a stethoscope. These same people, however, may be quite reluctant to pay for their own psychological well-being. A lot of statements like "I just can't afford it" come up when the costs of therapy are considered. However, the real thing to fear here isn't being out a few thousand dollars. Instead, you need to consider the negative impact that avoiding therapy will have on your life. The value of getting well much sooner — and of diminishing both the duration and intensity of PPD — is incalculable.

If you're a partner of a woman with PPD, and your own fears about money are arising, you should try as hard as humanly possible to not mention your fears aloud. Your partner, the new mom, is undoubtedly already feeling guilty about everything that she's "causing" you and everyone in her world to undergo, and she certainly doesn't need this added bit of worry about money. It would be all too easy for you to talk her out of seeking and receiving psychological treatment, and in almost every case, doing so would be a serious mistake. Whatever you do, don't be penny-wise and pound-foolish when it comes to PPD.

You and your family need to be willing to pay for the care you need and deserve. If you can't afford it, find a way to pay for it anyway. If a loved one can lend you the amount for an initial consultation, that would be a great start. For instance, when I speak to a woman for the first time, she always has an initial plan of action at the end of that very first session. Even if that's all the help she gets, she at least has a plan. Also, if it would help, it's worth it to ask the therapist if she will accept a payment plan. You have nothing to lose.

If there's a strong enough will, there's always a way. This therapy is an investment in the health of your entire family. And, remember, this is the time when families spend savings (if they have one) and take out loans if necessary. Even though getting specialized help is definitely more difficult without money, in most cities and counties, you can find low-cost mental health agencies that will refer you to a counselor. (There are also groups, but unless they're therapy groups, they don't replace individual counseling.)

When you're figuring out how to pay for your psychological care, remember to check with your insurance company (if you have one). Some insurance companies are willing to add a specialist in PPD to its provider list, or they'll otherwise be willing to pay for your therapy if you're severely debilitated by your PPD. For more information on insurance, flip ahead to Chapter 10.

Even if a practitioner is covered, however, what's most important is whether they're a good fit for you and will really be able to help you recover. Very often, you may find that in order to get the mental healthcare that you really want and need, you have to pay out of pocket.

Locating a Therapist or Counselor

Of course you want to see an excellent therapist, but you may not be sure where you can find such a person. Rest assured that there are a number of sources that can guide you. Here are a few:

- ✔ **Check the Postpartum Support International Web site.** Located at www.postpartum.net, Postpartum Support International offers a list of support groups and state and area coordinators who can help you locate an appropriate therapist from among the list of those who are members of the organization.

  Even though no official screening occurs through the site and no official endorsements or recommendations are given, the very fact that someone has paid to be a member of the organization shows that they at least have a real interest in working with women who are suffering from PPD.

- ✔ **Ask for referrals from other healthcare practitioners that you trust.** You don't have to ask a medical doctor. You can ask any healthcare practitioner whose judgment you feel you can rely on, especially one who knows you well and has already worked with you. You can directly ask this practitioner if he can recommend a therapist who has experience with PPD. Even if he can't recommend such an experienced therapist, he very well may be able to recommend to you an open-minded and compassionate therapist who's willing to learn about PPD.

Because the reputation of the healthcare practitioner you're asking is also at stake based on the quality of his recommendations, he'll probably give you one or more solid possibilities.

✔ **Keep your ears and eyes wide open.** General word of mouth may also generate a recommendation or two for you. If you know someone who has had PPD, she, of course, would be the best place to start. But if you don't know anyone who has had it, go ahead and ask your friends if they know anyone who specifically works with PPD, or if they know of any therapists or counselors who generally get stellar recommendations. Most professional service people generate a majority of their business through word-of-mouth, so if you really "work" this channel, you'll probably come up with something useful, even if it's only a lead or two.

✔ **Ask around at hospital maternity wards and public health centers.** More and more PPD support groups are popping up all over the country at hospitals and public healthcare centers. Try calling the maternity ward at the hospital where you gave birth, and ask if there are any resources for new mothers with PPD.

Assessing the Therapist You've Chosen

Assuming that you've found a therapist or counselor who, on the surface, seems qualified and appropriate, how do you know if you've really found the right person? It can be tricky, but by the end of this section, you'll know exactly how to do it.

If you're suffering from PPD, it's all too easy to doubt your judgment and want to give your power away to the first person who waves a license in front of you and says "Yes, I know all about depression and I can help you." So, it's important at this phase that you don't just accept the first doc you come across. Before accepting any doctor's help, make sure that you really feel comfortable with her. Part of getting over PPD is reclaiming your power of judgment, and there's no better place to start than with your choice of a therapist.

Even if your chosen doc seems qualified, competent, compassionate, and experienced at first glance, you should still ask her at least a few of the upcoming set of questions over the phone before you make an appointment. If the candidate won't let you ask any questions or becomes indignant, I suggest you drop her like a hot potato.

The first question is the most important, so definitely start with that one. If she passes the first question, go on to the second. If at that point you feel comfortable making an appointment, go ahead and do so. After you make an appointment, you don't necessarily need to run through the rest of the questions (which aren't in any order of importance). When you're having your first session, if you still want to ask the other questions, though, feel free to do so. Here are the questions:

- ✔ **What specific training have you received in working with women with postpartum depression?** If the therapist or counselor answers, "Depression is depression, and I have a lot of graduate training in depression and have worked with lots of postpartum moms," that's not good enough. PPD is a specialized area, and she either needs to have received specific training or know that she doesn't know about it and be open to learning about it.

- ✔ **I'd like to start reading more information about PPD. What books, audio programs or Web sites can you recommend for me?** If the therapist truly has expertise in postpartum depression, she should be able to name several relevant books or other resources. After all, you'd expect a grief counselor to be able to name some resources on grief, and a therapist specializing in trauma to be able to rattle off some trauma resources. This specialty deserves the same respect.

- ✔ **Do you have a favorite type of therapy?** Research has shown that the most effective types of therapy for PPD are cognitive-behavioral therapy and interpersonal therapy. For a woman who's experiencing a crisis like PPD, psychoanalysis isn't appropriate — so if the candidate you're interviewing answers this way, you probably want to go with someone else.

- ✔ **What are your general feelings about the causes of postpartum depression?** The candidate's answer here reveals whether she believes there are biochemical and other causal factors behind PPD or whether she holds to one of the outdated views that somehow the new mom is at fault for her own PPD.

- ✔ **Do you belong to any organizations dedicated specifically to education about postpartum depression?** Someone who's committed to offering therapeutic interventions in a field like postpartum depression should belong to Postpartum Support International or at least another postpartum organization.

Part III

Diagnosis Confirmed: Looking at the Treatment Options for PPD

The 5th Wave   By Rich Tennant

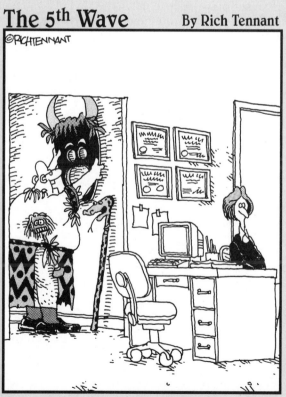

"Fortunately for you, Ms. Dobbins, at this clinic we firmly believe in alternative medicine."

In this part . . .

*B*ecause you're likely to use some kind of treatment as you head on down the road to recovery, I devote this entire part to the three major types of treatment for postpartum depression: psychological, medical, and alternative. I round out this part by addressing how and why you should create a comprehensive treatment plan that combines one or more elements from these three types of treatment.

Chapter 7

Venting Your Mind and Heart: Psychological Treatment

Therapy that addresses the psyche — that is, the thoughts, feelings, emotions, mind, mental state, and psychological state of a person — is a crucial part of working through postpartum depression (PPD). In this chapter, I introduce you to a general scope of psychological therapy: I tell you what to expect once you're there, how to make sure you get the most from it, how to end therapy but stay healthy in the process, and what types of groups can serve as a valuable supplement to your therapy.

Knowing What to Expect From Therapy

Knowing what to expect from therapy can, in some ways, be just as important as finding the right therapist (see Chapter 6 for tips on finding the right one for you). It's helpful to start out with realistic expectations and an understanding that the relationship between you and the therapist should be a partnership (not a one-sided chat). And, starting out with short-term therapeutic goals boosts your overall chances of recovering rapidly and fully. Even though every therapist and every therapeutic relationship will, of course, have unique attributes (not to mention the fact that you're a unique patient with your own special set of challenges and strengths), this section and the ones that follow are meant to give you some guidelines to maximize your chances of an extremely successful therapeutic experience.

The first point to remember: Keep your expectations realistic

It makes sense to expect a great deal from therapy. By setting high expectations (that you'll feel at least somewhat better very soon and that you'll then completely recover) you magnify the chances of achieving your recovery goals. For example, psychologists and students of human behavior talk of *self-fulfilling prophecies* (the tendency for what you believe to come true). And studies of high achievers in all fields of life consistently note that both having a positive mindset and having specific positive goals in mind tend to make the achievement of those goals far more likely.

Don't worry if you've temporarily lost your positive mindset — it will eventually come back. The depression is just stealing it away right now. And, please know that even if your belief in recovery isn't strong at this point, you'll still recover no matter how far in the dumps you are. Therapy will help you turn off the downward spiraling thoughts and bring about the positive ones.

Even though you do want to set high expectations for the therapeutic process, you don't want to set your expectations *too* high. To do so is to set yourself up for disappointment, and to make it more likely that you'll quit before the therapy has really had a chance to do you any good.

So, for example, don't expect that in your first therapy session you'll feel instant relief and that the whole thing will just go away. I keep a beautiful magic wand on my desk and often tell clients I'd love to be able to wave it and make their PPD disappear. But, more often than not, even though you may experience some relief of anxiety and you'll walk out of the therapist's office with a solid action plan and set of steps to follow, you'll still be deep in the throes of your condition.

With a few more sessions under your belt, you'll likely be feeling significantly better, but it's important that you stick to the plan and keep going back so that you allow the process to fully work. In short, it's entirely reasonable for you to expect that you'll feel like you're heading in the right direction from the very first session, but it's not reasonable for you to expect a miracle or instantaneous cure.

Partnering with your therapist

The best way to think of your relationship with your therapist is as a partnership. You both bring considerable — although different — strengths to the relationship. You, as the client, are responsible for bringing the following things to the partnership:

> ✔ Your willingness to be honest and vulnerable
>
> ✔ Your own wisdom of who you are and how you feel (you're the expert of your own experience!)
>
> ✔ Your capacity to work hard and to trust yourself, the therapist, and the therapeutic process

Your therapist brings to the table training, experience, knowledge, compassion, and guidance to help you do whatever it is you need to do in order to recover as quickly as possible. He also brings a sincere desire to see that you get well.

Because recovery isn't one size fits all, your therapist should also be open to trying new things with you that are directly suited to your particular needs. Your therapist should be eclectic and responsive in his *modalities* (methods of doing therapy) and techniques. If you're getting worse or your life isn't changing for the better, your therapist should change his treatment modality. If your therapist needs new tools, advice from a colleague, or better training in PPD, he should be willing to get it as soon as possible or refer you to another therapist with greater expertise.

You and your therapist share the responsibility for making sure that your therapeutic relationship is an effective and valuable one. If things aren't going well with your therapist, you may have to leave and try someone else (see the section "Deciding when to show or when to go" later in this chapter for more info).

Despite his credentials (even if the therapist has a PhD or an MD), despite the fact that you may be paying him a high hourly rate, and despite the fact that you're going to him as someone who is, in fact, suffering from an illness and quite vulnerable, don't feel intimidated by your therapist. Even though you generally do want to be as cooperative as possible, it's important to always keep in mind that the therapist isn't totally in charge. If, for example, the therapist comes up with an element of your wellness plan or a specific exercise or task that you just can't do (or don't want to do), it's up to you to say so as soon as possible. Ultimately, it's the therapist who's working for you (not the other way around). And, in any case, you both need to work together as partners.

A critical part of your partnership, therefore, is recognition that the therapist can't do all the work. For one thing, no therapist or counselor is a mind reader. He may be able to read your body language pretty well, tune in to your voice tone, and derive a great deal of information from what you don't say, but you have to be willing to speak openly and honestly, to tell the truth, and to reveal yourself. Your relationship with your therapist is legally protected for a very good reason: So that you won't feel tempted to hide sensitive information for fear of disclosing what you perceive as shameful parts of yourself.

Because you've actually made it to therapy, you might as well give it a chance to really work — and that may mean opening yourself up in a way that you never have before. The mere act of trusting a therapist deeply enough to open up like this can prove extremely therapeutic beyond whatever content you bring up.

The mechanics of therapy: Where, when, and how long

Having clear expectations and agreements about how therapy actually works is important to making the most of your sessions. So, here, I give you the basics on what you can expect:

- **Where:** Therapy usually takes place in the therapist's office, if you're local. Telephone sessions also work well for most clients, but many therapists are only willing to see their clients face to face.

  While a few old-fashioned or classically psychoanalytically oriented therapists may have you lie down on a couch where you can't look each other in the eye (not the most appropriate therapy for you), most therapists (if your session is in their office) have you sit in a comfortable chair while they do the same, sometimes with and sometimes without a table between you. You can also expect the therapist to have a notebook or pad of paper nearby for making notes or keeping some kind of chart or log on your progress.

- **When:** In the beginning, especially if you have a severe case of PPD, it's best to have sessions with your therapist no less than once a week. The key is that you're meeting regularly — whatever "regularly" means to you and your therapist (who may have his own feelings or policies about attendance).

  As your therapy continues, the number of sessions may decrease to once every two weeks, once a month, or even less frequently (see the section "Ending Therapy and Staying Healthy" later in this chapter).

- **How long:** Most sessions with therapists last for what has been labeled "a therapist's hour," which is fifty minutes. Some therapists prefer longer time periods, such as an hour and twenty minutes, especially for the initial assessment.

  Busy therapists (and most really good therapists will often be quite busy) need time to take a break, make notes, and reset between clients, which is why that ten minutes is slotted in there.

Grasping the length of the therapeutic process

Very often, especially near the beginning of therapy, clients ask their thera-pists when they'll be 100 percent better. The truth is that there's no typical amount of time. Each client is unique, and while a good therapist will work as fast as he can (which usually means as fast as the client is ready to work), it would generally be irresponsible for a therapist to circle a date on the calen-dar and tell the client that is when she'll be fully recovered. However, as a loose guideline, you can expect full recovery to take between weeks and months, but not usually years.

Because you're getting help and you're willing to work hard, your recovery will likely be sooner rather than later. What's most important, though, is that you're going in the right direction.

Deciding when to show or when to go

If everything is going well with your therapist, that's great and that's all there is to it. You're on your way to feeling like your old self, especially if you follow the other suggestions in this book. But what if things aren't improving? How do you know when it's time to move on to a different therapist?

For starters, if you don't think the therapist is helping you, he probably isn't. The quality of your life should improve after you start working with a compe-tent therapist with whom you have a good rapport. If he's the right therapist, then the very first time you leave his office, you should have both a sense of hope (which you may not have had before the appointment), as well as a starting plan of action for getting well.

Of course, there are some other clear signs that a therapist isn't the right one. For example, consider the following types of not-so-great therapists:

- ✔ **The insensitive therapist:** If the therapist says things, such as "Why are things so difficult for you?" or "It's too bad you're missing out on breast-feeding," you've got the wrong person. He may have hidden his judgmen-tal attitude from you when you were making your decision to try him, but within no time, his real colors came out.

  If the therapist is mouthing the myths of merry motherhood — "This should be the happiest time of your life!" — you certainly have the wrong person and you shouldn't go back.

✔ **The out-of-date therapist:** This therapist was trained at a time when PPD wasn't recognized as a real malady, and so he says outdated things like "What you're going through has nothing to do with the fact that you just had a baby."

Here's why the therapist would say things like this: In the old days, the fact that a new mom was depressed and just had a baby were considered completely unconnected and unrelated. The new mom's depression was thought to be the same as any other depression (and therefore therapeutic interventions were typically not as effective).

✔ **The biased or inappropriate therapist:** This therapist mishandles or otherwise shows a severe bias with respect to a particular issue you bring up.

For example, suppose a new mom with PPD tells her therapist that one of the things she's obsessing about is that she isn't producing enough milk to feed her baby, and as a result she's feeling horribly guilty. If the therapist attempts to give this woman detailed lactation advice instead of addressing her feelings about the situation and empowering her to feel good about herself regardless of how breastfeeding goes, he's probably the wrong therapist.

✔ **The blast-from-the-past therapist:** This therapist wants to talk only about past issues, such as issues the new mom has with her own childhood.

Of course, some things from the past may come up and get in the way of what's happening with the new mom in the here and now. (For example, if the new mom had a terrible issue with her own mother and if now that she's a mother the issue is front and center, it may indeed need to be dealt with now in therapy.) But if a therapist or counselor wants only to talk about the past and keeps returning to it, and isn't helping the new mom put one foot in front of the other in the *here and now,* he has shown that he probably isn't the right person to be working with.

✔ **The lackadaisical therapist:** If the therapist simply sits there with a pad of paper, occasionally taking notes and saying "Uh-huh," but not really giving any feedback, he's probably not the right person to be working with. Yes, in the first session you may be doing a lot of talking, but after that the therapist should be interacting with you, offering suggestions and verbal encouragement, and being truly present with you.

By now, you may be saying, "What about self-deception? How can I be sure whether it's time to leave, or whether I'm just fooling myself and not really giving the therapist a reasonable chance?" As a general rule, you should give your therapist at least three sessions before moving on. After those three sessions, you can ask yourself whether you feel comfortable with the therapist, whether you feel you can say anything you need to him, and whether you feel safe and not judged. If after three sessions you don't feel the therapist really "gets" what you're going through, you may want to try another one.

Ultimately, just like your initial choice of the therapist, your choice to move on to someone else is a gut call that only you can make. You can get advice from your partner, family members, and friends, but this decision is quite subjective because you're the only one who ultimately knows how it feels to be in therapy with this individual. If you want feedback from loved ones, fine. But, whatever decision you make will be another opportunity to practice trusting and validating yourself.

It's important that you feel no shame, no fault, and no need to second-guess yourself if you make the decision to leave your current therapist. You did the best you could. Instead, you can learn from what didn't work with your first (or second) choice, and move on. Life is a learning process. There are many course corrections, and having the courage to make the choice to move on is, in and of itself, a healing and empowering decision. (If you continually therapist-hop whenever you hear something about yourself that you don't like, that's a different story, which I won't get into here.)

Making the Most of Therapy

Earlier in this chapter, I give you a good idea of what to realistically expect from therapy, what a therapeutic partnership feels like, and what some of the mechanics of therapy (frequency and duration) tend to look like. In this section, I cut straight to the therapy itself, and I explain how to make sure that you make the most of it. This section concentrates on your initial needs assessment, why you want to focus first on handling whatever short-term crisis that you're in, and what it means to develop and be guided by a wellness plan.

Assessing your needs

Your therapist may already know a bit about you before your initial session based on what you've already told her. For instance, many therapists have you fill out a form before your first session that asks you about your past experience with therapy, your family history, and other pertinent items, such as whether you're currently taking any medications or actively receiving treatment from any other healthcare providers. The form usually also inquires about your current symptoms, such as your anxiety and stress levels, and whether you're suffering from insomnia, for instance. There may be a blank section on the form where you can spell out, in as much detail as you want, what you're currently going through and why you're seeking therapy.

A form, however, is only a form, and it will inevitably leave out info that's important or relevant. Many people also tend to be shy or reluctant when disclosing things on paper. The form, then, is only the first step in assessing your needs. The actual critical needs assessment happens during the first one or two live sessions with your therapist. Each therapist has her own way of assessing what's going on with you based on her training, education, experience, available tools, and overall preferences.

From your perspective, these first live sessions will involve you doing a lot of the talking — you may end up talking up to 85 percent of the session — while your therapist asks a few questions and takes notes (maybe mental notes, which she later writes down) about what you're saying. What the therapist is seeking is a well-rounded picture of what's really going on in your life so that the two of you can come up with a detailed wellness plan that quickly and effectively puts you back on the road to 100 percent recovery.

As partners with the therapist, and as someone who wants to get well as soon as possible, you should fully cooperate with the needs assessment phase of your therapy. Don't be shy, reluctant, or evasive. Tears — even waterworks — are totally acceptable. If you're in her office, tissues will probably be within arm's reach. The therapist knows why you're there, and she's there to help you. Help her really understand what's going on with you by including the following information:

- Present and past experiences that may be relevant
- Your current situation with respect to your partner
- Whether you're self-medicating with over-the-counter or street drugs
- How things are going with your new baby and your other children (if you have any)
- Any situations that may be going on with other people, such as friends, co-workers, and so on.

If you're up-front with your therapist, you'll likely get what you need a lot faster.

Putting out the fire before rewiring the house

Suppose your house has caught on fire because of an electrical wiring problem. The following question has an obvious answer, but it proves my point well: Would you rewire the house first and then put out the fire, or would you put out the fire first and then rewire the house? Obviously, you need to put out the fire first. This same logic holds true for psychological and emotional life crises just as well as it does for fires. In other words, you have to handle the crises in your life before you can move on to fix any long-term problems whether or not they're related to the crisis at hand.

If you're so symptomatic during your first therapy session that you can barely sit still, it probably won't be useful to discuss how you were embarrassed during your third grade play. But, after you've handled (at least addressed and come up with a reasonable plan of action) the real-time difficulties that are at or near crisis stage, you can then consider spending time on issues stemming from the past. At first, when a client is very symptomatic, I only address those issues from the past that absolutely need to be looked at in order to relieve the symptoms. Otherwise, I stay completely in present time so my clients can first put one foot in front of the other and survive this difficult period.

Continuing with the analogy, this kind of deep rewiring, which can be thought of more as "regular" therapy, can play an important role in your 100 percent (or better!) recovery. For example, if perfectionism has plagued you for years, and that perfectionism has seemingly played a role in making your PPD worse (for example, "Why can't I breastfeed my baby better?" or "I should have a spotless house."), eventually, during the course of therapy, you may want to address it.

It makes sense, then, especially in the beginning, for a therapist to engage you in one of two kinds of therapeutic modalities that are designed for, or are particularly well-suited for, dealing with crisis management and putting out real-time fires. There are other types of short-term therapies available as well, but the following two have been shown to be particularly valuable for a woman suffering from PPD:

- ✔ **Cognitive-behavioral therapy (CBT):** This kind of therapy is based on the concept that the distorted thoughts that you frequently repeat to yourself in the privacy of your own mind can frequently reinforce feelings of depression. By bringing these thoughts into conscious awareness, and then changing them (even if that simply means saying a different, opposite, much more positive thought both aloud and to yourself), your moods and feelings can radically and rapidly be changed for the better.

- ✔ **Interpersonal therapy (IPT):** This kind of therapy focuses on the role changes that you're going through. Typically, IPT is a structured type of therapy that focuses on the significant real-time relationships in your life and how they've had an impact on your ability to function. The purpose of IPT is to strengthen your relationships and communication skills so that you have better interpersonal relationships and can make your life work better.

Many therapists work mainly with one of these types but are open to using what works for you. Some therapists, on the other hand, work exclusively with one or the other. You'll be okay either way, but I suggest that, if possible, you work with someone who can take the best from each of these (and other therapies not mentioned here) and tailor your therapy to suit you and your specific needs.

Whatever the combination of therapies, the therapist should provide you instruction and help in changing your behavior even before you feel ready. It sounds scary, but it really isn't. Let me explain: Sometimes people, especially therapists trained in the "old school," believe that your feelings need to change before your behavior can change. What your therapist will hopefully help you understand is that the behavior can change first — thank goodness!

If, for instance, you think you need to wait until you feel less guilty or anxious before you hire a babysitter and take a break, your child may be 18 years old before you're actually ready. It often takes *doing it* first, changing the old behavior, and then the desired feelings follow. After you see that your baby is okay when you hire the sitter, you calm down and feel good about yourself for conquering that fear — and then it's easier to take another break.

Developing a wellness plan

Early on in your therapy — at the same time or right after your needs assessment, and often as part of addressing any real-time crises — you and your therapist should develop a *wellness plan*. This plan spells out what you need to do in order to get well, including the following:

✔ Where the new mom is now

✔ Where she hopes to get to

✔ How she'll report in with the therapist

✔ What homework assignments she's responsible for

✔ Any other unique features a therapist may come up with

Taken together, all these elements of the wellness plan represent a guiding map or document that both the new mom and the therapist can rely on. (You'll find Chapter 10 particularly helpful regarding how to create a comprehensive plan.)

Of course, to get started, you have to first determine what wellness means for you. In short, you begin to craft a wellness plan by spelling out the short-, medium-, and long-term goals of therapy so that both you and your therapist know when you're completely better (and when you're therefore done with therapy).

ANECDOTE

Breaking through the terror

My client, Annette, expresses in the following paragraphs what it took for her to push through her emotions to get the help she needed:

"I don't think it's fair to call it fear. Calling it fear diminishes the feeling, which is nothing short of a quiet terror that crawls through your veins. You're isolated even while you're surrounded by happy people — every one of them full of smiles. You play along. You go through the motions and match those smiles because you're afraid not to. You're afraid someone may see through the veneer. The charade, for me, went on for a long time, too long, because I hid it so well. Then one afternoon my husband dressed me and my son, put us both in the car, and drove us to the park. My husband and toddling son went out and began to kick a ball around. Even though I was in love with my husband and son, I couldn't move from the car to join them. The only restraints were in my mind, but they paralyzed me nonetheless. I sat, watched, and sobbed. Later, I feebly reached out for the only help I could think of — help from a counselor who had helped me years earlier.

I remember being scared and confused when I went to my first PPD appointment. During my initial call, the counselor had listened on the phone. It sounded as if she might understand, but the PPD made it hard to have hope. At the appointment, my darkest thoughts and fears spilled out. I was afraid to let go, but I was more afraid not to. My illness was real, she said. More importantly, it was physical. There were medical terms to explain it. I embraced her words. I left believing there was hope, but I had no confidence that I could survive the journey. My therapist believed I'd recover. I became determined. I held onto that knowledge and it propelled me through the darkest days. No matter how long it took, how expensive it may become, what kind of criticism I'd face from those people who didn't understand, I was going to get well. I was going to be the mother I wanted to be, and more importantly, I was going to be me — whole and alive once again."

Often, when planning out her goals, a new mom with PPD will say something like, "I just want to be me again." But what, exactly, does that mean? And how will you and your therapist know when you've reached that point? It's important, then, to spell out in some detail signs or markers of what full recovery will look like for you. Will you be smiling more? Will you be singing in the shower again? Will you resume certain hobbies or sports that you truly loved before you became depressed? For each woman, these objective signs or markers will be different.

The way the therapist will check up on the progress of the therapy regarding these signs will also differ. So, talk with your therapist and spell out whether she'll regularly inquire as to how you're doing, or whether you'll be responsible for self-reporting. It's usually a combination.

A good therapist, in many ways, is like a travel agent who gets people from here to there. For example, a woman with PPD goes to the therapist and together they agree that she's at Point A, and then the therapist helps her determine the Point B that she's attempting to get to. Finally, together, the therapist and the new mom can set out a plan, a psychological itinerary, for getting the new mom to Point B. To get her to Point B, the wellness plan can include a variety of daily or weekly "homework" assignments that can help her reach her ultimate destination.

These homework assignments shouldn't be overwhelming — that would be self-defeating. Instead, these assignments are exercises that build self-esteem and focus. For example, one woman's assignment may be to say "Thank you" whenever someone spontaneously pays her a compliment. This may not seem like very much, but for someone who's suffering from PPD, it can represent a significant breakthrough because she hasn't been feeling deserving of anything lately — including compliments. The more she practices, the easier it will become, and the feeling of "I'm worth it" and "I deserve it" will surface more quickly. Another assignment may be for the women to tell a trusted support person at the end of each day at least one thing that she accomplished during the day, no matter how small it may seem.

Therapists have different styles, and not all of them will give the practical suggestions that I call "homework." If you find yourself working with a therapist who doesn't offer this structure, you may find that it works fine for you. But, if not, you can always ask her for some homework (or make up some steps for yourself).

My colleagues and I find that, especially with PPD, it's a combination of discussing feelings, changing old, destructive thought patterns, and suggesting specific next steps that helps women most effectively. When a woman sets her goals, no matter how small the assignments are, it's empowering for her because she has taken measurable steps to get well.

Letting the nature of therapy take its course

There is a very human tendency for people in general to want to quit therapy after they start feeling better. For example, you may attend a dozen sessions and then say to yourself, "Well, really, I'm much better than when I started. I'm not in active crisis, and this is probably as good a time as any to quit therapy." Or after a few months you may say to yourself "You know, this has been going on for quite a while already. I wonder if I really need therapy any more."

In some cases, women begin to feel substantially better after just one or two therapy sessions. It should be noted, however, that there are very few women who only go to one therapy session, get the direction and wellness plan that they need, and are then off and running. Such women are usually mildly depressed, and typically they're already seeing a doctor, taking medication, and enjoying a robust support system. But again, this is unusual.

The issue here is that even though you may feel somewhat or significantly better, it's not a good idea to stop therapy until you feel 100 percent recovered — or even better than 100 percent (that is, you've worked through issues that predate your PPD). If you stop too soon, without having developed a really solid psychological foundation and without a substantial toolkit under your belt, you may have a slip of some kind.

One way to keep tabs on your recovery progress is with your wellness plan (see the previous section). In discussion with your therapist or counselor, you should be able to tell whether you've really met the markers that you set for yourself to indicate a 100 percent recovery. Another way to check on this is to simply ask your therapist if she thinks you're ready to stop therapy. Based on her experience and training, a therapist will be a much better judge of how other factors, such as medication, fit into the bigger therapeutic picture.

Keep in mind that after you come out of your crisis phase, you may want to consider continuing regular therapy with your therapist. Often, when I'm working with a woman who's in crisis, an issue will come up that I can tell is important — possibly even pivotal to her ultimate well-being — but it's just not the right time to discuss it, and so instead I merely make a note of it on my chart. In other words, when she's in crisis, I only work through this particular kind of issue as much as necessary to get through the crisis. But later on, if she chooses, we can focus on those issues that have been bothering her for a very long time — in this case, we try to get rid of "it," whatever "it" may be, once and for all.

PPD-related issues and preexisting psychological issues are often intertwined and difficult to tweeze apart. So, if you've developed a good relationship with your therapist, continuing to unravel and work through a wide variety of issues may prove incredibly valuable to you, both with respect to finishing off any PPD-catalyzed issues as well as older, preexisting, issues.

At a certain point, however, you may not need to attend therapy quite as often. In consultation with your therapist or counselor, you may decide to drop attendance down to once every two weeks, four weeks, or even six weeks. If your therapist is local and you've been seeing her face to face the entire time, it may also work for you to begin sprinkling in phone sessions among the face-to-face visits.

Eventually, the time will come when, in fact, you're done with therapy. You will have worked through all of your PPD-related issues and maybe even some preexisting issues as well. While you, and not your therapist, have the final call on when you're done, ideally the two of you will be in agreement that your therapy is complete.

Ending Therapy and Staying Healthy

Just as you want to start therapy in the right way (finding the right therapist, having the right realistic expectations, and so on), you also want to end therapy in the right way. So, make sure that you keep on doing whatever it was that was working for you during therapy even after therapy stops and even after you feel as if you've completely recovered.

Suppose, then, that you've reached all of your wellness plan goals and you've checked them off of your list. You're ready to end therapy — or at least the current phase of therapy with the therapist you've been seeing — and your therapist is in agreement that you're ready to stop. Here's what I want you to remember: It's extremely important that you don't get cocky at this point about what has helped you and that you don't stop doing whatever has helped you get well. If you suddenly stop doing what you've been doing, you may very well start suffering again and fall back into a negative spiral.

For example, if you've put into place a system of taking regular breaks every day to recharge your batteries, you shouldn't stop taking such breaks just because you're now feeling 100 percent.

In fact, you've probably taken many healthy steps as part of your healing process. So, why would you want to reverse these healthy steps, such as eating nutritious food, regularly exercising, or making regularly scheduled time with your partner to ensure that your primary relationship is as solid as it can be? There's no doubt at all that finding a way to get at least five to six hours of uninterrupted sleep every night is something that's important for all mothers, not just moms with PPD (see Chapter 12). So don't think you can stop making sure that happens just because you're generally feeling better.

Attending Groups

On the one hand, attending any of the different kinds of groups can be a very positive experience for a new mom with PPD. On the other hand, while groups can be helpful, they're usually not enough. Even if a group is wonderful, almost all women with PPD need a level of individualized support and treatment that a group just isn't designed to provide. So, if and when you have your own individual therapy, and you feel inspired to check out a group, by all means do so. Just don't to it prematurely or try to have a group take the place of the individualized psychological treatment that you need and deserve.

How can you tell when you're ready for a group? You probably aren't ready if you haven't sought out and found appropriate individualized therapy. Many women say things like, "All I need to do is talk to some other women who are going through what I'm going through, and I'll be fine." Unfortunately, this isn't usually true. Even though speaking to others who are going through PPD can be tremendously therapeutic, you need to have a plan in place that's designed just for you. You'll be cheating yourself if you don't receive the full, one-on-one attention of a trained professional therapist. You need your own individualized, professionally managed wellness plan, and a group simply isn't designed to create that for you.

Attending a group — no matter how well-run it is — before you've started down your own therapeutic path, can actually damage you. Suppose there's an issue in your life that you're barely coping with and not yet ready to think about (not to mention discuss), and then a group member brings it up. Being in a vulnerable or an agitated state of mind already, this situation could drop you even deeper into the well. Also, if you're obsessing about scary things or you just have really high anxiety, you could find yourself traumatized by what you encounter in a group setting. Wait until you're more stable and less impressionable ("It took her almost a year to recover! Oh no! Will that be me too?")

Luckily, your therapist or counselor, after you have chosen one, can help you identify when you're ready to attend a group. As a general rule, though, you ideally want to be psychologically stabilized and past the worst of the crisis, and you want to have in place an individualized wellness plan before you pop into a room with other women and their worries. Chapter 14 explains the types of groups available, so head there for a brief review when you feel ready.

Chapter 8

Counteracting a Chemical Cause: Medical Treatments

· ·

In This Chapter

▶ Understanding the benefits of medication

▶ Consulting with a psychiatrist

▶ Dealing with worries about medications

▶ Discovering the many medical treatments and their side effects

▶ Deciding the best time to begin treatment

· ·

*W*hen it comes to treatment for PPD, antidepressant medications are some of the most commonly prescribed medications. They're frequently used to treat depression, anxiety disorders, pain, and sometimes other conditions as well. Just as in the case with any medication you would take for any physical disorder, medications for depression can have both risks and benefits. Because of these risks, many women are confused or have mixed feelings about medication. However, other women feel more afraid of antidepressants because of the perceived stigma about needing to take this type of medication. If you're nervous about beginning an antidepressant, please note that they aren't meant to change you — they're meant to help you recover from depression and anxiety. They're meant to help you be you.

This chapter starts off by considering the many benefits of medication and then covers some of the typical concerns that new moms with PPD (and their partners and families) may have. I also pay special attention throughout this chapter to the issue of nursing while taking medication and emphasize the importance of having the new mom's thyroid evaluated (a thyroid imbalance can cause depression or anxiety). Finally, I round out this chapter with the six major categories of medical treatment (five types of medication plus electroconvulsive therapy). I cover these one by one, including who they're for, when they're best used, and what side effects are possible.

Recognizing the Benefits of Medication on Depression

There's no doubt that prescribed, pharmaceutical grade medication can have substantial benefits for a new mom with PPD. Whether it's antidepressants, antianxiety medications, sleep aids, mood stabilizers, or antipsychotics, each of these groups of medications is targeted at helping a different kind of problem or disorder. And, in combination with other types of treatment, these medicines can rapidly propel a new mom with PPD into a much healthier place and put her well along the road to complete recovery.

A mom with PPD doesn't always need medication in order to recover, though — sometimes all she needs is support, education, and psychotherapy. But when her particular symptoms or situation warrant the use of it, medication can be a blessing. A woman doesn't have to be feeling horrible to be prescribed and to take medication. As a matter of fact, catching and stopping PPD before the woman feels horrible is the goal. Often the mom worries that if the doctor or therapist thinks she needs medication, then she must be pretty far gone, so to speak. Not so at all. The doctor will prescribe medication if he believes that the symptoms may respond well to medication, not based on how severe the symptoms are. Some of the symptoms of PPD that often respond well to medication include the following:

- ✔ Anger
- ✔ Anxiety
- ✔ Depression
- ✔ Hopelessness
- ✔ Insomnia
- ✔ Loss of appetite
- ✔ Scary thoughts (see Chapter 3)

Moms also worry that if they start taking a medication then they'll always need it. This isn't true either. Often my clients take an antidepressant (and possibly an antianxiety or other medication as well) temporarily to help them get back on track, and then they're slowly weaned off and they go on with their happy lives medication-free. It depends on each particular woman's history, reasons for the depression, and a host of other factors. I discuss this in more detail later in this chapter.

Who You Gonna Call? A Psychiatrist, That's Who

When medication is suggested to you, the professional that you should consult if at all possible is a psychiatrist. If you're worried about stigma, remember that if you broke your arm or needed a cavity filled you'd see the properly trained professionals for those ailments. For this ailment, optimally you should see a psychiatrist — in this section, I give you the full scoop on why.

Understanding why a psychiatrist is essential

Ultimately, psychological meds make up a detailed and specialized scientific area, and because of the great amount of detail, even your regular medical doctor isn't always fully up-to-date and informed for purposes of PPD (unless, of course, she's specifically following the literature on antidepressants, antianxiety, and other medications as they relate to new moms suffering from PPD). So, if you need or otherwise are seriously considering prescribed medication, work with a psychiatrist, especially one familiar with PPD, if at all possible.

The confusing world of pharmaceuticals

Even though prescribed medication can be enormously beneficial, it can also be a confusing area to understand because you have to take many factors into consideration. For example, you have to consider the following questions:

- ✔ Which medication is the right one?
- ✔ What should the dosage be?
- ✔ How do you best use the medication?
- ✔ What side effects should you look out for?

Unless you've taken a medication earlier in your life that's worked well for you, you'll be doing some trial and error when starting a medication for the first time. Most often, though, the first medication prescribed will work well with your body chemistry, because the psychiatrist is trained to make an educated guess regarding what may work well for you, based on your symptoms and family history.

What makes this confusion even worse is the fact that PPD is a scientific area that's constantly changing. It seems that every time medical science declares a particular medication safe for breastfeeding, another report comes out a few weeks, months, or years later that raises a question. Or as soon as the best scientific evidence shows that a particular medication is just fine for a depressed woman to take during her third trimester, new research comes out that implies a possible risk to the developing baby. This so-called "research" may not be good research at all, but in the meantime it causes alarm among moms trying to make the decision about whether or not to take the medicine. Also, sometimes research findings are blown out of proportion by members of the media, who like to shock readers and viewers.

As one example, the media announced a study reporting that taking an anti-depressant in the third trimester causes symptoms in the newborn, and it scared women into not taking badly needed medication. The researchers and practitioners I know and trust who devote their professional careers to study-ing this specialized area continue to prescribe in the third trimester, because they don't believe that these "symptoms" in the newborn are damaging — they're transient and mild. In the meantime, these children have mothers who are enjoying them and can care for them.

Not only is research and evidence on existing medications constantly chang-ing and evolving, but the medications themselves keep changing. New med-ications keep hitting the market, and as time goes on you can expect new substances to emerge that may be more effective and that have fewer side effects than anything available right now.

Two great benefits of working with a psychiatrist

Working with a psychiatrist has advantages in addition to the wealth of trust-worthy information you'll receive:

- ✔ **Psychiatrists are best at — and best trained at — prescribing the right medication, including the right starting and follow-up dosages.** To help determine these dosages, they're trained to think about certain patient background information and to ask questions that elicit other relevant information.

  Compared to most general practice MDs or even MDs who are OB/GYNs, a psychiatrist is likely to inquire about any blood relatives of the new mom (or the new mom herself) who have previously and successfully taken any antidepressants. Knowing about past successes may help determine which medication should be tried first. Similarly, a psychia-trist is far more likely to inquire into whether there's any bipolar illness anywhere in the new mom's family history, which demands a specific medicine combination.

> ✔ **Psychiatrists are best at monitoring your progress and following up with you.** As wonderful as many MDs are, very few are as conscientious as psychiatrists about follow-up on the impact of prescribed medications. This lack of follow-up is mainly because they don't have the background and training to know how — they're excellent at performing the tasks pertaining to their own specialties.

Knowing where to go if you can't get to a psychiatrist

If you feel you need (or might need) medication and no psychiatrist is available, do whatever you can to find one anyway — even if you have to travel to go see one. If there's absolutely no way for you to get to a psychiatrist, see another MD or nurse practitioner who can prescribe medications. Try to find one who either specializes in or has substantial experience with PPD.

Don't underestimate the knowledge of PhD psychologists or other psychotherapists if they have experience in PPD. As one of those psychologists, I can tell you that frequently I receive calls from obstetricians and other medical professionals who ask my opinion on what to prescribe for various patients and at what dose. They know that I follow this highly specialized area and know the data well. Psychologists can't give you medical advice or prescribe, but if they're specialists in the area of PPD, they can educate you (and your doctor) about what the research says.

Addressing Concerns about Taking Prescribed Meds

The potential benefits of taking prescription medications, especially when they're properly prescribed, dosed, used, and followed-up on, are clear. But there are also some concerns that should be considered, some of which can rightly be dismissed, and some of which have to be cautiously watched for and monitored.

The most common general worries

Many people, from new moms with PPD to ordinary folks encountering depression for the first time, are wary about taking prescribed medication for their condition. I address a few of the most common worries in the following sections.

"Taking meds means I'm a weak person"

Never buy into the self-reliant myth that says you should be able to pull yourself out of your PPD on your own without any outside help. Admittedly, given the backwards thinking about PPD that's still far too common, there may be some stigma attached to seeing a doctor (especially a psychiatrist) and receiving prescribed medication as a result. But here's what I have to say about that: So what? It would be sad to let other people's ignorance stop you from being placed firmly on the road to recovery.

"I'll become dependent on or addicted to the drugs"

It never fails to amaze me how often women with PPD refer to prescribed medication as a "crutch." When someone with a broken leg ambles past you on crutches, you don't say, "Look at that sad excuse for a human being — I can't believe that she has stooped to relying on crutches." If you need crutches to help you get stronger until you don't need the crutches any longer, then so be it. And if you need prescribed medication to give you a boost until you're well enough to wean off, do it.

Unfortunately, women with PPD also have the fear that if they start using antidepressants, they'll become dependent on them. Well, just as crutches are used as a temporary support until you no longer need them, the medication that you're prescribed is meant to restore the normal functioning of your brain chemistry so that you no longer need the medication. When you have felt like yourself again for a few months — the length of time will differ depending on your history and other factors — the psychiatrist or other MD will make sure that you successfully begin the process of weaning off of the medication. And if it turns out that you need to stay on the medication longer, try to count your lucky stars that there's something you can take to help you enjoy your life.

Never stop a medication, especially an antidepressant, cold turkey because your body will have gotten used to it (not addicted to it, just used to it). Typically, if you abruptly stop taking an antidepressant you can experience bad side effects, sometimes amounting to severe dizziness and queasiness for a number of days. These side effects are other reasons why you want an experienced doctor in your corner — one who knows how to gently and steadily decrease your dosage until you're medication free.

Even when you wean appropriately off the antidepressant, you still may experience some unpleasant effects as your body gets used to continuing without the medication. Or, at the very least, you may experience a bit of a bumpy ride. Often, though, there are little to no negative effects.

"I'll suffer horrible and long-lasting side effects"

Mild side effects are common, and I cover them in some detail in the section "Side Effects: You Can't Always Get Just What You Want" later in this chapter. The important things to note about medications are that

- ✔ Side effects, if any, are usually mild and of short duration — they generally subside after a few days to a week or two of beginning the med therapy.

- ✔ If you experience a really uncomfortable side effect, your doctor won't continue prescribing that particular medication. But, if the side effects are mild, weigh them against the benefits. Most women decide to stick it out, because some temporary stomach upset is better than feeling hopeless and withdrawn.

"Is taking meds while nursing safe?"

For the mom who isn't pumping or breastfeeding her baby, her body is hers alone, and the entire psychiatric treatment arsenal is open to her without any reservations whatsoever. However, for those who are breastfeeding or pumping, a sensible worry is whether taking medications will affect their babies.

The growing modern consensus is that the benefits of breastfeeding seem to far outweigh any risk of harm to a baby when their moms take medication. For many years the research emphasis has been on whether there might *possibly* be any harm to the baby from a nursing mother who's taking medication. Over time, however, the research (especially with respect to antidepressants, the most important category of medication for PPD) has consistently shown no harmful effects. Researchers and practitioners agree that it's time to change the general way this issue is framed — from one that emphasizes potential harm to the baby to one that emphasizes the great deal of overall good that comes to new moms (and therefore to their babies) when they take the appropriate medication.

Most antidepressants are virtually undetectable in a baby's system. Sometimes tiny amounts are detected, but without exception, the infants and children whose moms were taking medication while they were nursing have, to date, been completely normal across all tested behavioral and developmental parameters.

It's worth repeating, however, that if you have PPD and you're pumping your milk or breastfeeding your baby, you have no reason (with respect to your child's health) to not take advantage of the medication that your doctor feels is right for you. Pediatricians are becoming more and more aware of the literature regarding the safety of antidepressants and breastfeeding, so it's becoming less confusing to women in need.

Ironically, often a breastfeeding mother who's anxious about taking medication while she's breastfeeding finds that as soon as she starts on the medication, she calms down completely with respect to this issue. Her anxiety may be an indication that she'll benefit from the very medication she's anxious about taking.

If you're *that* concerned about taking an antidepressant when you're breastfeeding, though, talk to the psychiatrist about "pumping and dumping." In this tactic, you pump and discard the feeding that follows the time that the particular medication peaks in your system. Instead, you can use a bottle of previously pumped milk or formula for that feeding.

"How do I know I'm not dealing with a thyroid problem?"

At least 10 percent of women, after delivering a baby, develop some kind of postpartum thyroid disorder or *thyroiditis* (inflammation of the thyroid gland). And many times, these types of disorders mimic PPD.

If a new mom is depressed *and* has a problem with her thyroid — which will typically be an underactive thyroid, or *hypothyroidism* — then all the antidepressants in the world won't make her feel completely well.

It's important, then, that the thyroid be treated if there are any signs that it isn't functioning well, including unusual tiredness, lack of energy, inability to get warm, ongoing sore throats, weight gain, dry skin, low sex drive, constipation, anxiety, and, not surprisingly, depression.

Because many of these symptoms are also symptoms of PPD, you probably want to know how you can determine whether they're just due to the PPD or are also in part due to a thyroid disorder of some kind. Not surprisingly, you really can't tell and really can't rule out a thyroid problem without seeing a medical doctor who can perform a blood test to check your thyroid. If I had my way, all postpartum women would be screened and tested for potential thyroid disorders. If you do have a thyroid problem, it can usually be addressed fairly quickly, either with thyroid supplements or through natural remedies. The optimum time to test your thyroid postpartum is two to three months after delivery.

If you have a personal or family history of thyroid imbalance, usually the MD will make sure you get tested. If not, you may need to convince him that you want to rule out a thyroid problem before starting on an antidepressant. *Subclinical hypothyroidism* (meaning that it doesn't show up on the thyroid test because it's so slight) can make PPD worse. So, many doctors will give a woman a bit of thyroid medication to boost the antidepressant if it's not working 100 percent. Sometimes this addition is all the woman needs to confirm that a thyroid imbalance was lurking.

Specific Types of Medical Treatments for PPD

After you decide to try a medication to recover from your PPD, you and your doc have another decision to make: What medicine is best for you? The six major types of medical treatments available for women with PPD — five of which are prescription medications — are shown one by one in this section.

Antidepressants

A woman suffering from PPD is, by definition, depressed, so it makes sense that the first line of treatment for PPD is an antidepressant. There are two main types of antidepressants used for PPD:

✔ **Tricyclics:** Tricyclics (TCAs) have been available since 1958 and, although they're generally less popular today than they used to be (because they have more side effects than the newer group of meds), they're still useful for many women and for particular symptoms. Tricyclics work by beefing up the brain's supply of *norepinephrine* and *serotonin* — two important brain chemicals affecting mood if they're low. Some of the more commonly used tricyclics are amitriptyline (Elavil), desipramine (Norpramin), nortriptyline (Pamelor), and imipramine (Tofranil). Some psychiatrists like to prescribe these meds during pregnancy and breastfeeding because they're considered to be tried and true, having been around for so long. These meds are also prescribed for women who don't respond well to the newer antidepressants, SSRIs (see the next bullet).

✔ **Selective serotonin reuptake inhibitors (SSRIs):** These substances work the brain's serotonin levels, and have become increasingly more popular since the original SSRI, Prozac, was introduced in the late 1980s. Fluoxetine (Prozac), sertraline (Zoloft), paroxetine (Paxil), citalopram (Celexa), escitalopram (Lexapro), and fluvoxamine (Luvox) and other SSRIs are the first line of treatment for most women with PPD.

A mom with PPD commonly worries that an antidepressant will change who she is or will alter her in some way. If this is you, remember that the PPD has already altered you — you're already changed by the illness. The antidepressant simply helps you get your real self back. So, in fact, you better hope it changes you — back to you!

A woman with a personal or family history of bipolar disorder should be monitored very carefully if she's given any amount of an SSRI, because an antidepressant may increase the risk of a manic episode in moms whose depression may actually be part of a bipolar disorder (jump to Chapter 3 for a description of a manic episode). Usually these moms are prescribed a mood stabilizer as well, (if they're accurately diagnosed), which I discuss later in this chapter.

Antianxiety meds

Anxiety is a frequent and major symptom of PPD (see Chapter 2 for a list of all the other symptoms). Sometimes women who have PPD identify more with anxiety than with depression. To address anxiety and to help the new mom gain control over the wheels in her mind that are constantly spinning, a psychiatrist will often prescribe antianxiety medications (also called *benzodiazepines*) such as lorazepam (Ativan), diazepam (Valium), clonazepam (Klonopin), and alprazolam (Xanax).

To make matters confusing, though, some of the best medications that treat anxiety are the same medications that treat depression (see the preceding section). But sometimes an antianxiety medication is needed temporarily just until the antidepressant kicks in. You don't necessarily need to take these meds every day (unlike antidepressants). They help you come down a couple of notches so you can relax enough to remember to breathe, affirm yourself positively, and take the other steps you're working on in therapy.

One common result of anxiety is insomnia. It's not that the new mom isn't tired or that she needs something to sedate her, it's that she has so much anxiety that she can't settle her mind and stop it from racing. The benzodiazepines are also very helpful for insomnia.

Antianxiety medications are also prescribed to stop or, better yet, prevent the onset of panic. Generally speaking, you want to prevent your body from going into a full-blown state of panic whenever possible because with a panic disorder, the more often you enter into a state of panic, the easier it becomes for your body to return to that panicked state. So, you want to do everything you can to prevent yourself from getting there in the first place.

Antianxiety medications, therefore, can either be taken on an "as needed" basis — when the new mom with PPD feels a panic attack potentially coming on — or on an ongoing basis (as long as the potential for panic remains). An antianxiety medication like alprazolam or lorazepam is often prescribed to be taken on an "as needed" basis. The longer-acting antianxiety medication called clonazepam (Klonopin) is frequently used if the mom has more persistent anxiety that lasts night and day.

Often, women with a history of substance abuse are extra wary of taking a potentially addictive medication such as the benzodiazepines. It's important to mention that sometimes these meds are abused, even by women with PPD, and the biggest risk factor for someone abusing them is a history of substance abuse. If you've ever had a problem with alcohol, illicit drugs, or prescription medication abuse, make certain you tell your doctor — this information is crucial for your medical care! Make sure that you stick to the regimen as prescribed by your doctor.

Doctors, trying hard to be responsible, sometimes prescribe only a few of these antianxiety pills at a time, and ironically, a mom starts obsessing about running out, which only adds to her anxiety. The psychiatrists I work the closest with have no problem extending the prescription of antianxiety medication as long as they know the moms are taking them responsibly.

Sleep aids

Needless to say, sleep is a huge issue for new moms with PPD. Nothing is more frustrating for a new mom than working with her support system to set aside the time to sleep (as described in Chapter 12), and then being unable to actually take advantage of it. Imagine lying there for hours thinking "I should be sleeping. I should be sleeping. I should be sleeping. The baby will be up soon and it will be my turn." To get over this particular hump, a sleep aid can prove very useful.

Sleep aids, including medications such as zolpidem (Ambien), trazodone (Desyrel), and many of the benzodiazepine medications, help new moms with PPD obtain the good rest that they so desperately need. However, a woman often needs a separate medication for sleep only until her main antidepressant kicks in.

Tricyclic antidepressants with sedative effects, such as nortriptyline (Pamelor) or amitriptyline (Elavil), are frequently prescribed as sleep aids as well.

Mood stabilizers

Mood stabilizers are used mainly for women with bipolar illness, so that both their "high highs" and their "low lows" are moderated. Quite often, mood stabilizers are used to boost the effect of an antidepressant — even for women who aren't bipolar. So, if your MD or psychiatrist recommends a mood stabilizer, don't necessarily take this as a sign that you're also bipolar.

Atypical antipsychotic medications, despite the name, are some of the most frequently used mood stabilizers. But, again, just because a doctor prescribes one doesn't mean that a patient has a psychotic disorder. Two of the mood stabilizers, valproate (Depakote) and carbamazepine (Tegretol), are anticonvulsants, and both of them are approved by the American Academy of Pediatrics for breastfeeding mothers. Lithium, another mood stabilizer, however, is *not* recommended for breastfeeding mothers but is the mood stabilizer of choice during pregnancy.

Antipsychotic meds

The most important use for antipsychotics is for women who have postpartum psychosis (PPP). PPP isn't just a really bad case of PPD, but rather, is an entirely different kind of animal (see Chapter 3 for more on the distinctions). PPP can have tragic results, as in the infamous case of Andrea Yates, the Texas women who drowned her five children in 2001. About two out of a thousand new moms are thought to suffer from PPP. For new moms who want to continue breastfeeding, certain high-potency antipsychotics, such as haloperidol (Haldol), are often recommended.

Antipsychotics can also be used in other ways. For example, because it tends to really knock people out, the antipsychotic medication olanzapine (Zyprexa) is occasionally used for powerful insomnia that isn't responding to any of the other sleep medications.

Electroconvulsive therapy

Often used when psychotherapy and medication are ineffective with an individual, electroconvulsive therapy (ECT) is in some ways similar to rebooting a computer that has started to malfunction, because it temporarily alters some of the brain's electrochemical processes. ECT, also known as "shock therapy," has proven to be an effective treatment for severe PPD and postpartum psychosis and can be used safely by nursing mothers. It's also useful in treating postpartum bipolar illness. ECT is also used during pregnancy to treat severe depression and psychosis. It isn't, however, an appropriate treatment for anxiety, panic, or obsessive-compulsive disorder. Interestingly, sometimes an antidepressant that didn't work before suddenly starts working after the woman has had one or more ECT sessions. It's also suggested when a mom is on the verge of committing suicide, since ECT works much quicker than antidepressants.

Unfortunately, this kind of treatment has an undeserved negative reputation that often prevents the effective deployment of ECT. This is in part because whenever ECT is brought up, the Ken Kesey book *One Flew Over the Cuckoo's Nest* (or the 1975 movie of the same title) is what people often picture. In this book and movie, ECT was presented as a terrible type of therapy akin to torture, and so people tend to believe ECT is associated with screaming people holding on for dear life.

This view of ECT is a truly antiquated and distorted version of what goes on with ECT. As a clinical psychologist, I accompanied a client of mine as she received ECT. I saw the entire process from start to finish, and I can unequivocally say that this is an extremely humane process that isn't scary or painful at all. In fact, a short-duration general anesthesia is given to the patient, and the treatment itself takes only seconds.

In the United States, because of the prevailing negative view towards ECT, it's usually considered the treatment of last resort. In other countries, however, depending on their history, ECT is often the first line of treatment for some depressed new moms. Healthcare providers in these other countries wonder why women in the U.S. are so cruelly deprived of ECT, and why they're allowed to continue to suffer, going from one medication to another, instead of receiving something that only takes a few seconds and often provides relief even after the first treatment is given (sometimes women undergo a series of treatments).

Understanding the Fact that Finding the Right Med(s) Is a Process

Quite frequently, after a mom with PPD has made up her mind that she may benefit from medical treatment and wants to try it, she'll ask, "So, what's the right type of medical treatment for me?" Unfortunately, there's no one right treatment for all women because every woman is unique. So, a doctor may present various options and may discuss them with the woman before the two make a decision. This discussion usually happens in one office visit, but the woman may want to think about the options and discuss them with her partner or other supports. Different factors go into this important decision-making process, and I outline them in this section.

Identifying the important health-related differences among women

Although this decision is usually left up to the doctor's expert opinion, you can and should still have a say in the matter — after all, it's your body. When you're weighing out the information your doctor is giving you regarding different medication options, remember that you're unique in so many different ways — from your emotions and situations all the way up to your physical makeup. For example, not only do you have a unique medical history, but you also have your own special body chemistry that works better with some medications than others. For one thing, each woman metabolizes medications differently, and in most cases both the correct diagnosis and the correct dosage can only be approximated at first.

In short, the answer to "What's the best medical treatment for me?" can't be determined until you do the following:

- ✔ Meet with a competent psychiatrist or other medical doctor.
- ✔ Have your symptoms brought to light and your history taken.
- ✔ Have a blood test administered if your doctor needs information about your thyroid or other hormone levels.

After these steps are taken and the tests are returned, an assessment is made and one or more prescriptions are given. When you've finally received a prescription from your doctor, don't play what I call "the milligram game." Remember that each person metabolizes medication differently. A higher dosage doesn't mean that you're more ill than the next mom who's taking a lower dosage (and it wouldn't be shameful if you were). A few women with the same level of depression may be given the exact same dosage of the exact same medicine, and each may respond differently. So, take whatever you need to reach the therapeutic dosage that's right for you.

Keep in mind the fact that the first prescription may not be the best or the last one you try. Medicine is an art, and you may go through a succession of treatments — or dosage changes — based on how you respond. Usually the first medication chosen will be a good one for you, but not always. Think of it this way: Prescribing medicines for PPD is an educated trial and error system.

Staying the course after you receive a prescription

It's crucial for you to stay on your prescription until your doctor tells you to stop. Undertreating can lead to chronic illness and to an increased chance of relapse. "Treat to wellness," therefore, is the mantra that you need to follow here. Never, ever quit cold turkey because you think the medicine isn't working right or because you're experiencing side effects. Your opinion counts, however, so certainly bring up the topic and discuss the possibility of stopping the medication if you're thinking about it. This is your health, and your opinion is important, but trust that the psychiatrist has knowledge that you don't, so her reasoning about your staying on the medication should be taken seriously. If you want to get a second opinion, do so.

Many women say, "I stopped taking my medication because I felt better." Most psychiatrists would recommend a period of wellness, so that a woman feels like her normal self for at least a few months before stopping the medication, to decrease the risk of the depression returning. Also, don't forget that the reason (at least a big part of it) that you felt better is because of the medication. The last thing you want to do at that point is stop what's working.

Because your body quickly adapts to and gets used to the substance being there, even if it's the wrong medication for you, you're far better off (in most cases) if you gradually wean yourself off of it with your doctor's help. The opposite is also true: If you need more of a substance, you need to gradually increase the amount you're taking — but only with your doctor's guidance. The bottom line is this: Dose up slowly, dose down slowly, and make changes only when your doctor or psychiatrist says you should.

Needless to say, after you receive a prescription medication, you need to take it exactly in the manner that has been prescribed for you. Take your meds regularly, and don't skip a dose. If you forget to take it (forgetfulness is a symptom of PPD, as you probably know), ask your doctor how to proceed. You may want to come up with a simple system for yourself, such as marking a calendar after you've taken your pill or getting a pill holder with the days of the week imprinted on it.

To make staying the course a bit easier, remember not to be shy with your doctor. If you feel like you're having an adverse reaction to a medication, you need to let your doctor know pronto. It's her job to listen to what you have to say and evaluate your situation. If you think you may need a different medicine, it's up to you to make sure you get that across. And the same goes if you feel you need to increase your medication — talk to your prescribing doctor and see if it's time to take more.

Side Effects: You Can't Always Get Just What You Want

All of the medical treatments listed in this chapter can have side effects, which are, of course, unintended (and generally unwanted) symptoms that can be experienced physically or psychologically. As you know, the thigh bone is connected to the knee bone, and as soon as you start adjusting one part, system, or biochemical process in the body, it can easily have unexpected and unintended consequences on other parts, systems, and biochemical processes that are related to it.

The good news is that most side effects are mild, and few tend to persist after the patient stops using the treatment. In some cases, though, if you have a severe side effect, you may want to stop using the treatment in question and try something else. But, this should only be done in consultation with your psychiatrist or other prescribing MD.

Table 8-1 shows the most common side effects for the various types of medicine (and ECT) discussed in this chapter. More detailed information on the side effects of the particular medications you're prescribed can be found on the labels and inserts that come with the medication. But, if you're anxious, please don't read those — they'll only make you more anxious. Ask the pharmacist to throw the labels and inserts away before giving you the medication (I'm not kidding).

Table 8-1	Common Side Effects of Medicine and ECT
Type of Treatment	*Side Effects*
Antidepressants	Different categories of antidepressants can have different side effects.
	SSRIs can cause gastrointestinal problems (most common are nausea and diarrhea) and a lowering of libido (the main one that doesn't go away with time). It can also make you feel jittery or either tired or wired. Some individuals gain clarity, while others get "fogged out."
	Tricyclics can cause weight gain, dry mouth, constipation, dizziness, or heart palpitations. (The better tolerability of SSRIs explains why they're more commonly used.)

Type of Treatment	Side Effects
Antianxiety meds	Benzodiazepines can be habit-forming or addictive and can make patients lethargic (proper dosing is critical here).
Sleep aids	These aids can be habit-forming and can leave patients feeling a bit "drugged" in the morning if the substance hasn't been thoroughly "slept off."
Mood stabilizers	Mood stabilizers often increase appetite and slow metabolism, so weight gain can result. Some individuals with bipolar disorder (or tendencies of bipolar) miss the "high" side of their unmedicated cycle, which they consider to be a negative side effect. Some are sedating (and can help with sleep if taken at bedtime).
Antipsychotic meds	These meds have a very sedative effect, which can be helpful for sleep purposes but can also make patients feel "drugged."
Electroconvulsive therapy (ECT)	ECT is often accompanied by memory loss, which is usually short-term in nature (for example, the patient may not remember the day she came to the hospital for treatment). Her short-term memory generally comes back after a few weeks or a couple of months.

Knowing When to Begin Med Therapy

If your particular situation clearly suggests that you should at least seriously consider taking prescribed medications, you want to get on it right away. This decision may depend on a few factors:

 ✔ **The reasons for your depression:** Causes of depression are quite individual. If, for instance, your therapist evaluates you in the initial assessment and discovers that you're totally isolated, you're up every night for hours with a screaming baby, and you were just diagnosed with a low thyroid for which you'll be receiving treatment, it may make sense to wait and see what happens with your depression in the next few weeks after you start your new plan of action with social support, sleep, and thyroid treatment. If, on the other hand, your support system and sleep are in place, but you have a history of depression and an antidepressant has helped you before, you should probably start your treatment immediately (and use the medication that's helped you in the past).

✔ **Your level of functioning and level of depression:** If you're suicidal, your doctor will want you to take medication right away (and possibly have you hospitalized if you're in imminent danger of harming yourself). If you're having really scary obsessive-compulsive thoughts (see Chapter 3), you probably want to begin medication right away.

✔ **How you feel about your treatment:** If you have mild to moderate depression and prefer not to take medicine, if at all possible, waiting a few weeks (assuming you don't get worse during that period) is an appropriate option. Sometimes psychological treatment, increased support, and better self-care are all you need.

The whole point of medical treatment is for you to get well as quickly as possible. Getting well sooner rather than later is far better for you, your entire family, and your future prognosis. In general, the longer PPD hangs around, the longer it's likely to stay with you and the more difficult it is to get rid of.

Some therapists and MDs believe that every woman with PPD should start medication as soon as possible. That's not my opinion. I believe it's an individual choice — some women should definitely use it right away, others don't need it at all, and many fall in the gray area ("It could help but it may not be necessary").

Chapter 9

All Things Natural: Alternative Treatments

*W*hen you're suffering from postpartum depression (PPD), it may be helpful for you to consider alternative treatments and healing methods. Many of the alternative treatment options seem to work, at least some of the time, and some of them seem to be helpful most of the time (but none of them are helpful all the time, as Bob Dylan might say). They're generally less costly and invasive than what conventional medicine recommends, and for the most part (with some important exceptions), they're unlikely to harm you. Ultimately, though, whether or not alternative treatments do you any good depends on many factors, including the specific alternative treatment you're pursuing, the practitioner or supplier that you're relying on, and the specifics of your situation — for example, your physical condition and your frame of mind.

No alternative treatment takes the place of a thorough evaluation from a health professional who's knowledgeable about PPD. Alternative treatments can be excellent additions to an overall plan, but they aren't to be used as substitutions for good overall care. No matter what types of treatment you're using, you need and deserve the help of a caring and observant professional to determine what's working and when it's time to try something else.

This chapter begins by exploring alternative treatments in general, as compared to other forms of treatment. I then break down a list of the most common alternative treatments into two categories: Ones that are proven to have benefits and ones that aren't proven (but are still worth considering). As always, remember that no book, including this one, is a substitute for working individually with a qualified medical practitioner, and you should always consult with one before undertaking any significant treatment, conventional or alternative. To help get you started on your walk with alternative treatments, I include a whole section to clue you in on the types of professionals you may consult as well as how to assess — alongside a professional — whether a treatment is working or whether you need to throw it along the wayside and pick up something else. And for those of you with insatiable appetites for options galore, I fill you in on the warning signs you absolutely have to consider before jumping on the Web — a lot of what's out there won't do you a lick of good (and may also set you back quite a bit financially).

Introducing the World of Alternative Treatments

Alterative treatments have been growing in popularity ever since the 1960s, when "back to the land" lifestyles, vegetarianism and natural foods, and Eastern meditation techniques and spiritual practices were all taken up in various combinations by an increasing number of young people. Some of the alternative practices that were tried back then have since been proven ineffective or even harmful, but many others have found their way into mainstream consciousness and practice (however, these same practices haven't necessarily made their way into mainstream *medical* consciousness and practice).

In some cases, treatments that conventional medical doctors thought were impossible have been unquestionably proven, such as the ability of acupuncture to control pain or the ability of certain trained meditators and yogis to control physical functions and processes that were formerly thought to be beyond conscious control. In other cases, the sheer number of people reporting positive success with alternative treatments have brought these options into the domain of the medical establishment. Bestselling authors, such as Andrew Weil and Deepak Chopra, have also helped to popularize alternative possibilities and have brought them to the awareness of tens of millions of people. In fact, at times the line between conventional treatment and alternative treatment is blurred. So, many practitioners prefer the term *integrative medicine* to reflect a style of treatment that's open to all options that have evidence for benefit.

Looking back on the rise of alternative treatments

How popular are alternative therapies and treatments? Just take a look at some numbers:

✔ In 2005, Harvard Medical School researchers found that 35 percent of Americans used at least one form of alternative medical treatment in the previous year.

✔ Around the world, the numbers are even higher than those in the U.S. The World Health Organization (WHO) has estimated that between 65 and 80 percent of the world's population relies on alternative medicine as its primary form of healthcare and that 80 percent of the world's population uses herbal remedies as a major constituent of its primary care.

Everything from the spread of yoga studios to the popularity of the supermarket chains specializing in organic foods indicates a rise of interest in alternative treatments and perspectives. There is, then, no question that alternative and holistically medical approaches and perspectives are more popular now than ever. Why? Because they work for many, many people (just the idea that something's "natural" is often appealing as well).

Having said that, I'm sure you have questions: "What does it mean to say that an approach "works?" "Who judges what is and isn't effective, and how are such judgments made? And how does this all play out for the new mother who's overwhelmed by PPD?" And finally, "How can I possibly determine which alternative approaches I should try or how to go about trying them?" As you can imagine, this is a tough enough endeavor when a person is not overwhelmed by PPD. The remainder of this chapter will address each of these questions.

Sorting out basic treatment-type terminology

Before going any further, it may be helpful to get a bit clearer about the medicine labels. First off is the kind of presumably no-nonsense medicine that's practiced in modern hospitals and medical centers. This type of medicine can be referred to by any of the following names:

✔ Conventional medicine

✔ Western medicine

✔ Standard medicine

✔ Allopathic medicine (in contrast to homeopathic medicine)

✔ Modern medicine

The U.S. government's response to alternatives (therapies, that is)

Recognizing the growth of interest in alternative therapies, treatments, and modalities, in 1991, the U.S. government formed the Office of Alternative medicine, which was later renamed the National Center for Complementary and Alterative Medicine (NCCAM). Overseen by the National Institutes of Health (NIH), NCCAM's job is to explore alternative practices scientifically and to spread the word about their effectiveness both to professionals and to the public. Its four main focuses are research, training and career development, outreach, and integration (that is, ways of bringing alternative medicine's best practices into conventional medicine and into the medical curriculum of medical, dental, and nursing schools).

Conventional medicine is practiced by medical doctors, is associated with the use of pharmaceuticals and surgery, and is basically the starting place for most Westerners in regard to a medical concern of any kind. It's good to note, however, that medical doctors in training today usually receive education about alternative treatments as well. For purposes of clarity, in this chapter I use the term *conventional medicine* to represent the standard, conventional, allopathic, Western approach.

The alternative to conventional Western medicine also goes by a number of different names:

- Alternative medicine
- Complementary medicine
- Holistic medicine
- Indigenous medicine
- Integrative medicine
- Natural or naturopathic medicine
- Traditional medicine

The most popular of the terms for alternative treatments are *holistic medicine* and *alternative medicine*. *Holistic* refers to an approach that takes the whole person into account, including mind, body, and spirit. Because this book is meant to bring women back to wholeness and is also concerned with effective alternatives, in this chapter I refer to nonstandard medical approaches as both holistic and alternative.

Complementary medicine is also a useful term because alternative treatments complement standard medicine. As such, the medical community (especially in conventional medical literature) often uses the acronym *CAM* to refer to "Complementary and Alternative Medicine."

Note that the term *traditional medicine* is somewhat confusing because people use it to describe both sides of the treatment coin. Sometimes it refers to medicine the way native people have practiced it for hundreds or even thousands of years, for example, by using herbal medicine and the laying on of hands. But sometimes people use it to refer to what has been traditional in the United States for 100 years or so — that is, the conventional medicine practiced by MDs and hospitals.

Combating the negative stigma of the alternative route

Moving up the ladder of proof, there's a relatively tiny amount of clinical and strict experimental evidence about alternative and holistic approaches for PPD. Generally, because of the cost of performing clinical or experimental studies (a study can cost tens or hundreds of thousands of dollars to undertake, especially if a large sample of clients is to be studied), these are only done when someone with a considerable economic stake in the outcome is willing to fund it. Without meaning to criticize the U.S. economic system, many alternative and holistic treatments are inherently unprofitable, and therefore those who can afford to test them aren't interested.

The rise of the alternative: A story that spread the news

One way that alternative treatments become popular is through anecdotal stories. One of the most famous anecdotal reports concerns Norman Cousins, the long-time editor of the Saturday Review. In 1964, experiencing severe joint pain and fever after a trip to Russia, Cousins was diagnosed with a very serious disease, a collagen illness that attacks the body's connective tissue. He was put in a hospital bed and given high doses of painkillers.

But Norman Cousins had surmised that a different kind of treatment — laughter — might be more effective. He took himself off of the painkillers (don't do this without your doc's approval) and hired a nurse to read him funny stories and show him lots of Marx Brothers movies. The ensuing hearty laughter that he experienced relieved his pain and enabled him to sleep.

Twenty-five years later, in 1989, an article in the Journal of the American Medical Association (called JAMA for short, and taken as the single-most authoritative medical journal) stated that laughter therapy could immediately relieve the symptoms of chronically ill patients and help improve their quality of life. In this case, it took science a quarter-century to catch up with an innovative and courageous magazine editor!

As a result, there's relatively limited scientific proof for many holistic and alternative treatments, regardless of how strongly they're backed up by anecdotal or even clinical evidence. And even for those alternative treatments where good, widely acknowledged scientific evidence exists, it seems that a new study will always come out either completely questioning or substantially rearranging what was previously accepted. Just because a study says that eating cooked tomatoes is good for you doesn't mean that the next year's study won't come out and say just the opposite. At minimum then, it's important to constantly be on the lookout for the latest evidence regarding any approach or treatment.

But even though establishing unquestioned scientific proof is difficult or impossible for many holistic and alternative treatments, there's still a great deal about many of these approaches that obviously works, obviously makes sense, and is obviously worth trying. For example, if your dietary habits are quite poor, it makes sense that a partial or complete change in this part of your life may make a real difference to your physical and mental health (refer to Chapter 12 for ways to boost your mood with food). Likewise, if massage feels good to you (and you can afford it), even if there's no proof that it helps women with PPD, you may want to get a massage regularly anyway. (Interestingly, at least one study shows how massage may help PPD!)

A lot of the effect that a holistic or alternative therapy may have for you will come from the personal power and excitement (the oomph) of the alternative practitioner you choose to see. Never underestimate the powerful effect that another human being can have on your healing, especially if that human being is both knowledgeable and caring. Sometimes, all you need to get to the next level of recovery is a tiny bit of acknowledgement and encouragement, and such human treatment may be a lot more likely to come from an alternative practitioner than a licensed MD who's embroiled in a big medical practice with a variety of institutions. That's not to say there aren't great, caring MDs out there — because there most certainly are — but there are also many great alternative practitioners who may have more time to spend with you, and the fact that they don't have a license to prescribe drugs or authorize surgery doesn't mean that they aren't capable of helping you through your struggle with PPD.

Alternative Treatments that Make the Cut for Their Success

This section reveals a list of alternative treatments that may be useful for treating your PPD. However, remember that this list isn't by any means complete. A complete list would be impossible to put together because scientific knowledge — whether anecdotal, clinical, or experimental — is always moving forward. Treatments that years ago would have seemed ridiculous may very well prove to be useful, and other treatments (both conventional and holistic) that were commonplace fade away over time.

Here, then, in alphabetical order, are some holistic and alternative treatments that women with PPD may find useful.

Energy work

Many different types of *energy work* have delivered a great deal of value and comfort to those receiving them. It may just be that, as with massage, the patient is receiving the loving and warm touch of another human being, which in and of itself tends to have a healing effect. But some who practice energy work look at it as more than this. They claim that they can channel energy from their body and through their hands into the body of the receiving patient.

Therapists now know that sometimes the old-fashioned "talk therapy" doesn't help with trauma and that it can actually end up re-traumatizing the client. Energy work has proven to be extremely helpful with many of my clients who experienced postpartum post-traumatic stress disorder (see Chapter 3 for more on this disorder). For example, with some types of energy work, the "grip" of the person's trauma is released so the person is no longer experiencing the terror, nightmares, or flashbacks.

Here are a few of the many energy therapies that have provided relief for women suffering from PPD. Although healthcare professionals don't always know exactly what is working or how, these methods certainly seem to be making a difference:

- ✔ **Reiki:** Meaning "universal life energy" in Japanese, *Reiki* is one system of healing. Reiki is said to go through the practitioner as electricity goes through a conduit, healing only what it finds most pressing in the body of the patient. Because the intervention is noninvasive, there are no defined contraindications. Reiki supposedly helps the energy channels of the body to flow, stimulating the body to heal itself. Many of my clients report feeling very calm after a Reiki treatment — it seems to alleviate their stress and anxiety. It's used to reinforce the effects of any other method of therapy. (Check out *Reiki For Dummies* to get more in-depth info on this healing system.)

    Reiki has been used for stress reduction and deep relaxation. One lengthy study investigated the effects of Reiki on depression and found it to be a successful treatment method.

- ✔ **Polarity therapy:** An interesting blend of Ayurveda and both chiropractic and osteopathy, *polarity therapy* is said to balance the positive and negative energies that make life possible, and it also involves bodywork and nutrition.

- **Emotional Freedom Technique (EFT):** EFT is similar to acupuncture, except needles aren't used. Instead, you stimulate energy meridian points on your body by tapping on them with your fingertips. The process is very easy to memorize. And, because all you need are your hands, you can do this anywhere.

- **Eye Movement Desensitization and Reprocessing (EMDR):** EMDR is a therapy that researchers believe works through stimulation of the two sides of the brain. This technique, which involves a back-and-forth motion by the practitioner that the patient's eyes follow, has tremendously helped many of my clients with postpartum post-traumatic stress disorder. Although clients still remember the traumatic event after the treatment, the emotional distress associated with it is gone (or at least dramatically reduced). After the distress subsides, the therapist is able to do psychotherapy with the client.

  EMDR has been tested carefully in the treatment of trauma (no fewer than 24 research studies), and the results have been impressive. The American Psychiatric Association in 2004 reported that EMDR was given the highest level of recommendation (the category for robust empirical support and demonstrated effectiveness). In 2004, both the Department of Veterans Affairs and the Department of Defense placed EMDR in the "A" category as "strongly recommended for the treatment of trauma."

- **Therapeutic Touch (TT):** Developed in the late 1960s after researchers observed how healers of ancient healing practices prepared and performed treatments, *therapeutic touch* is a light touch that's now performed in hospital settings. TT is used to balance and enhance the flow of human energy and it helps with healing and relaxation. It's taught in colleges around the world and has a substantial base of formal and clinical research.

Exercise

For simple suggestions on incorporating exercise into your busy life, see Chapter 12. There's a lot of research on the benefits of exercise for relieving depression and anxiety (if done correctly).

Guided imagery

Guided imagery is a form of focused relaxation that helps create harmony between the mind and body. It works by helping the patient or client use the power of her own imagination to explore a particular area of concern. The process provides an opportunity for her to allow an image to form that in some way holds significant information or knowledge of the area being addressed. Guided imagery — often supplemented with beautiful music — creates calm and peaceful images in your mind. Basically, it's a mental escape for therapeutic purposes. The use of guided imagery can prove to be a powerful psychological strategy for enhancing your coping skills. It can help you cope with — and possibly overcome — stress, anger, pain, depression, and insomnia. After you meet with a practitioner one or more times, you can use this process at home.

Light therapy

It's well established that *light therapy* — purposeful exposure to bright light — can have a positive impact on those who suffer from seasonal affective disorder, or SAD. It can also help individuals realign and get their sleeping patterns back in synch. One study of pregnant women suffering from SAD found that light therapy helped lessen their depression. Another study reported in the *American Journal of Psychiatry* (2000) found positive impacts on women with PPD. Recent advances in light therapy generally show that a particular spectrum of light in the blue range has the greatest effect and can be used at lower light intensities. This treatment is showing a great deal of promise, and more studies are being set in motion.

To implement light therapy, clients use special lighting or a light box in their houses or in a professional's office. The light box is just what it seems: A box that emits a very bright light. Patients are instructed to position the light box in a specific way where their eyes are open (but not staring directly into the light). The exposure times that a professional prescribes range from 30 to 90 minutes daily, six to seven days a week in the morning.

Massage

Massage tends to make almost everybody feel better. Look for a massage therapist who does the kind of work that you like. Some people prefer light sweeping strokes, as in Swedish massage, while others prefer deep tissue work.

In 1996, a study of 32 depressed teen mothers found that compared with just receiving relaxation therapy, the mothers who received massage had statistically significant changes in their behavior as well as significant decreases in overall depression, anxiety, and stress scores.

Meditation

Meditation, which is sometimes described as an altered state of consciousness, is a form of relaxation that, unlike sleep, is entered into purposely. Meditation is usually practiced regularly, for at least 10 to 15 minutes each day. You can meditate in many different ways, but one of the most common ways is to clear your mind by focusing on your breathing or on one thought, word, or phrase (which is called a *mantra*).

If you suffer from anxiety, meditation may be difficult because your mind will probably be flitting from one thought to the next. If you try meditating a few times, but it's too frustrating to sit still, you may want to wait a couple of weeks before you attempt it again. For instance, even though many wonderful meditation tapes and CDs line store shelves, I know all too well that when you're suffering from PPD, sitting still long enough to listen to one is torturous. It's too frustrating, and feels like one more failure. If you just can't meditate, don't. And don't sweat it. The whole idea is to help yourself feel better, not worse!

Omega-3 fatty acids

Please see Chapter 12 for an in-depth description (and suggestion for a particular supplement) of what this remarkable essential fatty acid does for your body and mind. I highly recommend this supplement, and evidence shows its success in relieving depression and PPD.

SAMe

SAMe (short for S-adenosylmethionine and pronounced *sammy*) is a nutritional supplement that helps control the functioning of brain chemicals, including serotonin and dopamine (both of which are tied to your mood). In healthy brains, amino acids produce enough SAMe, but this isn't so for women with PPD. Numerous controlled studies have found SAMe to be one of the most effective natural antidepressants, and it's better tolerated and works faster than many antidepressant drugs. It has been widely used in Europe for at least 20 years, but it's newer in the U.S.

Alternative Treatments that May Add a Bit of Benefit

Many alternative treatments can help you recover, some of which have more research and "proof" of alleviating PPD than others. I have listed some of the most popular ones in this section, but they aren't necessarily proven to work.

Acupuncture

Acupuncture is an ancient Chinese method of healing that prevents and cures specific diseases and conditions by sticking very fine, solid needles into specific points on the body. This method stimulates the body's ability to resist or overcome illnesses and chronic conditions by correcting imbalances. Acupuncture also prompts the body to produce chemicals that decrease or eliminate painful sensations. Acupuncture has also been shown to increase melatonin, which reduces anxiety and insomnia.

In 2004, the American Psychiatric Press published a study by D. Warren Spence, Leonid Kayumov, Adam Chen, Alan Lowe, Umesh Jain, Martin Katzman, Jianhua Shen, Boris Perehman, and Colin Shapiro (phew!), where 18 anxious adults who reported insomnia were administered acupuncture to examine its effects. Five weeks of acupuncture was associated with a significant increase of melatonin secretion at night as well as the quality and quantity of sleep, as anxiety was reduced. These findings are consistent with the clinical reports of acupuncture's relaxing effects.

Acupuncture has a long and varied history, and over time it has won the confidence of an increasing number of MDs (some of whom have themselves decided to study acupuncture and incorporate it into their practices). However, its ability to fight depression, and specifically PPD, remains scientifically unproven. Nonetheless, in my own practice, I have seen numerous women suffering from PPD who benefit from acupuncture, both emotionally and in their sleeping habits. Acupuncture is showing promise as a safe, effective, and acceptable treatment of depression in pregnancy, but more studies with a greater number of subjects are needed.

Applied kinesiology

Applied kinesiology (AK) is a system that evaluates structural, chemical, and mental aspects of health by using manual muscle testing along with other standard methods of diagnosis. AK is based on the *Triad of Health,* which uses chemical, mental, and structural factors to balance the major health categories. In order to fix a problem, a practitioner must evaluate all sides of the triad for the underlying cause, because a health problem on one side can cause an imbalance on the other sides. Usually the patient lies on a table while the practitioner muscle tests the patient (pushing down on her arm as she resists) to see what strengthens her and what weakens her. From the assessment, various treatments will be prescribed and either carried out right then or in a series. From my simplistic description, AK may sound pretty "way out there," but I have personally benefited from this method and have witnessed my clients regain sound sleep and a sense of wellbeing.

An *applied kinesiologist* is a doctor who's licensed to diagnose and treat patients and who has extensive training and certification in the field of kinesiology. MDs, chiropractors, dentists, osteopaths, and others can all be trained in this field.

Ayurveda

Ayurveda is the ancient Hindu science of health and medicine. Popularized by Deepak Chopra, MD, Ayurveda is a complex and comprehensive system that has its own unique take on depression generally and PPD in particular. Ayurveda operates on the assumption that various materials of vegetable, animal, and mineral origin have some medicinal value. The medicinal properties of these materials have been documented by practitioners and have been used for centuries to cure illness and to help maintain good health. Ayurvedic medicines are made from herbs or mixtures of herbs, either alone or in combination with minerals, metals, and other ingredients of animal origin. If you choose to pursue this alternative therapy, consult a qualified Ayurvedic physician.

Chiropractic therapy

Chiropractic therapy uses adjustments to the spine and joints to relieve pain and to balance the overall health of the body's nervous system. These adjustments assist in establishing better coordination between the central and peripheral nervous systems. A major strength of this treatment approach, which many believe has helped their depression, is that it tends to be relatively safe. Although the research is sparse regarding chiropractic therapy's benefit in treating depression, chiropractic is nonetheless often used as a part of an overall health plan to reduce depression as well as an appropriate maintenance plan to reduce the likelihood of a relapse.

Herbs

Herbal medicine is used by more people throughout the world than virtually any other type of medicine. The helpfulness of herbs with PPD isn't entirely clear and remains up for question in scientific literature. Despite the uncertainty, in my practice, I've seen numerous positive effects in my clients who take certain herbs. Because the changes happen within a few days of beginning the herbs, I'm assuming there's a cause and effect relationship operating here. But, my observations can't be taken as proof.

Herbs are powerful medicines and should be taken with caution. Because herbs can cause serious drug interactions, you need to consult with your physician if you're taking an antidepressant or other prescribed medicine. Also, if you're pumping or breastfeeding your baby, check with a knowledgeable professional before taking any herb, because "natural" doesn't necessarily mean "safe."

Herbal medicines aren't generally produced in a standardized way. That is, it's often unclear exactly how they're produced or whether certain preparations contain substandard or less-than-therapeutic dosages. This fact is yet another reason that you should be monitored by a health professional to make sure you're getting what you need.

If you have moderate to severe PPD, you need to have your condition addressed by a qualified psychotherapist or physician. However, if your PPD is more on the mild side, an assessment is always good, but trying certain herbs on your own (if you aren't breastfeeding) may improve your condition. You can typically find all of the following herbs in health-food stores and in other stores selling natural remedies.

Ginkgo biloba

Ginkgo biloba, which is made from the leaves of one of the oldest living species of trees in the world, is thought to be the most frequently recommended herbal medicine. It's known to stimulate mental clarity, alertness, and memory. Most people tolerate ginkgo well, but anyone on an anticoagulant therapy should use it with caution.

Kava

Kava (Piper methysticum) has a long history of use in reducing anxiety but has only recently been used for the treatment of the anxiety that often accompanies PPD. Several European countries have approved Kava for the treatment of insomnia, anxiety disorders, and depression. In the U.S., Kava is available as a dietary supplement. Since 1999, some individuals using products with kava in them have reported liver problems, so I'm staying tuned to find out more.

Passion flower

Passion flower (Passiflora incarnata) is used as a sedative and for insomnia and can relieve anxiety, nervousness, and PMS symptoms, all without side effects. When combined with St. John's Wort, passion flower can help calm you and possibly reduce high blood pressure and nervous tremors.

St. John's Wort

St. John's Wort (Hypericum perforatum) is a wild yellow flower used to treat depression, anxiety, and sleep disorders. Named for St. John the Baptist (because it blooms around the day of his feast), St. John's Wort is continually being studied to try and validate its alleged benefits.

Over 30 clinical studies have been conducted over the past 22 years to evaluate the effectiveness of St. John's Wort. The active ingredients in the herb are thought to boost serotonin levels, which are usually lacking in depressed people, including those with PPD. The most recent scientific trials in the U.S. show that it's effective for mild depression but not for more severe cases of depression. The experiences I've had with my clients support these findings.

Research from the National Institutes of Health has shown that St. John's Wort may reduce the effectiveness of several drugs, including birth control pills and some heart disease medications. The long-term effects of its use in breastfeeding (on babies) are unknown and need more study. Watch for possible side effects of St. John's Wort, including the following:

- ✔ Increased sensitivity to the sun
- ✔ Increased blood pressure
- ✔ Upset stomach
- ✔ Allergic reactions
- ✔ Fatigue and restlessness
- ✔ Cataracts (after long-term use)

In some countries, such as Germany, the sale of St. John's Wort is greater than the sale of many of the major prescription antidepressants.

Homeopathy

Homeopathy is typically quite difficult for conventional medical practitioners to accept because according to homeopathic theory, the more times a remedy is diluted, the more powerful it gets — to the point that supposedly the most powerful doses statistically contain less than one molecule of the original substance. Nevertheless, homeopathy has been around for quite a while, and it's very popular in Europe. Even though you can sometimes simply consult a homeopathic book to find the right remedy, a good homeopathic professional will spend a great deal of time interviewing you in detail to determine which remedy is the right one for you. After the professional determines the appropriate remedy, he or she will tell you what dosage to take and at what frequency you should take it.

Most homeopaths undertake three or four years of training, which includes case analysis so that they learn the finely honed skill of matching remedies to specific symptoms. Most naturopathic colleges have programs in homeopathy. In fact, many naturopathic doctors (NDs) use homeopathy in their practices. Homeopathic practitioners who have attended a school of naturopathy also fulfill medical school — like training and clinical application.

Many homeopathic practitioners also are MDs, chiropractors, NDs, and doctors of osteopathy. Unfortunately, a few people practice homeopathy even though they have little formal training. Your best bet is to ask whether the practitioner you're consulting is certified in homeopathy.

Hormones

The most common theory regarding the cause of PPD is the sudden and precipitous drop in the reproductive hormones following birth. You would think that by replacing the estrogen and progesterone lost at birth, PPD could be prevented. However, even though there are some promising studies using forms of these two hormones to either treat or help prevent PPD, there's still limited scientific support for this treatment, especially since risks are associated with hormone replacement therapy.

The data does provide evidence that estrogen and progesterone are involved in developing PPD in some women. The confusing fact is that no one actually knows why some women react to the hormone shifts while others don't. Some women report feeling much better with estrogen or progesterone, and others report feeling much worse (especially with progesterone).

Hypnotherapy

Depression can be lifted substantially if the depressed person can relax her mind (which is pretty tough with PPD). When your mind is relaxed, you sleep better. You become more confident and motivated and are able to bring about positive shifts in your perception and turn negative thought patterns into positive ones, which is very much needed as you recover from PPD. Hypnotherapy can help you do just that.

During a hypnotherapy session, you'll either sit in a comfortable chair or lie down on a comfy table. Different practitioners use different methods to help you into a state of relaxation (commonly called a *trance*). (As a hypnotherapist myself, I basically bore my client into a trance; my voice eventually sounds to her like a droning TV in the background that she can't wait to tune out.) The hypnotherapist will then help you get information from your subconscious (which inherently knows what you need) by guiding you through different exercises and asking questions of the subconscious. You may be fully aware of everything during the session, or you may be so relaxed and tuned out that you don't remember much of anything. To find a qualified practitioner, check out the Web site of the American Council of Hypnotist Examiners (ACHE) at www.hypnotistexaminers.org.

Reflexology

Reflexology, which is related to acupuncture (they're both based on the Chinese system of *meridians,* or energy channels), is a technique in which a therapist applies pressure to specific points on the hands and feet. Reflexologists, like chiropractors and osteopaths, believe that the body has the capacity to heal itself. For example, by manipulating the nerves in the hands and feet (which are related to various parts of the body), reflexologists think that the healing process is stimulated.

Yoga

If you're wracked with anxiety, concentrating on anything may prove to be too frustrating right now. On the other hand, taking your mind off of your troubling thoughts and focusing on a yoga position may be exactly what the doctor ordered. Choose a type of yoga that you'd enjoy. Bikram yoga, or "hot yoga" may be too intense for you right now (you don't need to be in an extra-warm room when your hormones are already making you sweat!), but a nice, light "Hatha," or health-focused yoga could be just the ticket. You can learn and practice yoga from a book or tape, but as with most types of exercise, being in a group environment means you'll probably get more value from it. Check out *Yoga For Dummies* by Georg Feuerstein and Larry Payne (Wiley), *Power Yoga For Dummies* by Doug Swenson (Wiley), or *Yoga with Weights For Dummies* by Sherri Baptiste and Megan Scott (Wiley) if you want to delve into the wonderful world of yoga.

Administering Alternative Treatments: You and a Pro

When picking your alternative medicine practitioners, you have to consider many factors: their qualifications, your rapport with them, and what types of treatments you have chosen. This section introduces you to many of the common professionals.

Who's who in the name game

Licensing requirements for the many alternative medicine professionals vary across the board. Some are pretty strict and others are nonexistent. So, as always, use your instincts to evaluate what's being offered. Look for local practitioners who have references, and be wary of individuals who promise too much or who are too eager to sell you some miraculous product or device.

Medical doctors and naturopaths

As for who's who, I start, of course, with MDs. These traditional medical doctors and specialists, who serve as the practitioners of modern conventional medicine, are the gatekeepers of medical science and are the anchor points in the entire medical delivery system. Hopefully you won't have to work too hard to find an open-minded MD who's both good at what he or she does and open to the possibility that alternative treatments and therapies can be quite effective as supplements to conventional medicine.

On the natural side, the rough equivalent of an MD is a naturopath, or ND. *Naturopaths* are medical practitioners who receive an ND degree after four years of intense schooling. These practitioners use holistic or alternative medicine to treat patients, but they aren't licensed to practice unlimited medicine like medical doctors and osteopaths can. In the United States, whether a naturopath can prescribe any controlled or prescription drugs (and which types), differs from state to state. Naturopaths have a substantial focus on nutrition as well as a wide range of alternative therapies and treatments.

Chiropractors and osteopaths

Chiropractors focus mainly on addressing spinal misalignments by "adjusting" clients so that a free flow of nerve impulses and bodily energy can be restored, enabling the body to self-regulate, and in turn heal itself. Chiropractors are abundant in many areas. They often prescribe nutritional supplements and holistic therapies to their patients.

Doctors of Osteopathy (DO) are similar to chiropractors in that they have a primary focus on the musculoskeletal system of the body — that is, the nerves, muscles, and bones that make up two-thirds of a person's weight. They practice a whole-person approach, meaning that they consider both the physical and mental needs of their patients. According to the American Osteopathic Association (AOA), osteopathic medicine is a complete system of healthcare with a philosophy that combines the needs of the patient with the current practice of medicine. Interestingly, just like an MD, a DO is licensed for the unlimited practice of medicine in all 50 states. In other words, a DO can prescribe drugs, authorize surgery, and so on. Remarkable healings are often attributed to osteopaths, who, among other things, work to realign and rearrange the plates that make up the human skull. Although osteopathy is growing in popularity and seeing a bit of a resurgence, it's typically more difficult to locate an osteopath than a medical doctor.

Acupuncturists

Acupuncture has gained increasing recognition as being effective in treating pain, infertility, and other conditions. MDs with an unconventional orientation sometimes study acupuncture and add it to their offerings. But, a serious study of acupuncture can take many years, so your best bet for acupuncture, if you can, is to find someone who became a doctor in China.

The U.S. has national licensing boards for acupuncturists. If you want to check to make sure a practitioner is board certified, you can contact the National Certification Commission for Acupuncture and Oriental Medicine (NCCAOM) by going to www.nccaom.org. Another organization to check is the American Board of Medical Acupuncture (www.dabma.org).

Other alternative-therapy professionals

Besides the main alternative medicine professionals described earlier in this section, many other individuals deliver holistic and alternative therapies, from massage therapists and herbalists to those who prescribe color therapy and those who undertake different types of energy work. Many of these talented practitioners use essential oils as part of their various treatments. Among your options are the following:

✔ **Massage therapists:** These healers may be trained in a variety of massage techniques. An experienced massage therapist can be an important person on your team. Many of my pregnant and postpartum clients regularly schedule massages and put them high on the priority list of expenses. Your massage therapist should be certified. The American Massage Therapy Association (www.amtamassage.org) recommends that you ask the following questions of a massage therapist to find out whether he or she is trained and qualified:

  • Are you licensed to practice massage?

  • Are you a member of the American Massage Therapy Association?

  • Where did you receive your massage therapy training?

  • Are you Nationally Certified in Therapeutic Massage and Bodywork?

Another good organization for checking certification is the National Certification Board for Therapeutic Massage and Bodywork (www.ncbtmb.com).

If you're pregnant, make sure that your massage therapist is experienced in working specifically with pregnant women. This area is a specialty because certain positions are more comfortable (those where you lie on your side), and certain areas of the body should be manipulated very carefully or not at all. These practitioners are usually the same ones who are experienced with new moms with loose ligaments and muscles that are still sore and healing.

✔ **Herbalists:** These practitioners treat the whole person and not just the symptom. Two people could visit the same herbalist, with apparently the same condition, but leave with totally different prescriptions. Your herbalist should be registered with the organization called The National Institute of Medical Herbalists.

Searching for Other Alternative Treatments: Be on Guard!

Be wary of Internet searches, especially on the topic of holistic and alternative treatments (and if you're anxious, remember to stay away from the Internet in general). A mind-boggling number of Internet sites pop up when you search for alternative treatments, and many aren't neutral — they're trying to convince you that their miracle product will cure you. Some of the sites are better than others, of course, but it's difficult to determine who has the real scoop (and who's pushing bologna).

You also may run into a lot of haphazard information about what happened to different women when they used various treatments. This load of lyrics may be interesting (if in fact it's even true), but don't count on it — this stuff isn't scientific data. A lot of these anecdotal reports are happenstances, treatments, or alternatives that just happened to work for the woman in question, for whatever unknown reason, but may not be applicable to your situation. If, for instance, you go online and find a random support group and you read a discussion where one woman raves about eating red licorice and how it really made all the difference to her, it's difficult to tell how seriously you should take her advice. You can try it, if you want, but maybe you'd be better off eating healthful food or trying something that we know works (like dark chocolate!).

If you're planning on searching the Internet, I suggest you start by going to NCCAM's Web site at nccam.nih.gov. This federally funded Web site provides current research and solid information about complementary and alternative medicine.

Chapter 10

Creating a Comprehensive Treatment Plan

*E*very professional has a bias, and I'll state mine here. As you'll probably gather when you read Chapter 12, I believe in helping pregnant and post-partum women heal without pharmaceuticals whenever possible, and that can frequently be accomplished. Although healing naturally with alternative therapies (along with psychotherapy) is my bias, I'm no fanatic. My strongest belief is that you need to use whatever works in order to completely recover.

A comprehensive treatment plan refers to one in which the whole person — body, mind, and spirit — is focused upon, instead of just one part or symptom. For instance, even though an antidepressant can often alleviate the symptoms of postpartum depression (PPD), the trauma of a mom's delivery will most likely cause her to need therapy of some sort. The bottom line is that a new mom is much more than the sum of her body parts and symptoms.

Many times, healthcare providers combine different treatments to create a comprehensive plan. Consider why: Is it, for example, really possible to treat a new mom's anxiety and depression without looking into her physical and biochemical condition and whether that can be helpfully addressed through medication? With that in mind, I always give a new client a full initial assessment. Like any experienced practitioner, I want to obtain a well-rounded picture of what's happening in my client's life — types of stressors, feelings, physical complaints, relationships and support systems, preferences of treatment, and beliefs — before I create a treatment plan with her.

Because every client's life and experiences are different, no one plan of action will work for every woman — the plan needs to be individualized. For one woman, a combination of psychotherapy and conventional medication may work great. For the next woman, acupuncture and enlarging her support network may be the bulk of what she requires in order to get well. Most importantly, though, a treatment plan should continually be assessed and updated as needed. If one piece of a woman's puzzle isn't being addressed adequately, she and her healthcare practitioner should create a plan that includes a different treatment method or combination of methods.

In this chapter, I cover all the basics of creating a comprehensive plan. So that you know what to expect, I also offer guidance on how you and your healthcare practitioner can adjust your plan as you go through treatment. And because I know what a pain it can be to deal with insurance companies when all you want is help to get better, I give you a rundown of how insurance typically works for such comprehensive treatment, and I provide some tips on getting the most out of your money.

The Three Components: Finding the Right Balance for You

Because handling your psychological and physical needs and knowing who can take care of what can be confusing, in this section I outline for you how these essential pieces of the recovery puzzle fit together. Please remember to be open-minded as you read, because the methods of treatment you may have in mind may not end up being the ones that actually work for you.

Last year, I had a client who, for the first six months of treatment, was quite rigid regarding her willingness to try various treatments. Based on her cultural background, she was open to using only Chinese herbs, which helped her — but only to a point. Eventually she tried a low dose of an antidepressant along with her herbs (with her MD approving the combination as safe) and she became 100 percent better quite quickly. As you can see, it pays to strike a thoughtful balance, keep an open mind, and attempt to gain the most benefit from both conventional and alternative medicine.

Here's a rundown of the three different treatments:

✔ **Psychological treatment:** Psychological therapy is a conventional treatment that encourages you to stay conscious of your negative thought patterns (such as when you mentally beat yourself up) so that you can switch them to affirming, supportive ones. Psychological treatment also helps you adjust to your new roles and communicate better when you're feeling lousy. If any issues from your past are getting in the way of your life now, at some point in the therapy, you can learn to release them.

Basically, the role of psychological treatment within the whole treatment plan is to guard your mental and emotional well-being. Psychological treatment is sometimes used without the other two — medical and alternative — and can, for some, be all it takes to recover.

✔ **Medical treatment:** With the term *medical treatment,* I'm referring mainly to conventional medicine. If your evaluation results in a recommendation for medicine, this piece of the puzzle, which concentrates on balancing your brain chemistry, enters.

Medication without therapy isn't recommended. Many people think that all they need to do to heal is take what comes out of the prescription bottle. Oh contraire — they may be fine chemically, but not psychologically. Doing both forms of treatment gives you the clarity to process what's happening to you and also helps you move through the emotional pain deliberately and consciously.

✔ **Alternative treatment:** Alternative treatments are wonderful adjuncts that can boost both the psychological and the medical treatments, but they aren't a must for many people. Some women use alternative treatments without conventional medicine and do well, but if you're one of these women, please make sure you're getting psychological treatment too.

Conventional Therapy or Alternative? A Quick Comparison

It's the million-dollar question that everyone's dying to know the answer to: Which is better, conventional medicine or alternative medicine? The answer: It depends on so many different factors — most of which have to do with your beliefs about both forms of treatment and your chemical makeup, which determines how your body will react to them.

Like it or not, there's no way to know ahead of time what the "right" answer for you is. In other words, there's no way to know whether you should stick with only conventional medical treatments, whether you should try a combination, or whether you mainly want to try an alternative approach. But regardless of what you initially decide, you can always make a course correction if necessary.

To become a savvy and effective (even if depressed) healthcare consumer, it is useful to consider the pros and cons for both conventional and alternative approaches. Table 10-1 summarizes quite generally what's good and what's bad about both sides of the equation.

Table 10-1	A Comparison of Conventional and Alternative Treatments	
Factor to Consider	*Conventional Treatments*	*Alternative Treatments*
Overall effectiveness	Treatments are very effective in some situations, but less clear in others.	Treatments are effective in some situations, but not really appropriate in others.
Amount of scientific proof available	More proof is generally available, but not always.	Less scientific proof is generally available.
Cost	Treatments are generally more costly, but they're usually covered at least in part by most health insurance plans.	Treatments are generally less costly, but they can also be expensive. They're often not covered by insurance.
Focus of treatment	Conventional medicine is often criticized as focusing on symptoms rather than causes, but psychotherapy looks at more of the whole picture.	Treatments often focus on deeper causes, but they may not be as good at relieving symptoms.
Side effects and interactions	Treatments can have strong side effects and interactions, but they're generally well mapped out. Monitoring by healthcare providers with expertise can minimize risks.	Treatments often have no side effects but can have some side effects and interactions that are sometimes not well-known.
Fraud and quackery	Treatments include limited outright fraud and quackery, but some overselling occurs. It's easy to check the reputation of providers through licensing boards.	A good deal of fraud, quackery, and overpromising exist with alternative treatments, because licensing boards don't always oversee alternative practitioners.

With respect to overall effectiveness, there's some dispute as to whether conventional or alternative approaches are the winner. With some sorts of things — a bursting appendix or a broken arm — there's no question that conventional medicine is irreplaceably valuable. However, with other conditions that affect the emotions (such as PPD), especially those that insidiously creep in (or hit like a Mack truck), alternative approaches may be quite helpful. But the decision regarding both forms of treatment isn't an either/ or choice. A combination of conventional and alternative often works beautifully. For instance, Emotional Freedom Technique or Eye Movement Desensitization and Reprocessing (see Chapter 9) can help dramatically with emotional trauma, which may accompany physical trauma — as is the case with a scary delivery.

Understanding how researchers determine the success of a therapy

With respect to science in general, and medical science in particular, how do we know what works? Consider aspirin, which most people would agree works pretty well. As it turns out, the ancient Egyptians (and later the ancient Greeks) knew about and used aspirin-related compounds way back in the day. (Hippocrates, said to be "the father of medicine," prescribed a compound made from willow bark, which contained salicin, aspirin's natural cousin.) But how did the Egyptians and the Greeks know about these compounds?

Presumably, some early ancient Egyptian just so happened, by chance, to make up an infusion of dried myrtle leaves (containing salicylic acid, which is related to aspirin), and that infusion just happened to relieve back pain. Typically, scientists find out what works through a process of trial and error. Their trials fall under three umbrellas:

- ✔ **Epidemiological studies:** Scientists use this type of study for several reasons, such as for looking at risk factors of a particular disease or for looking at a disease's rate of occurrence. Epidemiological studies help generate ideas about what causes certain problems or helps with their treatment, but it doesn't prove cause and effect.

- ✔ **Case study:** This study is an analysis of the results of treatment for one patient or a small group of patients and is useful for generating ideas about what deserves further study. For example, if a small group of patients are all given the same treatment and the results are noteworthy, this interesting information can serve as the basis for research. Only with more experimentation and with a greater number of subjects can the treatment be proven.

- ✔ **Clinical trials:** A clinical trial is a scientific study requiring a research design and criteria about which patients are selected to participate. In an *open trial,* researchers and patients know what treatment the patient is getting. In a *double-blind trial,* neither the researchers nor the patient knows which treatment the patient is getting.

For a prescription antidepressant medication to come to market in the U.S., it usually needs to have several of these studies showing that it works better than a placebo (such as a sugar pill or another substance that doesn't provide benefit) for depression.

There's actually another kind of (very important!) proof: proof-in-the-pudding! When you've tried something and it works for you and made a real difference, the rest of the kinds of scientific proof are pretty much irrelevant. Validate what's working for you, whether or not anyone else has ever heard of it working before.

As mentioned in Table 10-1, fraud and quackery is something to watch out for, especially when dealing with alternative treatments. Even though most alternative practitioners are good people who are well-trained and who accept their patients' well-being as their primary concern, many so-called practitioners are out to make a buck by selling the latest "miracle" product or unproven healing approach. You may encounter a great deal of over-promising and overselling with alternative medicine, so be on the lookout for promised cure-alls and panaceas. It's easy to fall prey to miracle products when you feel desperate to get better — and most women feel at least a bit of desperation with PPD.

On the conventional side, even though relatively little outright fraud is reported, a good deal of overselling and overpromising still occur. Some conventional doctors treat everyone who comes to them in the same way, regardless of what's really going on with the patient. Consider it a bad sign if you hear something such as, "I treat all my patients with the same medication because it always works within two weeks." You don't need to drop the doctor like a hot potato if you hear this, but take this statement with a huge grain of salt. A particular medication, therapist, or type of therapy may work well for one woman but not at all for the next.

Coordinating the Plan

Organizing anything right now — even the contents of the diaper bag — can be daunting. So I imagine that hearing that a plan must be organized for your recovery may seem completely out of the realm of possibility at the moment. I assure you, though, this plan doesn't need to be complicated, and it will serve you well to make sure your treatment is happening in a coordinated fashion. Most often you can leave the coordination of your recovery plan to one of your practitioners (often the therapist), and all you need to do is show up and follow through.

After the practitioner performs an initial evaluation and finds out your medical history (including your obstetrical history), your family history, your social situation regarding supports, and whatever else may be impacting your life, she can help figure out what you may need to recover. At this stage, you and your practitioners can outline a plan with whatever treatments may help you — whether conventional, alternative, or a combination of the two.

Letting a good doc guide the way

For each woman, the main practitioner who's coordinating her care may be different. For one woman, it may be her primary care doctor. For the next woman, it may be her psychologist. And for yet another, it may be her psychiatrist or OB/GYN. I've found that because PPD is a mood disorder and the woman is almost always seeing a therapist, most MDs (OBs, primary care physicians, and other doctors who are in charge of the medical aspects of treatment) consider the therapist as the primary coordinator. Your therapist, however, should also relay any pertinent and relevant pieces of your psychological well-being to the other doctors currently providing your care. Later in this chapter, I explain how this important teamwork can work beautifully.

The relationship you have with your therapist is a partnership. She uses her expertise to guide you, but you're dealing with your health and your plan, so your willingness to follow through is crucial. For more about this partnership with your therapist, jump to Chapter 6.

I frequently receive calls from a woman's OB/GYN, psychiatrist, and primary care doctor (sometimes from other specialists if her care requires it) just to update me on the various treatments and changes in medications she's receiving. These smart and caring docs not only want to keep me informed, but they also know that these changes may affect their patients psychologically, and I'm the one in charge of that. If a woman is seeing a psychiatrist for both therapy and medication, those two are rolled up into one.

Meeting with a psychiatrist

Many psychiatrists will prescribe medication for someone only if the person is going to them for psychotherapy as well. On the other hand, other psychiatrists are fine with being in the role of only prescribing and monitoring medication, if the psychiatrist knows the woman is seeing another therapist. If you want to consult a psychiatrist only for meds (because you're seeing another person for therapy), make sure you ask her if she's willing to give you a medication evaluation, and tell her you're seeing another person for therapy. Depending on what the psychiatrist answers, either make an appointment with her or call another psychiatrist.

Working with two therapists

It can be confusing to see two therapists for therapy, and usually I don't recommend it, but sometimes this arrangement works well. If you've been working successfully with a therapist (maybe that therapist is a psychiatrist) until your PPD hit, and the therapist realizes that PPD isn't her expertise, she should refer you to a therapist who specializes in PPD to help you through the crisis. You have a choice at this point. You can either continue meeting with your original therapist on the weeks that you don't meet with the other therapist, or you can temporarily meet with the specialist until the crisis passes and then continue with your regular therapist. It's probable that after the crisis passes, you won't need the specialist anymore. Sometimes, though, it's a good idea to check in with the specialist a few weeks or even a couple of months down the road, just to make sure the PPD is on its way out.

When I'm working with a woman, if I know she is or will be working with her regular therapist on certain issues, I point out those issues as we go along and defer them to her work with the other therapist. I tell her that I won't focus too much on subject *x* because I know she'll be working on it with her other therapist. Doing so frees up our time to zero in on the areas that specifically pertain to the postpartum period and PPD.

Sometimes it's confusing for the woman to have more than one therapist, especially when the therapists' orientations are too different and the advice given conflicts. Trust your gut. Ask yourself which professional would be able to help you more *right now* in your life (not which one is the best therapist). You'll get an answer — listen to it, and go with it.

Doing a bit of research

If you're thinking about discussing other conventional or alternative treatments with your doctor or therapist, you can go to your plan-creation session armed with a bit of knowledge about what's available, what interests you, and which practitioners you may be interested in seeing.

If all you can do is show up (or call in, as the case may be) for your appointment, fine. You don't have to have any information at all. Often it's enough just mobilizing yourself to follow through with the appointment. In this section, I just give you more information in case you're able and want to be more involved with creating your treatment plan.

If you do decide to research some treatments, you don't necessarily need to be the one finding the information. As a matter of fact, especially if you're anxious, obsessive, or overwhelmed (all are typical with PPD), I suggest that you designate a support person who's eager to be put to work. (For your purposes, though, Chapters 8 and 9 give you a solid rundown of the most common medical and alternative treatment options.)

No matter who's doing the research, it's always important to know where to look. The most common resources are a library, a bookstore, or online sources, such as the Internet. One particularly helpful online resource is the U.S. Government's National Center for Complementary and Alternative Medicine, whose Web site can be found at www.nccam.nih.gov. On this Web page, along with a full-scale search engine, you'll find a further link to an A to Z list of clinical trials by keyword. You can also browse popular health topics (including depression).

If you're anxious or obsessive, I strongly suggest that you don't go to the Internet to do research — the Internet will almost always increase your already high anxiety level. If you think that going on the Web is necessary to find your practitioner, delegate someone else to do it for you. The Internet generally, of course, pulls up thousands of hits for a single search on postpartum depression. So, as you (or your support person) trudge through the material, always keep in mind who's writing and what his or her bias is (everyone has one).

Deciding whether meds are right for you

Making a decision regarding medications that could potentially make you feel better may seem like a difficult one — each of them carries benefits and risks of side effects. So, listen carefully to the professionals on your healthcare team and ask all your questions before making your decision and coming up with a plan about where medication may or may not fit for you. Sometimes you need to trust their expertise even though you may not be entirely comfortable at first with the plan. And at other times, the opposite is true — your doctors may not be entirely comfortable with your preferences but may need to adjust. For example, they may want you to start on an antidepressant right away, but you may want to instead use the nutritional suggestions (see Chapter 12) and make other changes in your life first and see how you do. As long as your life or anyone else's isn't in imminent danger, your team of doctors should respect your decision. However, they should reserve the right to bring up the topic of medication after a few weeks if you aren't better — it's important that you and your doctors constantly reevaluate your plan to make sure you're headed in the right direction.

On occasion, you may find yourself being dissuaded by a therapist or other healthcare professional from taking medication or even consulting with a psychiatrist or other MD simply for an evaluation. My feeling is this: If you think that a consultation to gather more information may be useful to you, do it. Even if you receive a prescription (which you probably will) and then decide not to use it, at least you have another point of view from a medical professional, including some pros and cons of taking it versus not taking it.

If you choose not to take medication (at least for now), be honest with yourself and determine whether you made that choice for the right reasons and not the wrong ones. (A wrong reason would sound something like this: "I'll be weak if I take meds.") Making even the littlest of decisions while you have PPD is challenging, and so this huge one can feel overwhelming to many moms. Remember, you can always get the prescription and then think about it.

Picking an alternative treatment or two

If you're considering taking alternative treatments along with your medication, be sure to choose a cooperative MD. A smart and open-minded MD is a great resource for an objective opinion when it comes to alternative treatments, because she can alert you to possible dangerous interactions with your meds as well as side effects. Such an MD may also have her own suggestions of holistic and alternative therapies that you can try.

If you have a doctor who's at least reasonably open-minded, consult with her about what it is you want to try. Not to mention the fact that she can potentially help you find a good balance with your overall treatment plan, having a discussion about alternative therapies is a good idea just in case a dangerous interaction could occur between, for instance, a drug you're already on and an herb you want to try. Or, you may find out that because of complications resulting from your pregnancy and delivery, certain types of bodywork may be harmful to you.

Frequently a client will casually mention to me that she's thinking of trying or has already started using SAMe, St. John's Wort, Chinese herbs, or other remedies. If she's taking conventional medication, I tell her she needs to let the prescribing doctor know about these additions to make sure they're okay and will mix well with her other medicine. If she's not up to making the call, I either make sure a support person calls the MD or I relay the information myself (obviously with her permission).

When it comes to alternative treatments, many doctors say to their patients, "Well, go ahead and try one if you want, but I don't think it will do any good." Even though that response isn't optimal, it's okay. (If your doctor is unwaveringly against them, head straight for the "Reacting to a doc who stands her ground" section later in this chapter.)

After you do a bit of research and spend some time thinking about which alternative therapies to pursue, you may find that because you're frustrated and unhappy and desperate to get well sooner, you're tempted to jump in and start trying all the alternative treatments at once. For example, maybe one book you read says that a select lot of herbs work well while another one says you should try homeopathy. And then there's the book that says you should put special magnets under your pillow. In this case, you might say to yourself, "I think I'll try them all tonight!" Needless to say, overindulging in alternative therapy isn't a good idea. Consider the following reasons:

> ✔ **Trying too many things at once can be exhausting.** Both in terms of energy and resources, you can easily burn yourself out by going from appointment to appointment and shelling out considerable dollars each time you do.

> ✓ **If you try multiple treatments at once and you feel better, you won't be able to distinguish which ones are really working for you and which ones aren't.** This uncertainty is confusing and makes it difficult (if not impossible) to manage your treatment plan effectively.

Instead of going whole hog, choose one or two alternative techniques or treatments that you feel most strongly about. Stick with them for a few weeks, and then you can always drop one, or add another, and see what happens. You should undertake any alternative treatment in a well-thought-out and methodical way, not haphazardly.

Making sure you're on the same page as your doc

If you already have a trusted healthcare practitioner who's recommending a particular type of treatment, you can be sure that her suggestion is a good bet, because this person knows you and cares about your well-being. Especially when you're at your lowest, assuming of course the recommendation makes sense to you, simply trusting the good judgment of this practitioner and going forward with the suggestion is usually fine. Even so, it would be wise to ask if there are any known risks to this type of treatment (if you aren't already familiar with it).

Whatever the case, it's important that you agree with your treatment plan. If you're in disagreement with your therapist, doctor, or other practitioner, make sure you say something. Don't leave the office with a plan you're not willing to follow, or else you'll be much less inclined to stick with it (and you need to get on the road to recovery as soon as you can).

Get thorough explanations regarding why the professional thinks this particular piece of treatment is important so you can make an educated decision for yourself. Discussing your plan with the practitioner can help you discover the other options that are available (some of which you may be more willing to do). If you need help making a decision, you may consider asking a close support person for input. It's important that you feel supported and respected in your choices, so don't be afraid of choosing to forego your practitioner's suggestion. If you evaluate what the practitioner suggests and decide not to follow that suggestion, ask if she's still willing to work with you. The answer will probably be yes. But if not, be prepared to find a different person.

I'm not saying that each treatment step should feel comfortable. Sometimes your recovery will require you to stretch yourself and go outside of your comfort zone. But, I promise it'll be good for you. Whatever you do, don't let your comfort level with a certain treatment task be the sole determiner of whether that task is valid and good for you.

If your practitioner's suggestions really aren't feeling right to you, you may want to seek other opinions. Keep in mind, though, that every professional will give different advice. The variety of options can be good, but it also can be confusing.

One of the biggest problems with PPD is that many times women don't follow the treatment plan — whether it's with medication, therapy, or something else. So, after you're clear on the plan and agree that a certain step is important, commit to it and follow through. If you need an accountability buddy to help you stay on track (for example, a friend or your partner), get one.

Reacting to a doctor who stands her ground

What if your primary care physician, OB/GYN, psychiatrist, or therapist is completely closed-minded to any holistic or alternative treatment? This is never a good sign. In fact, in this case, you should probably run fast and try to find another doc. (If you receive care from some kind of large medical establishment, try to have yourself assigned to someone else, preferably someone with a reputation for being open-minded.) The goal, after all, is to get you well. So, you want to work with a practitioner who wants you to get the best and most effective care you can regardless of how odd it may sound to her.

Sometimes, a formerly closed-minded MD will come around to the idea of alternative treatments based on her actual experience. In one case, I had a new client whose husband was a well-regarded MD. Like him, she was steeped in the medical model, and even though she had tried six antidepressants over a period of two years without much improvement, she was very reluctant to try any alternative treatments. Eventually she was willing to listen to my advice and try both acupuncture and major shifts in her diet (see Chapter 12 for more on diet changes). Sure enough, in just a few weeks she felt dramatically better. It took her husband a while to admit that these two changes had made the difference. But the proof was in the pudding, and he couldn't deny that where a half dozen antidepressants had failed, acupuncture and nutrition had succeeded.

Adding Professionals to Your Treatment Team

If you're considering a technique or therapy, such as acupuncture or massage, you need to find a practitioner. You may find magazines and catalogs that list practitioners by specialty, but an even better idea is to rely on the recommendation of someone you trust. Nothing beats knowing that you're going to someone who has already helped a friend or someone you know. If you know the type of treatment but don't know a practitioner, often the therapist or doctor can give you a couple of names.

After you find a practitioner, you want to know how he works, whether he provides a free initial consultation, and what kind of results you can expect. I suggest asking the following questions, but ask only what's relevant and what you're interested in knowing. For instance, a massage therapist isn't covered by insurance, so don't bother to ask. Be sure to ask these questions of alternative as well as conventional practitioners:

- ✔ What's your expertise working with postpartum women?
- ✔ What's your expertise treating depression? What results have you seen?
- ✔ Are you licensed? (Each state has its own licensing requirements, depending on the specialty. So if it's not required, an excellent practitioner may not be licensed.)
- ✔ What's your fee? Do you have a sliding scale?
- ✔ Are you covered by insurance?
- ✔ What is your cancellation policy?

Be sure to ask for references, and make sure to follow up on them (or ask a support person to do so for you), especially if you aren't coming to the practitioner based on a word-of-mouth recommendation.

If a practitioner answers your questions but you sense any defensiveness, be wary. The professional still may be excellent (he may just be having a hectic day) so don't rule him out yet, just watch for other hints of a bad attitude (and if you see them, drop him). Most professionals expect and welcome questions and will gladly answer them. Also, particularly in the area of alternative practitioners, there are those who practice psychotherapy without a license — a serious offense. Some of them innocently and unknowingly do so, and others don't seem to give a darn. Their attitude is, "I'm helping my clients, so what's the big deal?" The problem is that without knowing what they're doing due to a lack of training, a hypnotherapist, acupuncturist, massage therapist, or other practitioner can psychologically damage their clients without even knowing it. They confuse the therapeutic aspect of their practice with actual psychotherapy. A nearby acupuncturist in my area is notorious for giving his patients marriage counseling advice as they're lying on the table, and he gives this advice while probing into his patients' minds and trying to diagnose their issues (he's usually wrong, but that's not the point). So, when you see a practitioner, take what information he can offer within his specialty and throw the rest away.

Because I'm writing this chapter specifically about psychological, medical and alternative healthcare, I'm not mentioning other wonderful professionals such as doulas. These professionals can aid a great deal to your recovery. (Chapter 14 gives you suggestions about professionals you may consider adding to your team).

The breasts of Venus (and her difficulty feeding, which added to PPD)

From Mary L. Marine, BA, IBCLC, RLC:

"Long before I became a lactation consultant, I was a depressed mom. I struggled with adjusting to motherhood, and with each new baby, initially, with breastfeeding. So, as a lactation consultant I empathize with the challenges of new mothers.

I feel strongly about the need for new mothers to receive support in general, because the process of becoming a mother is a stressful life event, made much worse with the addition of PPD. On top of that, experiencing breastfeeding difficulties is also stressful — so a mother experiencing breastfeeding difficulties needs to be assessed by the lactation consultant as a whole person; including the mother's physical and emotional health. Then the consultant and mother can prepare a care plan together that helps her address her concerns and achieve her goals.

New mothers sometimes have questions about others feeding or caring for their babies so that they can sleep. So, my duty is to find a solution that's as unique as the mother and her circumstances. The mother needs to understand all her options and the advantages and disadvantages to each. And my job is also to preserve the breastfeeding relationship when that's the mother's goal.

When I assess a mother for breastfeeding difficulties, I also assess whether she's at risk for depression or other mood disorders, and I refer her to a mental health professional for further assessment and treatment if necessary. I also share information with her about the research on the effects of medication on nursing infants, reassuring her that healthcare providers can help her find the medications that are best for her and are safe to take while breastfeeding. By giving the new mother support and help finding the appropriate resources, I'm able to help her feel successful. I'm also able to empower her to care for her child and herself and to nurture their relationship."

Getting Your Team Members to Huddle

You want your professional team members talking about you — in all the right ways, of course. The process of coordinating your care should be a collaborative team effort, and more and more, this is exactly what's occurring. Unfortunately, what sometimes happens instead is that one professional gives a mom one piece of advice and another professional gives her a conflicting direction. These contradicting directions are difficult enough to follow without PPD, let alone with a condition that makes it difficult for a woman to process information and make decisions. So, especially if you're taking a medication, make sure that good collaboration is occurring between your psychiatrist and your therapist, if it isn't already happening. Ask your practitioners to be in touch with each other, and provide them contact information. Give the appropriate team members your official permission to speak to each other (sometimes practitioners require this permission to be in writing). You can be sure that only the pertinent pieces of info will be shared.

The professionals often take care of updating each other on their own. For instance, a psychiatrist may increase a woman's dosage of an antidepressant. He calls the therapist and leaves her a voicemail about the reasons why he made the change. The therapist, who's always watching carefully for changes in mental health in either direction, then calls the psychiatrist a week later to say that his patient seems to be responding well to the increase. By the time the woman is back in the psychiatrist's office for a medication check, the doc already has received helpful feedback from the therapist. Many benefits are occurring simultaneously: The doctor is being updated on how the med changes are working, the therapist is clued in to watch for changes, and the patient feels taken care of and secure that her team is on top of her treatment.

In order to protect your privacy, e-mail and fax typically aren't used as communication methods among your healthcare providers. If they are used, and even if someone other than the intended professional sees it, your identity is fairly impossible to determine. For example, one OB/GYN sometimes shoots me an e-mail with cryptic language such as "the woman that we were discussing last time on the phone" or "the person I just referred to you with the initial S." So, if anyone was to somehow see that e-mail, he or she would have a heck of a time figuring out whom the doctor is talking about.

As You Go through Treatment . . .

The team you've assembled will (either regularly or just as necessary) call each other on the phone to update each other and to check in. As you continue with your treatment plan, you'll likely need to adjust your treatments to achieve the maximum effectiveness for you so you start feeling better as soon as humanly possible. This section provides a brief idea of what you can expect in regard to making adjustments along the way.

Determining what's working

You'll know fairly quickly whether your psychotherapy and your therapist are right for you (refer to Chapter 6). Regarding your conventional and alternative medical treatment, on the other hand, it can get a bit tricky. For one, conventional medicine can take a couple of weeks to start working — sometimes fewer and sometimes more, depending on the medicine and how quickly your body absorbs it. And in the meantime, you may experience some side effects (skip back to Chapter 8). If you do, you'll need to be in close touch with your MD and therapist to help you determine whether what you're feeling is normal.

The trickiest therapies to gauge are often alternative treatments, because they often take the longest to work (with plenty of exceptions, of course). Homeopathy often uses remedies that increase your symptoms before they decrease (believe it or not, that's a good sign), and the process can be slow. Likewise, some herbs need a few weeks before you can fully tell if they're doing what you'd hoped. So, for each of the particular methods of treatment you choose, make sure you know the reasonable amount of time to wait before you stop and try the next one. (Your practitioner will clue you in.)

When women finally decide to use a particular treatment, whether conventional or alternative, they often become impatient pretty quickly. Although your eagerness is understandable, you must remember that improvement isn't immediate. The medicine or remedy takes the same amount of time to start working no matter how quickly you decided to try it. And actually, if in the meantime you became more ill, the treatment may take longer to start working. The biggest mistake you can make at this point is to stop the treatment prematurely (this is especially true for acupuncture, applied kinesiology, or any treatment that may require a series over a few weeks). Keep on trucking, and following the recommendations of the individual practitioner who understands that specialty.

Knowing when it's time to try something else

It's time to try a new form of treatment when either your practitioner of that treatment says it's time or when you feel you've given it enough time (evaluate carefully because the amount of time differs dramatically depending on the individual treatment).

If a treatment makes you worse, doesn't improve your condition at all, or improves it only a bit no matter what the dosage, it's time to either stop the treatment and try something else or add something else into the mix. (Remember, too, that side effects of conventional medication can take a couple of weeks to subside — see Chapter 8.) One example is when an antidepressant takes a woman to about 85 percent wellness and she's doing all other parts of her psychological, nutritional, and environmental plan beautifully. Instead of pulling her entirely off the med, though, the doctor may add in a bit of another treatment, such as thyroid medication or another antidepressant, to bring her to 100 percent wellness.

Ah, the Good Stuff: Dealing with Insurance

Insurance is great if you never need to use it. But when you get sick and have to start plowing through the red tape, you realize how frustrating it is to get your claims approved. Some companies are better than others, but generally they all have no problem taking your money and seem to have great difficulty giving it back. (If you haven't noticed, I'm not a fan of them!) I've seen what's happened to so many of my clients at the most vulnerable time in their lives — one denied claim after another. Depressed moms often become much more depressed due to the company that's supposedly there to help them. Nonetheless, I present the following sections to you in as unbiased (yet honest) way that I can, because ultimately, you have to deal with them whether you like it or not.

Putting a price on happiness

As for cost, conventional medical approaches are generally more costly than alternative treatments, but luckily, at least part of the cost is often covered by health insurance. The types of services and therapies that are typically covered by insurance (and which you may rely on for PPD treatment) include the following:

- Check-ups
- Chiropractic adjustments (many companies cover them, but not all)
- Conventional medicine office visits
- Conventional medicine
- Emergency care
- In-hospital care
- OB/GYN care
- Psychiatric visits (including psychotherapy, although usually a limited number of sessions are covered)

Making the grade: Understanding the "in-network" mumbo-jumbo

Just because a professional is on an insurance panel (in layman's terms, she's "in network") doesn't mean she's good or bad. It just means she's licensed. MDs accepted on insurance panels need to be licensed in their particular specialty, but you need to evaluate whether they're the right docs for you by asking the questions in the "Adding Professionals to Your Treatment Team" section earlier in this chapter and by following your intuition when you speak to them.

Regarding psychologists, marriage and family therapists, and other psychotherapists, many times insurance companies claim that they have therapists with specific training in PPD on their panels. But, with a few good exceptions, that usually isn't the case. For example, many therapists think that if they've had experience in the fields of women's health or depression, they're qualified experts in PPD — not so! You'd be shocked to know that in order to be considered an expert in the eyes of the insurance companies, all it takes is a check in a box on the application form to become a provider. In other words, a practitioner doesn't have to provide *any* proof of expertise in a particular subject area to the insurance company. If the therapist deems herself an expert, the insurance company simply enters that information into the computer — no questions asked.

Literally hundreds of women throughout the years have tried all the so-called experts in the insurance companies, and have subsequently ended up in my office or a colleague's office to finally get real help. This isn't to say that these other therapists weren't good therapists; it just drives home the point that women with PPD need therapists who are specialists in that field.

When you call the therapists that your insurance company recommends, interview them with the questions provided in Chapter 6. If you then determine that none of them has appropriate training, call your insurance company back (or have a support person call) and ask if a case manager can help you find a solution. Occasionally, if the insurance company acknowledges that it doesn't have an expert in PPD, the case manager can help you by setting up some kind of payment for a PPD specialist outside their network.

If you're seeing a therapist or other provider from outside your network, especially if you have a PPO, there's a chance that some reimbursement can come to you from your insurance company. If there's a possibility, ask your therapist to give you an invoice to submit. The reimbursement can then be sent directly to you. Depending on your energy level (and the importance to you), you can either call your insurance company in advance to inquire about coverage or just get the help, submit the invoice, and consider it gravy if you receive a reimbursement.

Part IV
Traveling the Road to Recovery

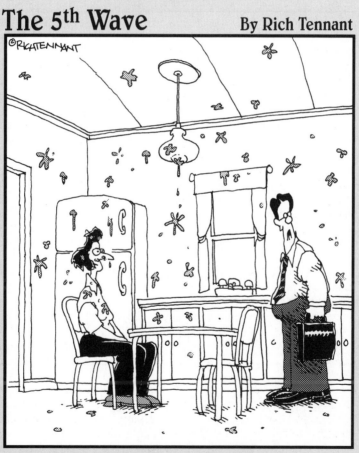

The 5th Wave   By Rich Tennant

"Bad day at the office...You're so lucky that you get to just stay home with the baby."

In this part . . .

Because you picked up this book, I'm guessing that you're looking for some advice on how to get back to your old self — the self before postpartum depression (PPD). So, in this part, I show you how to quickly and effectively travel the road to recovery, including how to get the most out of your treatment, how to handle the many feelings swirling around your head, and how to create the perfect support team. The final chapter in this part is written specifically for your friends and family. It gives them the basics on how to best help you as you recover.

Chapter 11

Getting the Most Out of Your Treatment

*I*t's easy to become discouraged when your recovery doesn't go as fast as you want it to (and, believe me, it never does). You're probably seeing a therapist and maybe even some other professionals and you're still depressed. Don't despair. You'll eventually feel better. Just remember that even though postpartum depression (PPD) can sometimes disappear quickly, it usually dissipates in layers and takes time — anywhere from a few weeks to a few months.

The key to recovery is accepting the fact that you have PPD. After you've accepted your situation, the recovery process has begun. Your next goal, as you form and work through a treatment plan with trusted professionals and loved ones (refer to Chapter 10), is to find ways to remind yourself that you're moving in the right direction, no matter how painfully slow it may seem.

You can expect this chapter to help you with all these things and more. I make sure you know exactly how to make your way through these layers of recovery and I discuss some concrete tips on how to speed things up a bit. And, finally, I show you how to handle your team of treatment professionals, from when they're not communicating with each other to when they're treating you in a way that doesn't work for you.

Recognizing the Stages of Recovery

Wouldn't it be great if you could catapult from the moment you're in the doctor's office hearing your PPD diagnosis to the finish line where you feel like your old self again? I have a pewter wand on my desk — I call it my magic wand — and I tell clients that if I could wave it over them and make their PPD go away, I would in a hot second. But, unfortunately, PPD just doesn't work like that. Instead, you have to maneuver through the stages of recovery, just as with other conditions such as grief. Although they're loosely formed, the major stages of recovery for PPD are

✔ Accepting your diagnosis and handling the reality of what may be ahead of you

✔ Overcoming fear

✔ Overcoming impatience

✔ Seeing the glimmer of light at the end of the tunnel

✔ Recognizing the old you returning

The progression through the recovery stages isn't at all linear. You'll come across ups and downs, and you'll notice that some levels are passed through quickly whereas others move more slowly. Sometimes you may even think that you're done with one stage only to find yourself still dealing with it a day later. And, often you're in multiple stages at the same time. Don't worry — this is all normal. Recovery isn't supposed to be a tidy process. In fact, just like there's no "right" way to have a baby, there's also no "right" way to recover from PPD.

Being familiar with these stages is helpful because they can validate that you're not the only one feeling this way. Knowing that you're not the only one suffering doesn't instantly take away your PPD, but it's always comforting to know you have company. Also, recognizing where you are in the process can help you measure your success. Especially when you feel like you're crawling through at a snail's pace, you'll be able to see that your feelings are expected, which in turn gives you a perspective that helps you hang on for the long haul.

Accepting PPD as a force to be reckoned with

PPD is very real. Despite what anyone tells you, it's not in your head. Okay, well, brain chemistry is technically in your head, but what I really mean is that your PPD is not imagined. Because many women (and many times their families) have this idea that PPD is "just in my head," they have a tendency to ignore it. Like ostriches, they put their heads in the sand and hope that if they simply pretend that it isn't there, it'll somehow just disappear.

The opposite is true. If PPD goes untreated, all kinds of relationship difficulties can arise, and most times this condition can fester and become worse. PPD rarely goes away on its own, and even if it does, it can take a very long time — sometimes even years, like it did with me. Meanwhile, the quality of your life and the lives of those around you suffer tremendously. The ripple effect of not seeking treatment is painful at best and tragic at worst.

Understanding why you need to accept your lot

Because PPD can continually get worse if not treated, it's important for you to quickly seek treatment. But, remember, to fully receive treatment, you have to first accept the fact that you have PPD. Accepting this fact requires getting diagnosed and adjusting to the news (flip to Chapter 5). The sooner you accept what's going on, the easier your entire recovery will be because

- ✔ **You'll be motivated to find help.** One of the most interesting (and unfair) parts of PPD is that the common emotions of guilt, shame, and embarrassment — the very things that may make you resistant to accepting PPD — are actual symptoms of the illness. And ironically, these symptoms are what often get in the way of a woman reaching out and getting the help she needs.

  If the PPD (which may be triggered by a combination of unrealistic expectations of motherhood, low brain chemical serotonin, and so on) is making you believe that you're a weak and incompetent person for not bucking up and handling your life, chances are you're embarrassed about coming forward to get support. After all, who wants to be associated with an inadequate bunch of people? (Flip to Chapter 14 for info on recruiting your support people.)

- ✔ **You'll stop questioning and resisting your rollercoaster of feelings.** After you fully accept that you have PPD and understand the up and down nature of how it behaves, it will be much easier for you to explain your constantly changing moods to yourself (and others).

- ✔ **You'll find it easier to accept and use the suggestions and directions of your therapist, doctor, and support group.** The guidance of your support team may be simple, but important. If you're thinking that the PPD doesn't need attention and is no big deal, it will be easy to disregard these simple suggestions about, for instance, sleeping, eating, and taking breaks.

  But, don't confuse simple with easy. A suggestion to take regular breaks isn't complicated. But, it will involve some logistical planning and maybe pushing through some myths about mothers not needing breaks. Similarly, a suggestion about taking medication is simple, but it may take some energy to make that decision (which isn't necessarily easy).

Accepting the reality of your PPD doesn't mean that you have to be happy about it. Instead, accepting your PPD means that you're ready to play with the cards that were dealt to you. Likewise, it's totally up to you how much energy you want to waste being resistant to the fact that you have PPD. Just know that the sooner you understand and accept it, the easier your recovery will be.

Taking steps to accepting your PPD

When you resist the fact that something exists, moving through the situation can become much more difficult. So, as the preceding section shows, it's crucial for you to come to terms with your illness. Here are some concrete steps to help you on your way:

1. **Let the information sink in, especially if it's unexpected.**

   If you already suspected that you were suffering from PPD, it will most likely be less of a surprise.

2. **Try to put words to your reaction.**

   If you're in a professional's office, he can help clarify what you don't understand and can answer questions you may have.

3. **Practice removing any judgment or negative emotion if it surfaces.**

   Check out Chapter 13 for ways to deal with your negativity and other judgmental feelings.

4. **Say to yourself, "Okay, I have PPD, and I'll be fine. This illness doesn't define me — it's just something I have to deal with."**

   Instead of fighting the fact that you have PPD, which is futile and a waste of energy, just deal with it matter-of-factly. You don't have to like the fact that you have PPD, you just need to come to terms with it.

Fear: Feeling the weight of self-doubt

At this stage you know intellectually that women recover from PPD, but you may still fear that you don't have the ability to achieve it. During this stage, I almost always hear my clients say, "What if I'm the only one who doesn't recover from this?" What I tell them is that almost every mom with PPD feels the same way. I know that these words won't take the PPD away, but I hope they're validating to you. Remember that with proper help, you *will* recover. Take it from me: I have yet to work with anyone who, when given proper help, doesn't recover. And that's saying something — I've worked with over 15,000 women in person, by phone, in groups, and with teleclasses.

When almost every task feels difficult, the thought of working on anything this big can feel daunting. It's like standing at the bottom of a steep mountain and looking up at the top wondering how you'll ever get there. But all it takes, and all you should focus on, is moving ahead, little by little. Eventually, you reach the top, and the view is awesome. In addition, you'll be able to share with others (if you want) how the climb was and what you saw, heard, and felt along the way. And of course, your self-esteem and knowledge will expand during the journey. One of the best parts is that you don't have to make the journey alone. You have support groups, therapists, other practitioners, and your family and friends to cheer you on, hold your hand, give hugs, and bolster your confidence.

During this stage, women also tend to have a fear of the unknown. They're afraid of not knowing what the recovery process will entail and they're afraid of being disappointed if the process takes longer than expected. Working with your therapist, you'll be able to tailor a recovery plan that suits you beautifully.

After you start down the road to recovery, sit down with your professional support (and doctor) and create a wellness plan for your recovery (see Chapter 10). Your plan is like a map that you can follow so you know where you're going and how you're going to get there (and what to do if you run out of gas). Don't set the plan in stone, however, because you and your practitioners won't be able to predict exactly how your progress will go. Rather, expect that your wellness plan will evolve and need updating as you and your support team continually assess how you're doing.

Impatience: Wanting to shove Father (or Mother) Time forward

No matter how quickly you recover, it never goes as fast as you want it to. Though it's impossible to know exactly when that moment will be that you'll feel totally normal, what's important is that you're going in the right direction. When you're making your way through the stages of recovery, make sure you keep taking steps — even if they feel like baby steps (and don't forget to congratulate yourself for moving toward your wellness goal either!). Each effort you make, even when you seem to be walking hip-deep in mud, puts you that much closer to reaching your goal.

When you hit the impatient stage, you'll likely entertain thoughts of giving up the treatment plan because the end is nowhere in sight. You may have only begun the journey two days ago, but nevertheless, you're understandably antsy and you want results *now.* But don't stop the plan. You really *are* getting closer to the light at the end of the tunnel; even if you can't see it, remember that it's still there. What you don't see is what is occurring as you walk through the darkness — the roots of healing have sprouted and are taking hold, and you just have to stick with the plan until you start getting the payoff.

As you continue to recover, expect to hit some dips in the road. Remember, though, that dips are just speed bumps — they're nothing to be concerned about. I get lots of worried calls from women who are back in a low spot and are frantic because they think they're suddenly dropping back to square one — to the bottom of the pit. But, when I quiz them about what they were able to accomplish, even during their dip, they're able to regain their perspective and realize that they're not at the bottom. The worst of their PPD is over.

You may also experience frustration about not having instant answers and solutions. Your therapist or doctor won't have all the answers, although you'll want him to. You're likely warding off nagging questions such as, "When will I be better? How long do I have to wait? Will my medication kick in by one week or two?" Just remember: Treatment for PPD, as with many other illnesses, requires trial and error. Your professional team will make educated guesses, but don't expect guarantees or promises when it comes to time frames for recovery. Frustration is normal at this juncture, and you can help yourself through it by occasionally venting to your close support people and by talking to others who have felt the same frustration and have come out on the other side.

Groups at this stage can be particularly helpful. In these groups, women in every stage will probably be present. It may be therapeutic for you to help those women who are still reeling from the initial diagnosis and who haven't fully accepted the reality of their illness. Similarly, those women who have been through this impatience stage and who have made it through can lend you a hand, bringing their belief and encouragement to you. If you want to explore this support system, head to Chapter 14 for a thorough discussion of the different types of groups.

If you truly feel that you're spiraling down in the wrong direction and aren't moving up at all, or if you think you're going way up and then way down, your wellness plan probably needs tweaking. Discuss your feelings with your health professional (refer to Chapter 10 for information on developing a wellness strategy).

Glimmers of light: Experiencing moments of feeling good again

At this stage, also known as the "light at the end of the tunnel stage," you begin to have returning glimpses of your old self. I call these glimpses *windows.* During these windows you experience feelings from your old self, whether that means feeling happy, relaxed, upbeat, or peaceful. Whatever feelings you've been missing will soon start making brief appearances.

At first, the windows may be so fleeting that they last only a short time —
perhaps just a millionth of a second. As soon as you recognize that they're
there, they're already gone. And initially, the windows may occur days or
weeks apart. But, here's what happens: The windows will get more frequent
and last for longer periods of time. From seconds they grow to minutes. From
five minutes they grow to ten minutes and from there to a half hour. After a
while, the windows show more than the depression. In other words, your situation reverses for the better. Instead of the windows being the fleeting
times, they become the majority and the depressed times get shorter and
happen less frequently.

Measuring the frequency and duration of your windows is a wonderful way to
gauge how well you're progressing. Even if you've had a rough few days, measuring your windows may allow you to see that you're doing better than you
thought you were. Your bad times now probably won't compare to the bad
times at the beginning. Even bad is getting better! At the end of your day,
mark down in your calendar your best guess about how many seconds, minutes, or hours you were having windows of happiness. Don't analyze them —
just write whatever pops into your head first. This task shouldn't feel like a
serious piece of homework — make it light and simple. If you skip a few days,
it doesn't matter. This effort is just another helpful way to help you gain that
precious perspective that you're moving up the mountain, where there's a
clearer, more expansive, and delightful view.

Recognizing the old you

The fantasy you may have at the beginning of your road to recovery is waking
up one morning (yes, you were able to sleep in this fantasy) and the PPD is
completely gone — your life is instantly rosy again. Sadly enough, an overnight
recovery isn't typical of this illness. The symptoms may go away quickly, but
usually not literally overnight.

So, I bet you're wondering how you'll know that you're "back." Interestingly,
the answer to that question is different for each woman who's reading this
book. Whatever means "you" to you is how you'll know. If you loved to cook
before your PPD and are now itching to experiment with a new recipe, take
that eagerness as a positive sign that you're coming back. If, before the PPD,
you prided yourself on your sales ability with clients, you'll see glimpses of
your sharp negotiation skills returning during this stage. Or, you may start to
enjoy being alone with your baby instead of dreading it. One of my clients
knew she was coming back when she started singing in the shower again.
Others around you may also start noticing and pointing these things out.
Your partner may perhaps notice that you're smiling more or getting your
feisty attitude back.

At the beginning of your recovery, you may have written down (or at least thought about) those qualities, personality quirks, and other things about you that you miss. If you haven't written them down yet, go ahead and do so now. In the following list, I get you started with some examples, but go ahead and fill in the blanks so that they specifically fit you. I'll know I'm getting back to my old self when I

✔ Feel like answering my e-mails

✔ Look forward to meeting my friends

✔ Can communicate with authority to the team I manage at work

✔ _____

✔ _____

You may want to ask your loved ones to point out these positive changes to you when they begin noticing them in order to boost your faith that you're moving forward. Sometimes you can feel the change before your supports notice, and other times they may notice first. Either way, you're moving on up.

Keeping the Faith: Ways to Foster Recovery

The speed of your recovery depends on a number of factors, with one of the biggest being the way you talk to and treat yourself. In this section, I help you strengthen and speed your recovery by describing simple ways you can keep track of your progress. Then I outline some steps to help you retrain your thoughts. It's one thing to have a therapist instruct you to "think positively," but it's another to actually figure out how. Read on, dear friend, to find out.

Staying in the present

Depression and anxiety make you want to dwell either in the past or in the future. You may tend to obsess about what you think you should have done differently or not done at all. For instance, "I shouldn't have had a baby — what was I thinking? My life was good before I messed it up." Or, you may anticipate each and every possible negative event that could happen in the future (especially with postpartum obsessive-compulsive disorder, which is discussed in Chapter 2). For example, "If she's crying this much and so difficult at two weeks old, what kind of a teenager is she going to be? It's going to be awful! She won't have any friends and she'll drop out of high school. Our lives will be miserable."

Good for you if you giggled at the last few sentences. You probably identified with at least some of it, and that's good awareness. One week after my daughter was born I was obsessing about not having enough money to send her to college. In a matter of a millionth of a second, I went from seeing two dollars in my purse — instead of the twenty I thought was there — to being convinced that my one-week old would never receive a bachelor's degree! By the way, my daughter, Elana, graduated this year from college without student loans.

So, you want to find a way to train your mind to stay in the present. Take it from me — you can spare yourself a ton of wasted energy! When you catch yourself fast-forwarding to an imagined negative future, follow these steps:

1. **Focus only on what's happening right this second.**

   Put on blinders like the horses in Central Park and just see what's in front of you *now*. If your baby is crying, instead of allowing yourself to worry about how long she'll cry, at what age she'll stop crying so much, and so on, tell yourself this: "All that's happening is that this minute she's crying. The next minute may be better."

   Anxiety comes from anticipating negative events, most of which never happen!

2. **Say to yourself, "I'll be able to handle whatever comes up in the future, if and when I need to. I trust I'll be able to find the resources I need to help me. Right now, this is all I need to deal with."**

3. **Ask yourself this key question: "What do I need to help myself right now?"**

   The answer to this question may be different each time you ask it. Other than escaping to a deserted island, here are some things that may help:

   - Eat something.

   - Drink some water.

   - Call a support person.

   - Schedule your next break.

   - Make a nurturing type of appointment for yourself, such as a massage, pedicure, or whatever you enjoy.

If, instead of dwelling in the future, you tend to obsess over the past — decisions you regret and mistakes you think you made — help yourself stay steady and in the present by saying these statements to yourself:

✔ When I'm driving my car forward, it's not a good idea to stare in the rearview mirror. I need to keep my eyes on the road ahead of me so that I'm steering in the direction that I want to go.

✔ There are no mistakes or failures. There are only learning opportunities. I'm learning, so that's good.

✔ The past has already happened — it's done. I'm now putting my energy on what's happening right now. Now is all anyone has.

✔ I need to figure out how I can help myself right now. What do I need to get through this particular moment in time?

Charting your progress to see success

I ask my clients to use a very simple system of percents in order to keep a perspective on their recovery. I suggest that you try using this method to chart your own progress. Grab a calendar and follow these guidelines:

1. **Turn to today in your calendar, and write down a number by today's date that reflects how you're feeling at this moment.**

    Use a scale of 0 percent to 100 percent, with 0 percent representing the lowest point in the illness — the worst you've felt with PPD — and 100 percent representing the point you're aiming for — the "happy you" who enjoys life.

    The process of picking a number can be healing in itself. As you already know, it's difficult to keep a perspective about how you're doing emotionally. But remember, you don't just feel bad or good, 0 or 100 — instead, many levels exist in between the extremes. Having to choose a number forces you to really evaluate where you are on that scale, and the action of choosing will help you build in that perspective.

2. **Go back in your calendar and write in the 0s as they occurred (approximately).**

    After you document them, you can see from week to week how far you've come.

3. **From here on out, around the same time every day, mark down in your calendar what percent you feel at that moment.**

    Your percents, of course, will fluctuate throughout the day, but pick one number that represents how you feel at that time.

Sometimes a client will call me and say, "Dr. Bennett, I'm back at zero!" I will then ask her, "Are you sure it's a zero — the worst you have ever been?" Without fail, after pausing for a second or two, she'll answer something like, "No, I was able to get up and get dressed and go outside today. I guess I'm about a 25 percent." Instantly she feels better with that perspective. She's not a 0, 10, or even 20 percent. She's a 25 percent! She's clearly getting better, and she recognizes that she's only in a dip.

Being kind to yourself

Are you quick to point out what you didn't do but should have? During these critical times, do you tend to kick yourself around the block a few times? Well, if you want to speed up your recovery big time, and I know you do, *stop kicking yourself.*

How you speak to yourself and act toward yourself is a major component to your well-being. In other words, the way you treat yourself can make or break your self-esteem and can therefore affect your happiness and adjustment in the world. I can't imagine anything more important than happiness and self-esteem.

For example, the saying about how you need to love yourself before you can believe anyone else will love you is true. And don't forget that your children's self-esteem depends on how you treat yourself too. In order for them to have a high self-esteem as they grow up, they need a role model (enter in confident Mom) who speaks respectfully to herself and who treats herself with kindness. Being kind to yourself also encompasses setting healthy boundaries so you respect your own time and the time you spend with those you love.

As you deal with PPD, remember that you're doing the best you can. You may say, "Yes, but that's not the best I can do, so I don't have a right to feel good about it." Well, pardon me, but you do have a right to feel good about what you're doing. Here's why: At any given moment, you're doing the best you can do given what you know and feel from moment to moment. You're probably wondering whether the "best you can do" changes as you progress. Of course! But, you need to acknowledge that the best you can do right now is the best you can do — period.

You're allowed to look forward to being able to handle your baby's crying or your sister's complaining (or whatever) with greater ease, but you must congratulate yourself for doing the best you can during your healing process. The more frequently you affirm the positive to yourself, the clearer your path will be.

The chatter that goes on in your head during PPD can be deafening. It's a miracle that others can't hear it. While you're recovering, this constant buzzing may be particularly negative and damaging. So, the quicker you remove the garbage that keeps hammering away at your self-esteem, the better off you'll be. Here's how you change the pattern:

1. **Practice catching yourself with the lies in your head.**

   When you feel low, I guarantee that you're telling yourself at least one lie. Try to hear what you're saying. The first step to making any behavior change is awareness.

2. **Congratulate yourself for becoming aware as you catch any negative messages in your head.**

   Some negative thoughts you may encounter are "I'm a bad mom," "I'm a weak person," blah, blah, blah. I know it may sound strange that I'm suggesting you commend yourself when you're speaking badly to yourself, so allow me to explain: You're congratulating yourself for *catching* the negativity, maybe even in the middle of a put-down. After all, the put-down session could've continued even longer, but you stopped it. Congrats to you.

3. **Apologize to yourself.**

   If you said something mean to anyone else you love, you'd say you're sorry, right? You get the point.

4. **Say the truth.**

   After you catch yourself saying negative things about yourself in your head, reverse the thoughts to positive thoughts. After all, you've already been doing affirmations (statements) — they've just been negative lies. If you're going to practice affirmations, say true ones, because whatever you reinforce in your mind gets stronger. Try these positive, true affirmations on for size:

   - "I'm a good mom." (instead of the lie, "I'm a bad mom.")

   - "I'm doing the best I can." (instead of the lie, "I'm a failure.")

   - "I'm taking good steps to help myself." (instead of the lie, "I'll never get well.")

The rule is that you counter each lie in your head with the truth. You may find a disconnect at first between what you know intellectually is true and what your emotional self will allow you to feel. For instance, you may realize intellectually that you're a good mom, but you may not be able to feel it yet. But, the more you practice the previous four steps, the more the positive statements will sink in. Those of you who tend to be perfectionists will probably try to perform the steps perfectly. Just remember that you're practicing, so you can't expect perfection. Besides, perfection doesn't exist anyway. Follow the steps I've laid out and be careful that you don't start kicking yourself for kicking yourself!

Your social support and professional support team can be quite helpful when it comes to self-talk. Ask the members of your team to point out when they hear you being hard on yourself. When they do, thank them, and rephrase what you said to make it positive or at least less judgmental. Remember, don't argue with them and don't try to justify or defend why you deserve to be mean to yourself! Being kind to yourself is a lifestyle change, not just a recovery issue. If you weren't very kind to yourself before PPD, you have more practicing ahead of you. But, you now have a chance to put yourself back together again even better than before. If you were kind in the past but lost some of it during the PPD, you're on the road to regaining your good habits and boosting your recovery.

Loving your body (and respecting yourself, too)

Having a baby is a life-changing experience, no matter whether you adopted or birthed a child. However, if you gave birth to your baby you get a double-whammy: Your body is different on the outside and on the inside. Body image changes are typical, both positive and negative, but unfortunately the negative usually feel much more prominent. Many new moms (even those without PPD) are taught by the multibillion dollar cosmetic industry that they should hate their changed bodies. Give yourself and your children a huge gift and don't buy into this dangerous nonsense. Remember that this industry can only get richer by making women in general, and new moms in particular, feel lousy about themselves.

My mom, thankfully, recognized this societal garbage. I have a small frame, and gave birth to large children. She taught me to rename my stretch marks as battle scars. She reminded me that these battle scars were proof that my strong body worked really hard to create this new life, and she told me that I should be proud of my body. Pretty empowering, huh? Her advice didn't stop me from having severe PPD, but it did spare me the extra negative body image layer that many new moms feel.

A myth that can be particularly hurtful at this time is the ridiculous one that expects new moms to snap back into their pre-pregnancy bodies after only six weeks. This idea is ludicrous, so please don't fall prey to it. And with PPD, many women often think that their depression would go away if they lost the baby weight.

Dropping weight at the appropriate time can help in the self-esteem department but it won't eradicate PPD. It's understandable that you're sick of your maternity clothes, but don't pressure yourself to lose weight or exercise irresponsibly just to fit an unrealistic image. Health is the priority, not looks.

Taking the steps to drop excess weight will be much easier as you regain your mental and physical health. When the appropriate time comes, contact me and I will give you a fantastic plan of safe and effective weight release options through nutrition (these plans are great for breastfeeding moms, too). In the meantime, follow the nutrition guidelines in Chapter 12.

I endured six days of labor and ended up with a C-section because I never dilated. In addition to being a special education teacher, I had been a professional dancer for many years before having a baby and my body had always followed my directions beautifully. In the past, whatever I told my body to do, it obeyed. Suddenly, though, I found myself in a situation where my body had a mind of its own and I was out of control. I felt as if my body had betrayed me and I was angry at it. I divorced certain parts of my body when I returned home. I averted my eyes from mirrors so I wouldn't see my abdomen, for instance.

If your labor and delivery didn't go the way you planned, you may be experiencing anger at your body, or maybe a sense of failure. Here's another opportunity to practice kindness. Remind yourself that your body did the very best it could. Tell yourself only those supportive statements that you would tell your best friend if she were going through the same thing.

Celebrating your successes

To enjoy healthy self-esteem, you must be able to acknowledge your successes and feel good about them. The whole deal here is to create an image of yourself that you're comfortable with and that you can present to the world. Because your sense of worth has taken a hit with PPD, this effort has to be a conscious one that you work on continually. The best place to practice celebrating your successes is with those closest to you. The family you're now creating should be a big part of your cheering squad.

You may have had parents who said just the right things to you — they complimented, encouraged, and supported you. They may have totally meant every word of this support for you, but not necessarily for themselves. In other words, your parents may have had completely different standards set for themselves than for anyone else. For example, if I received a B+ on my report card instead of an A, my parents would say, "Honey, we're so proud of you. You did the best you could." However, I would hear these very same wonderful parents berate themselves around the house if they did something less than perfect. "I can't believe I sewed that hem a quarter of an inch too short! How dumb!" Or, "My speech wasn't stellar — I used the same word twice in an hour. How could I have done that?"

If this is the case, guess what? Your parents probably had parents who modeled this same pattern to them. When children grow up with double standards they see straight through it. Kids are smart. As they're growing up they think "It wasn't good enough for Mom, so why should it be good enough for me?"

If you want your children to feel good about their accomplishments and about doing the best they can, you simply don't have a choice. You have to be their model. And here's the catch — you have to mean it when you compliment yourself! Acting just doesn't work with kids. Some moms say to me, "I don't say out loud in front of my kids that I'm ugly, so it's okay." I've got news for you — it's not okay. Getting rid of the poor body image is the goal. Just trying to improve your acting skills or secrecy won't work. As I said, kids are intuitive and they can tell how you feel about yourself through the subtlest of ways.

Here's an idea that has been successfully integrated into many families. I call it "The Family Game," but you can have fun choosing a special name that fits for you and your family. To play The Family Game, each evening when you're tucking in your children, have each member of the family take a turn (until the whole family has had a turn) to name one activity that he or she is proud of accomplishing that day. Until your youngest can participate for himself, do it for him. Here are the rules:

1. **One person speaks at a time, with no interrupting from anyone else. He or she says something like "I'm proud about making a difficult phone call today."**

   No task is too small to acknowledge, so don't censor what you think of first.

2. **After a person reveals his or her accomplishment, everyone else should cheer and make a big deal about it. They can say things such as "Hooray!" "Good job!" "That's great!" and "Good for you!"**

   Even before your very young children can cognitively understand what's going on, they'll be able to hear the "music" of what's happening and will happily join in when they're old enough.

3. **After the person shares and receives some hoots and hollers, he or she is only allowed to say (and needs to say), "Thank you."**

Moms report to me that they and their partners feel silly at first and don't want to play this game. If you fall into this camp, this game will be extra therapeutic for you. If you feel like you shouldn't need praise or that it's bad, wrong, or boastful to say your accomplishments out loud, I'm guessing this idea was taught verbally or nonverbally (or both) to you as you grew up. Because it's important to be able to compliment yourself and be able to receive praise, give self-compliments and share with their closest support people, so you must model this behavior to your offspring — it's a golden rule.

Playing your part in your treatment team

You're the star player on your support team. Even though you can respect a professional's expertise, don't be too quick to discount your own opinions. Your team is working for you — not the other way around. If PPD is making you feel weak or unworthy, it's easy to start belittling your own thoughts on matters. But, remember, your opinions count — this wellness plan is for you and your life. So, when you have a comment, question, concern, preference, or idea, say something. Be a partner along with your professional team in planning for your treatment and setting your short-term and long-term goals.

No matter how many academic credentials a member of your professional team may have, don't let him or her invalidate your feelings. You're the expert of your own experience, and you know better than anyone how you feel. For example, if a practitioner tells you that you can't be feeling a particular emotional or physical reaction, consider that an invalidation. If this happens, feel confident in correcting the practitioner. It's important that you speak up for a couple of reasons. First, it's emotionally good for you to assert yourself. Second, it's necessary that the doctor or therapist has the proper information about what's going on with you. A good practitioner will thank you for the correction. Please don't worry about her feelings — any practitioner worth seeing won't become defensive or take it personally. If she does, don't go back — find a different practitioner.

Also, if a professional says she has never heard of a particular symptom that you have, you're not wrong or weird. And remember, as long as it isn't said condescendingly, this reaction from a practitioner isn't necessarily an invalidation. You're just teaching that practitioner something new about what's possible in the realm of PPD.

Chapter 12

Setting the Supermom Cape Aside: Caring For Yourself

. . . .

In This Chapter

▶ Eating, sleeping, and exercising for your health

▶ Knowing how to take breaks

▶ Being social only when you're ready to be

▶ Making PPD easier with seven positive tips

▶ Asking for and accepting help

▶ Using lists and eliminating unnecessary chores

. . . .

*T*aking care of a baby is arguably one of the most difficult jobs on the face of the planet. If you have a partner, and especially if you have other children, it's easy for your needs to get lost in the shuffle. You know how the flight attendants always instruct you to place the oxygen mask over your own nose and mouth first? The same concept applies here. You must take care of yourself so that you're able to give your best to your child and your other family members. Sometimes new moms think that they should be plopped at the bottom of the list as if their own needs don't matter — that is, if they're even on the list at all. And when postpartum depression (PPD) is added to the mix, a mom often feels unworthy and unimportant. Her self-esteem is low. She thinks she's a bad mother, and she feels like she doesn't deserve anything that feels good. These thoughts don't set the stage for good nurturing.

In this chapter, I provide advice to help you pull yourself out of the deep pit of depression and get back to normal. I also give you a handful of ideas to help you take care of yourself.

Eat and Drink Your Heart Out, Baby! (The Healthy Way, of Course)

Feeding your brain properly is necessary if you want it to function at its best. New mothers have certain challenges with eating healthfully, even without a mood disorder such as PPD. Unfortunately, depression and anxiety make matters even worse. Because appetite is often low when you're depressed, your body may not be giving you the signal that it needs food. So, the whole eat-when-you're-hungry concept doesn't apply here. You basically need to force-feed yourself until you begin to experience the pangs of hunger again. Just remember that there are specific do's and don'ts when it comes to food — some foods may help you crawl out of the darkness, but some can send you back down the spiral.

If you notice a big change in your appetite — either an increase or decrease — this could indicate a thyroid imbalance. If this is the case for you, have your doctor check it out.

Boosting your mood with food

Often women with PPD crave sweets and carbohydrates. For example, you may find yourself unable to pass a cookie jar without indulging in a handful. You're having these cravings because your brain is low in serotonin and it needs the amino acid *tryptophan* in order to make more serotonin. However, to raise tryptophan, your body needs carbs — which is when you reach for a jelly doughnut or a handful of cookies. Even though you may feel a temporary lift in serotonin with a doughnut, shortly after eating it you'll feel a big drop when your blood sugar also plummets. Plus, consuming those unhealthy calories won't help in the self-esteem department either.

Food offers a much more healthful way of increasing serotonin than snarfing down a box of snack cakes. For example, you can combat depression and curb sugar cravings by

- **Nibbling protein:** Eat foods such as turkey, meat, chicken, fish, or eggs every time your baby eats — which is probably about every three hours. This protein will help keep your blood sugar even and your moods more stable.

- **Drinking whey protein shakes:** These shakes are especially helpful if you have no appetite. Many women find that drinking their meals is easier than trying to chew and swallow solid food.

✔ **Avoiding caffeine:** Caffeine is public enemy number one for anxiety so avoid it as much as possible. Instead, drink water, water, and more water. If it's the taste of coffee you desire, wean yourself by mixing some decaf in with your regular-strength stuff.

✔ **Eating legumes and grains, such as bulgur wheat and kasha (instead of white rice), pasta, and whole grain bread and cereals (for example, oatmeal):** Carbs from these sources can raise your serotonin and are much better for you than the simple carbohydrates you get from white bread and other refined snacks. Simple carbs only spike your blood sugar and increase anxiety and depression. Most grocery stores have at least two of these choices listed.

For women, the most important time of the day to generate serotonin is the morning. So, don't skip breakfast! Extreme dieting and skipping breakfast are the worst things you can do for your serotonin. A protein shake balanced in protein, fat, and carbohydrates is perfect. Also, don't eat a breakfast that contains only simple carbohydrates (such as toast, a bagel, or most cereals) because it can shoot your blood sugar levels way up, and mess with your moods. If you can't give up your morning bagel, always have some kind of protein with it. Eating the protein will help keep your blood sugar more stable, which therefore helps keep your mood more even. For example, if you want a piece of toast in the morning, eat an egg too.

The system that I follow

I've always had a deep interest in nutrition and feeding the body what it naturally needs for optimum functioning (including brain functioning). A health nut since the '60s, I've tried every way of healthful eating out there (a couple that were on the weird side, now that I look back!) I believe in nutrition — not diets. My incessant search for a complete, simple system finally ended a little over two years ago — I found it. Since then, I've been using this nutritional system and introducing it to my clients (and all others I care about). It's complete with high quality organic protein shakes, amino acids such as tryptophan (which raise serotonin), live enzymes, the essential fatty acids (Omega 3, 6, and 9) in the correct ratios, vitamins, antioxidants, and ionic plant minerals. The system, which consists of foods that you eat in addition to whatever healthful food you're already consuming, has a total body cleansing and detoxing component as well. The results have been quick and dramatic, and I'm thoroughly passionate about it. Some of the problems that I've seen either totally disappear or at least decrease significantly with this system are depression, anxiety, decreased energy, difficulty losing weight, insomnia, sugar cravings, low sex drive, and difficulty concentrating. (I'm not mentioning this system by name because I want to make sure you'll be ordering only what you need and should have, depending on whether you're pregnant, nursing, or finished with both.) If you're interested, feel free to contact me for more information by going to www.postpartumdepressionhelp.com or by calling 925-735-3099.

Hydrating your brain

You may already know that drinking enough water is essential for cleansing your body and for delivering nutrients to all your cells, but did you know it's essential for moods as well? For instance, dehydration can worsen your anxiety. You see, without sufficient water, your lymphatic system — which is responsible for flushing toxins out of the body — can't operate correctly. When your lymphatic system is on the fritz, the liver takes over and stops producing the amino acids necessary for the production of dopamine and serotonin — the brain chemicals needed for normal moods. New moms with panic attacks who go to the emergency room thinking they're having heart attacks are often given a couple of glasses of water by a perceptive staff person. Often the panic subsides immediately!

To make sure you're staying adequately hydrated, divide your weight in half and drink that many ounces of water every day. If you're pumping your milk or breastfeeding your baby, if you're sweating a lot from hormones, climate, or exercise, or if you're physically unwell, you may need to drink more. If you feel thirsty no matter how much water you're drinking, get your thyroid checked. One of the symptoms of a thyroid imbalance is continual thirst.

Well-meaning practitioners (doctors included) and authors sometimes advise women with PPD to drink some wine before bed to relax or to have a beer to help increase their milk supply. Neither is good advice. Alcohol is a depressant that disrupts sleep cycles and feeds your depression — two effects you definitely want to avoid. Also, alcohol doesn't help with milk production. On top of all that, babies eat less when their moms drink even one alcoholic beverage. So remember, the bottom line is that alcohol isn't good for you (or your baby) in any way and it can make you worse. If you're having a difficult time avoiding alcohol and you think you may be using it to self-treat, please speak with a medical or mental health practitioner you trust.

Taking nutritional supplements

Through my research in the field of natural healing and nutrition (especially regarding mood disorders), I'm now convinced that it isn't possible anymore to take in all of the nutrients your body requires just through food — even if you eat strictly organic food. Brain chemistry is affected greatly by what goes in your body, so it stands to reason that nutritional supplements are particularly helpful for PPD sufferers. Because this isn't a nutrition book, I've picked out just a few tasty morsels for you to chew on.

Minerals

One of the major reasons that you can't get your nutrition from supermarket foods these days is that soil is now depleted of minerals. And if the soil is mineral-deficient, food grown in the soil is also lacking. When you don't get the minerals you need, your body and brain chemistry can't be totally healthy. Among other things, minerals are vital to the production of hormones, including the reproductive hormones involved in pregnancy and postpartum. And, minerals also help your body use the nutrients taken in through the foods you eat. Most people already understand the importance of vitamins, but did you know that vitamins can't be used by the body without minerals?

Even though organic food has a higher mineral content, it's nothing like it used to be. Taking in high-quality ionic plant minerals, however, quickly remedies the deficiency problem. Even though you can get these plant minerals into your body in several different ways, the simplest one I know is part of the system I use, which you can find out about by contacting me through my Web site at www.postpartumdepressionhelp.com.

Essential fatty acids (EFAs)

Omega-3 fatty acids are essential fatty acids (EFAs) — good fats — that may help boost brain chemicals important in depression, such as serotonin and dopamine. However, your body can't make them on its own. So, if your diet is low in these fatty acids, all your bodily functions are negatively affected — including your organs, skin, and brain functions. And it's worth noting that most Americans, and especially pregnant and breastfeeding women, don't get enough omega-3 fatty acids in their diets.

With all the promising information about essential fatty acids helping depression, it's no wonder that omega-3 fatty acid supplements are being studied in pregnancy as a prevention for PPD. The more omega-3 you consume in the third trimester, the less likely you are to be depressed in pregnancy and up to eight months postpartum. When serotonin increases with omega-3, attention, concentration, sleep, and mood improve.

The following list includes many good sources of omega-3 for your body:

- Flaxseed or flaxseed oil
- Hemp seeds and hemp seed oil (these aren't marijuana!)
- Walnuts
- Pumpkin seeds
- Salmon, cod, cod liver oil, tuna, and mackerel (helps with mood)
- Kidney beans

The omega-3 foods that are known to specifically help with mood are types of cold water fish, such as Atlantic salmon, halibut, sardines, and tuna. They contain two omega-3 fatty acids that are shown to be most beneficial for mood.

Because these days you probably find it difficult enough to get dressed, let alone go out to buy cod liver oil, taking a high-quality supplement with the right balance of the omegas is probably the way to go. Choose an omega supplement that's high in the omega-3 fatty acids eicosapentaenoic acid (EPA) and docosahexaenoic acid (DHA). You should aim for the total amount of EPA and DHA combined to equal 1,000 to 2,000 mg per day. Also, brands vary by taste, so find one that doesn't have a bad taste. Keeping the pills in the refrigerator may decrease any aftertaste or fishy burps. If you want to try the one I use — which has no fishy aftertaste — contact me.

Multivitamins

If you're pumping your milk or breastfeeding your baby, talk with the pediatrician about whether to remain on your prenatal vitamins. If you decide to take a multivitamin instead, it should be a high quality one that can be easily absorbed by your body. The vitamin should never be in the form of a hard pill. Instead, choose one in the form of a powder in a capsule. Make sure the multivitamin has a full range of all the B vitamins, vitamin C, and folic acid. Folate is important for mood regulation (and it may also speed up the effects of antidepressants).

Without enough B-12 a person can become depressed because B-12 is required for the conversion of amino acids into dopamine and serotonin. Vegetarians are often deficient in B-12 because fermented soy products, such as tempeh and seaweed, or vitamin supplements are the only known nonanimal sources.

Making Sure You Get Some Winks

Even for moms with fresh buns out of the oven, sleeping is not a luxury — it's a medical necessity! This is the toughest time of the most difficult job you'll ever have. Sleep is your elixir.

Humans need 8.4 hours of uninterrupted sleep per night in order to function at their best (the key word here being *uninterrupted*). Broken sleep causes serotonin to drop and as I've mentioned before, PPD is often caused by a low level of serotonin. If broken sleep continues, depression and anxiety can get worse. You'll probably be able to handle the responsibilities in your day well enough with a chunk of five to six hours of straight sleep. The more nights per week you get these chunks of sleep, the faster your recovery from PPD will be.

Daytime sleep doesn't take the place of nighttime sleep. It's nighttime sleep that restores the brain and keeps the natural rhythms (biorhythms) of the body on track. Arranging to have good nighttime sleep when the baby comes is one of the best preventions for PPD.

Sleep problems are common with PPD. If you have trouble sleeping at night when your baby is sleeping, you may need a medication to help you. Consult your doctor if this is the case.

Starting with the ideal plan

Sleep deprivation is probably the most under-emphasized contributor to PPD there is. It's a serious issue, and it needs to be given the proper attention. Not all parents can set up the ideal plan, but I start with it here so that you know what you're shooting for. It's okay if you need to compromise it a bit (or a lot) due to extra challenges. Here's how thousands of new parents set up their sleep arrangements every night:

- **Split the night's baby duty with your partner.** Unless you've had a C-section or you have another medical issue at hand, only one person needs to be up with the baby. The other person should be sleeping. After five hours, when the baby wakes, your partner can wake you up and the two of you can switch.

- **Sleep in a separate area away from the baby and the adult on duty.** Use earplugs and a white noise machine, such as a fan or air purifier if necessary. The goal is to make sure that you aren't hearing the baby or other noises so you can achieve uninterrupted sleep.

- **Move the clock away from the bed so you can't see it.** Moving the clock is especially important if you tend to obsess. If a clock is nearby, you'll be tempted to check it and then obsess even more about not sleeping or about when the baby might wake up.

If you're breastfeeding or pumping, it's important to empty both breasts before bed so you won't be awakened engorged and in pain during your off-duty shift. If you can pump during the day, your partner can use your milk for the off-duty feedings.

Especially if you aren't breastfeeding or pumping at night and can take full advantage sleeping straight through the night, the following suggestions work great for enhancing the quantity and quality of your dream time:

- **Alternate nights with your partner.** This schedule means that you'll have one night completely on duty and the next night completely off.

- **Hire a night nurse or doula so you or you and your partner can both sleep (even if just for a couple of nights a week).** This plan is an investment for launching your new family. Because of the importance of sleep to mental and physical health, many moms and couples use up savings accounts or borrow money to be able to hire night help.

Making do with whatcha' got

Sometimes you won't be able to arrange your circumstances exactly the way you want, and your wonderful plan for heavenly sleep falls through. Just do the best you can to get more sleep and to enhance its quality, and allow yourself to feel good that you're continuing to work toward the eight-uninterrupted-hours-a-night goal.

I'm not a big fan of naps because after you're sleeping as you should at night, naps shouldn't be necessary (a bonus, maybe, but not necessary). But, many of my clients who still need naps or enjoy them find the following ideas to be mighty helpful for sneaking in naps throughout the day:

- ✔ **When your child is sleeping, sleep if you can.** Do remember, though, if you're anxious, sleeping may be really difficult at night, which means that sleeping during the day will probably be worse.

  If you find that you're just tossing and turning during the day, cross napping off your to-do list! It will be too frustrating and feel like one more failure. If you once enjoyed naps, but can't right now, don't despair. I promise you'll be able to nap again as soon as you recover. Your ability to nap may be one of the signals that your old self is returning.

- ✔ **If you're breastfeeding, lie down in bed or in a recliner while your baby nurses.** Doing so may allow you both to doze.

- ✔ **Nap while your baby gets some visual stimulation.** Secure your one-or two-month old (or any baby who's young enough to stay put) in a baby seat so he'll be safe, and turn on an educational baby video. Set your nap timer so you can sleep in the TV room for 15 to 30 minutes while your baby gets some enhancing stimulation.

- ✔ **Sleep in the parking lot as you wait for an older child at school.** During this time, your baby is in his car seat — hopefully also sleeping peacefully.

- ✔ **Put your baby in a front carrier and nap while you're in the doctor's waiting room.** Ask the receptionist to wake you when it's your turn.

- ✔ **Ask a friend, neighbor, or family member** (maybe someone you had at your baby shower) to watch your child while you take a short 15 to 30 minute nap.

- ✔ **Hire a babysitter or a mother's helper to watch your child while you take a nap.** A mother's helper, which may be less expensive than a babysitter, could be a responsible older child who comes to your home after school.

The ideal amount of time to nap during the day is in 15-minute increments (you can have more than one of these naps during the day). However, even if your situation permits, don't allow yourself to sleep for more than 30 minutes at a time. Napping for too long can throw off your biorhythms and mess with your sleep cycle, just like your baby's naps can with her sleep cycle.

If you find yourself resisting the idea of sleeping during the day because that's the only time you get to yourself, you're heading toward burnout. If this sounds like you, please refer to the section "Taking Regular Breaks" later in this chapter for help.

Working through the challenges

If you think that you have major sleep obstacles (no or little partner support) in your life, don't worry — you're not alone! Often with a bit of creativity, these obstacles can be easily overcome. You may relate to the following complaints my new clients sometimes present:

- ✔ **"There's no way my partner will get up with the baby."** Don't assume anything until you ask: He may in fact be very willing and it's your unnecessary guilt about asking him that's in the way. However, if he really is reluctant, usually when it's explained to him that he'll get his wife "back" quicker, he steps up to the plate.

  You're not asking if it's *okay* with him that you get sleep. That would be like asking permission to breathe. Instead, you're lovingly letting him know what you need. If he's still not willing to be a fully participating parent, you can tell him that you'll need to hire someone (if nothing else works, this step usually does the trick!).

- ✔ **"My partner works nights, so I'm all by myself."** If your partner sleeps during the day, split the childcare day shift with him and sleep for 30-minute chunks during the day. Or, invite an older child over to be a mother's helper while you nap during the day.

- ✔ **"I'm afraid my partner won't hear the baby crying. He'll probably just sleep right through it."** When he knows you're sleeping and he's on duty, you'll be amazed at what he, the seemingly deepest sleeper on the planet, can hear. Give it a try and you'll see. Place the monitor (or baby) right by his ear. If he takes a couple of minutes to get out of bed (as opposed to your half a second), don't worry. It's fine — your baby won't be psychologically damaged!

- ✔ **"I have no support. I'm a single mother and my family lives out of town."** Remember the friend or trusted neighbor who keeps offering to help? Call her up. Say something like, "I really appreciate your offer to help me with the baby. I'm ready to take you up on your offer." Your trusting her will make her feel great. If she's not able to relieve you during the nighttime, ask for a daytime shift. If the friend can come once a week and the neighbor can come another day, you have two solid sleep times you can count on.

  If you're financially able to hire a doula, do it (I discuss doulas in more detail in Chapter 14). If you brainstorm and still come up empty, try your local church, synagogue, or parent group. Often you can join a babysitting co-op. Remember, if you need to move in with a relative temporarily, that's no weakness. If you have the support, use it!

✔ **"We live in a one room apartment, so there's no other place for me to sleep. I hear everything."** If you have a couch in the living room, sleep there with earplugs and a fan on (or something else blocking the noise). Or, while your neighbor watches your baby during the day, go sleep at her house. If your helper can take the child out of your house, you can stay home. By the way, don't forget the local hotel in your area! Many mothers rent out rooms for a night, at least once in a while, to ensure a quiet night.

Shakin' It for Your Love

Exercise isn't just for the physical health of your body — it's also necessary for your emotional health. As you begin to incorporate exercise into (or back into) your life, your physical healing will be enhanced as well as your mental well-being. Many research studies support this fact that exercise has mood elevating effects. Regular exercise promotes the release of *endorphins,* which are feel-good chemicals that produce feelings of happiness and well-being and are known to relieve depression. Just remember that before you do any type of exercise, make sure your doctor has given you the go-ahead.

Make sure you accept whatever level of activity you can manage right now. As you probably know, today's society places a huge emphasis on exercise for many people — sometimes to the point of obsession. Some people may tell you that in order to recover you should go to the gym regularly. But here's what I (and numerous other healthcare professionals) say: You don't have to go to the gym at all to recover from PPD! Just getting out of bed and going through your day is a triumph. Most moms with at least a moderate case of depression can hardly get to the gym even once, let alone a few times a week — it's too overwhelming just *thinking* about it.

When you're considering exercise, make sure you keep the following facts:

✔ **Any physical movement is exercise.** If walking to the mailbox is all you can muster, that's great. Even just standing outside your front door and taking some deep breaths can help you get some air and sunshine and can lift your mood (even if you are still in your bathrobe).

✔ **Depression zaps energy, so any activity can feel like a lot.** But, keep in mind that your serotonin levels, which alter your mood, are affected by exercise — so taking two (or three, if you can) brisk walks every week for 30 minutes can increase serotonin and boost your mood. Don't push yourself too hard, though.

✔ **Exercising right before bed isn't a good idea — especially if your sleep patterns are already screwed up.** Right before bed you need to give your body the direction that it's time to calm down, not get going. Many women think that if they wear themselves out right before bed they'll sleep better. But, the opposite is typically true, depending on the exercise. For example, yoga and relaxing stretching may be an exception to this rule.

> ✔ **It's important to wait until you have at least a couple of weeks of good sleep before you begin a heavy exercise program.** Especially if you're prone to panic attacks, start your exercise program slowly and work your way up. I say this because lactic acid, which is released when muscles are worked too long or when they're not properly conditioned, causes soreness and panic.

When you exercise, your brain produces endorphins that make you feel good. If you feel a need to exercise for long periods every day in order to feel good, that's a signal that your brain chemistry needs some other help as well. It's easy to become addicted to overexercising when you're depressed, because the brain produces endorphins to reduce pain, and when a person overexercises, the muscles are stressed (in pain).

Fortunately, you have a built-in security system: If you overdo your exercise, your body lets you know by making your mood dip or by making your sleep problems worse (flip back to the section "Making Sure You Get Some Winks" earlier in this chapter for more information on disrupted sleep patterns). The difference between how much exercise you should try to do and how much is too much is a fine line. Experiment with the length of time you walk and with your pace. If it's right for you, you'll feel good. If you find yourself very tired and your mood is dropping, your exercise level was probably too high. Remind yourself that you're doing the best you can, and you'll recover regardless of the amount and speed of your exercising.

Taking Regular Breaks

When you work outside the home, no matter how rough your day is, you can look at the clock and say, "Just another hour and I'm outta' here!" Saying this makes it easier for you to hang on and not bite the head off the next person who approaches your desk, right? Well, this mom job is quite a bit different. Taking care of a baby is the only job where breaks aren't mandated by law. You must schedule breaks or they won't happen. And I don't mean just talking about taking breaks — you actually have to mark them in your calendar.

Avoiding burnout

Burnout occurs when you have nothing to look forward to. Wednesday may as well be Thursday because everyday feels the same. In fact, you probably feel like Bill Murray in the movie *Groundhog Day*. But, when your day gets tough and your moods are dipping, knowing when your next break will be makes all the difference. Having pockets of "you" time sprinkled throughout the week gives you something to look forward to.

If you're a full-time stay-at-home mom, you ideally need three or four two-hour breaks during the week to prevent burnout. Why at least two hours? Because you need about an hour to start relaxing and realizing that no one is hanging on to any of your body parts. Nothing is more disappointing than having to go home right as you start to relax. It's that second hour that will be the most enjoyable (or as close to "enjoyable" as you can get these days). These blocks of time should be as regular from week to week as possible.

Do the best you can. If your anxiety is so high that the mere thought of leaving your baby even for 20 minutes makes you short of breath, start with just 10 minutes. Leaving your baby will get easier and easier as you see that she's safe and as you realize that it's good for her to have experience with other loving caretakers. She needs a change of scenery too, don't forget.

If you have a partner who's home in the evenings and weekends, some of your break times can be during those times. But, it's wonderful for couples when the stay-at-home mom can get some respite before the partner returns in the evening. Then she has some energy left for the couple relationship.

Figuring out what to do with yourself

Are you wondering what you'd do with your time even if you had it? If so, you've just received a sign that you've been depleted of "you" time for way too long. To get started on regaining your "you" time, make a list of all those activities that gave you pleasure in the past. Each woman's list will be different. For one woman, shopping for herself or going to the gym are pleasurable. For the next woman those same activities may feel like chores. To each her own!

Tasks aren't allowed during this "you time." If you shop, make it exclusively pleasure shopping for you. If you find yourself in the baby aisle, laugh and say "Oops!" Then take yourself back to the women's section. If you add more time after your break, you can do other shopping chores, such as buying diapers or other baby toiletries — but only after you're done with your break and only if you add a half hour on to your trip. The point is that the "you time" must come *first.* Be honest — if, at the beginning of your break you said to yourself, "I'll just stop at these few stores and get these chores done so I won't have to think about them later," would the "you time" ever happen? Probably not. It's a trap. And that's often why moms get burned out and resentful. They put themselves last on the list — they only treat themselves if time is left over.

If you take breaks and you feel like you're just going through the motions — kind of zombie-like without joy — take them anyway. As you recover, you'll start experiencing the "up" feelings again. And, in this case, you'll already have the structure in place. The breaks also help boost your recovery, so don't wait to feel less depressed before you take them. If you're not up to leaving the house for every break, you can stay home, but be completely off-duty with chores and child care during that time.

It's a gift to your family when you recharge. Each member of your family benefits when you take care of yourself on a regular basis. No matter what anyone says, taking care of yourself first isn't selfish — it's a very important part of your job. If guilt pops up, remind yourself that you're a good and responsible mom, and that's why you're leaving the house right now.

Staying Social

Some women with PPD want to be with people a lot, and they want to talk about what's going on with themselves — sometimes to excess. They feel better when they're talking and sharing. There's nothing wrong with this at all, but if this describes you, make sure to give yourself a break from talking about PPD. Talk about other topics too. This will remind you that you aren't a walking case of PPD — you're a woman who happens to be dealing with PPD, but there's more to you than this illness.

On the other hand, some women with PPD hide away and don't want much social contact at all. If you're not answering e-mails, the door, phone calls, or invitations, you're in good company. Hibernating is very common with PPD, and it's not necessarily a bad thing. In this section, I explain how you can tell when avoiding other people is helpful to your recovery and when it can make you worse.

Cocooning versus unhealthy isolation

Sometimes you may want to curl up in a blanket, drink something warm, and watch TV instead of going out with friends. Staying in and comforting yourself can be a way of self-nurturing, and it's considered healthy. I call it *cocooning*. Even though your usual self, the self before the PPD, loved being social and getting out, now you feel otherwise.

Well-meaning loved ones may think that they should encourage or even demand that you join them at the neighbor's party. They may say, "You'll feel better if you just get out and do something." Here's how you gauge whether they're right, or whether cocooning is the best activity for you on that occasion: Ask yourself, "Would I feel better if I could just get dressed and go to the party?" If the answer is yes, ask someone to help you get ready. If your answer is no, because it feels too overwhelming or stressful, you should stay home. You can feel really good about tuning in to yourself and choosing what's healthy for you. The answer may be different each time an occasion arises, so listen to your intuition.

Sometimes you'll be involved in a personal tug of war — part of you will want to get out and part of you won't. At those times, tune in and ask what *most* of you wants to do. Listen for the answer and go with it. However, if you find yourself lying in bed or on the couch getting more depressed, lonely, or anxious, this is a clear sign of unhealthy isolation, and you should get up, and be active and social (maybe join your family at that party, even for just a half hour).

If you want to get out but don't have the energy to get yourself ready, ask for help. Unhealthy isolation will make you feel more depressed and you'll spiral down further, so learn to ask for support in getting up and out of the house or having visitors or phone calls. Becoming social again will take effort, but it will pay off.

Your choices of whether or not to go out may be confusing to your loved ones, since sometimes their encouragement looks like it pays off and other times it doesn't. Just tell them that at times you may join an activity and other times you won't, depending on how you feel. Tell them you understand if it's perplexing to them — it's perplexing to you too. Ask them to please trust and respect your decision, whatever it may be at any given moment.

If you push yourself to do an activity and it wasn't right for you, your mood may dip later that day or the next day. You can be sure that your body will let you know if you overdid it. But, don't be angry with yourself because you "knew better." Just learn from the experience. You'll get better at trusting your own wisdom and also at setting boundaries with others (for example, knowing how to say no).

Confiding in people you're comfortable with

Who you choose to socialize with and what you choose to talk about is important. It's good to confide about your PPD to a few close people. Disclosing how you've been feeling to your good friend, therapist, and spouse may be great for you. Sharing and feeling understood raises serotonin. That's one of the major theories as to why therapy works. But, if you're vulnerable to other people's reactions to PPD, protect yourself. Before you open up, ask yourself whether you trust this person and whether he or she is truly able to support you. If yes, go ahead and offer some information. Hopefully your chat will go well, but if doesn't, don't blame yourself (see Chapter 14). You did nothing wrong — it's the other person's limitations that caused the negative reaction.

It's also really important to talk to others about normal, everyday life stuff. You're not a walking illness — there's more to you than symptoms. Engaging in normal conversation will help you feel more like your old self. It's not that you forget you're dealing with this illness — it's just refreshing to remind yourself that you're a new mom who has regular new mom things happening as well.

Creating a Positive Ambience

Although it's always important to create an atmosphere that's conducive to your comfort and well-being, it's particularly important to pay attention to your surroundings now. Accommodating your specific needs during this time will enhance your progress. Your physical and emotional comfort are especially important right now.

For example, making particular alterations in your environment, choosing carefully what you read or watch on TV, and wearing certain clothing, can all make a positive difference. If you're dealing with rough clothing, loud, shrill noises, uncomfortable air temperatures, negativity blasting from the TV, and so on, this assault on your senses can drain your precious energy even more. And you need that energy to recover from this illness. You don't have to be obnoxious or demanding to those around you — just keep your awareness high.

Muffling the noise

You may be particularly sensitive to decibel level these days. Loud noises in general may affect your stress level, but the one that probably gets to you the most is your baby's wailing. Even though the pitch of your baby's screams may not bother other adults in your house, that sound may make those little hairs on the back of your neck stand straight up.

If you're not on duty, feel free to leave the vicinity. However, if you're the one in charge of your little one at the moment of her melt down, help yourself to a pair of earplugs or headphones. If you don't own a pair of headphones, invest in a pair today — you won't regret it. Even with the headphones or earplugs, you'll still hear all you need to hear in order to care for your baby, but at the same time you'll be protecting your stress level from climbing up your spine and shooting out the top of your head.

Getting away from cabin fever (without leaving the house!)

When you're waiting for your next break and it seems like ages since the last one, the walls may feel like they're closing in on you. The room actually feels like it shrinks. This claustrophobia is typical because depression makes everything feel dark and small. Consider the cabin fever that nondepressed people get when it pours or snows for days and no one can go outside — now multiply that by at least ten. Cabin fever will likely be much more difficult for you than the average person. When you start fantasizing about going out to buy diapers and it feels like a trip to the Caribbean, you'll know that you have a touch of cabin fever.

With PPD, you may start associating your furniture or certain locations in your home with feeling bad. You may grow to hate your bedspread or that couch in the corner where you cry a lot. Many women (I did this too) with PPD imagine living in another home — and they're sure they wouldn't be depressed there. "I bet I'd be happy in that house," I used to think.

If you start feeling trapped or depressed by your surroundings, try rearranging your furniture. Change the bedspread and move the rocking chair. Even though you know you're tricking yourself, it still works. You're changing the same old scenery to something new, which gives you a fresh start. Permit yourself to change the scenery as frequently as you desire.

Soaking in some vitamin D

Brightening your home with light — whether natural or synthetic — will also help brighten your mood and lift your spirits. Open your curtains, pull up the shades, and let the sun shine in. If it's gloomy and gray outside, just turn on lamps in every room. But, remember, this isn't the time to worry about your electric bill. If you're resisting these suggestions, ask your partner to do this for you. It may seem like too much energy and you may not have the motivation yet to do this for yourself. In any case, make sure it gets done for you until you can do it for yourself. You can even take care of two needs at a time by exercising near a window with the sun streaming in or by exercising outside. If you're more anxious than depressed, lots of bright light can be too stimulating. Experiment and see how you feel. If you need less light, adjust to your comfort level.

Trading the rags for britches

Every once in a while, get out of that sour milk- and drool-stained T-shirt and into a clean one! When you're just going to be spit up upon a second later, why is it worth it, you ask? You know why. Because feeling more like your old self helps your mood. You don't feel so lost in Babyland when you're feeling fresh. It'll be well worth the extra laundry, I promise.

When your energy is low and overwhelm is high, the first tasks that you'll probably drop are the ones for you. But those are the ones that can really lift your spirits. If you used makeup before the baby, get back in the habit (even just one part of your old regimen). When you go out (or stay in), take a shower, fix your hair (at least comb it), and dress well (that means get out of those big, baggy sweatpants). You count! You're not just a milk machine and a baby soother. You'll do better when you feel human and more put together. These suggestions may sound trivial, but you'll be amazed how well they work.

Shutting off the boob (tube)

Watching TV is damaging to your mental health even if you're not depressed or anxious. On every channel, at almost every moment, negativity of one sort or another is being shown. (To protect the obsessive readers, I won't start listing these instances here.) Especially when you're recovering from PPD, you need to surround yourself with all things positive. If you rent a funny movie, feel free to watch it. Otherwise, unless it's an educational children's show for your preschooler, turn off the TV. The TV just isn't your friend right now. If you're up in the wee hours of the morning and you want some mindless entertainment, put in one of those (funny) movies you rented. Just don't flip through the channels — that's bad news. And speaking of news — it's forbidden. The worst thing you can do right now is watch (or listen to) the news — nothing is more negative than that.

Reading airy fluff, not serious stuff

This isn't the time to read heavy-duty material on childrearing, illness (except this book!), or other serious topics. Stay away from newspapers, the Internet and all those parenting magazines. If you have a subscription to a parenting magazine, I suggest you stop your subscription, or at least ask your partner or other support person to temporarily remove the magazines from your mail pile. Most of those magazines are driven by the raising of a parent's (usually Mom's) anxiety. Good mothers see the headlines and think, "I better read this or I might miss something and my child will somehow be hurt by my lack of information." That's how magazines sell. Many books for new mothers — even some of the very popular ones with loads of marketing — are big guilt-trippers and anxiety-producers. Consider using them for other purposes — they make great door stops!

Instead, choose books and magazines with fantasies or some other light fluff. Basically, you want to choose something that you enjoy — something that can give you a mini-vacation away from the inside of your head. You might choose a mystery novel, a trashy love story, or a magazine on decorating. Motivational material is great too.

Giving Yourself Permission to Set Limits

Do any of the following thoughts sound familiar?

It's my job to take care of everyone else.

I shouldn't need help.

I should be able to take care of my baby by myself.

If I say "no," that's selfish.

They'll be disappointed in me if I refuse.

If even one of those statements rang a bell for you, I'm guessing that you're probably one of those people who put others' needs and wants ahead of yours, most likely at your own expense. You may have been taught that putting others first is the right thing to do. This way of thinking is an unhealthy paradigm that you need to shift. I don't mean that you should never do anything for anybody unless you're 100 percent thrilled about it — that's not reality. But, if you've been living your life from the bottom of the list, you have to make a change.

One of my clients, Emily, told me about the time that she had finally planned to spend some much-needed time with her preschooler (after a long hiatus because of her PPD). Her little girl was so excited to finally be able to spend some time with her mom. They were both looking forward to going to the park together and then to buy the little girl a new pair of shoes. But, just as they were about to leave the house, Emily's friend called and asked her to come over for a couple of hours to baby-sit so she could go shopping. Emily told her friend that she had plans to spend some time with her daughter, hoping that her friend would withdraw the request. When she didn't, and asked again if Emily could please come over, Emily agreed. Emily spent the day sad and angry with herself, and guilty about not fulfilling her promise to her daughter. She once again had put someone else's wishes above hers and above what she knew was best for her relationship with her daughter. Emily told me that she was worried that saying no to her friend would be selfish. But, during Emily's appointment she realized that her primary obligation shouldn't have been to her friend. She let herself and her daughter (and her relationship with her daughter) suffer because she had been programmed to believe that saying "no" made her a bad person.

Remember, your family is counting on you to set limits and healthy boundaries. If you don't, you'll burn out, and your family will suffer. Setting limits applies to everyone you interact with, including yourself. If you're taking on too much because of another person's expectations of you, this section is for you.

Reaching out and asking for assistance

Many women (and men, for that matter) believe that they should be completely self-reliant, and they feel that asking for assistance of any kind is a sign of weakness. The truth is, this baby thing does take a village, and the sooner you accept that you're part of the human race and that you need people too, the better life is for all concerned.

Have you ever said to yourself, "I wish I had help, but I don't want to burden my friends"? Put the shoe on the other foot, and think about how you feel when you help someone you care about. I'm guessing you feel pretty good, which means that your friends probably feel the same way. Don't ruin your friends' chances of taking advantage of the opportunity to feel good! Allow them to help you.

If you're thinking about how nice it would be to have just one person offer to help, you're on the right track. Now you just have to elicit the help you need. If your friends aren't offering, just ask them. You may be assuming that if an individual isn't coming forward, he or she doesn't want to or is unwilling to help. That assumption is completely wrong. Often these very people aren't asking if you want help because they don't want to interfere or appear pushy. They may be trying to respect your wishes and are waiting for you to approach them. The point is that you should never make assumptions. The worst that can happen is that you ask and they say they can't this time. That wouldn't be a tragedy, and you can pat yourself on the back for trying.

Accepting help when it's offered

You may have a number of people offering to help you in a variety of ways. Some may be offering to cook, clean, shop, or baby-sit for you. Others may come forward to keep you company and take you for walks. (Refer to Chapter 14 for suggestions on how to assign jobs to people so that you're well-covered and the jobs fit the strengths of the helpers.)

Whatever the offer, unless you have a good reason to refuse, always accept! And be specific so that you receive exactly what you really need. For example, consider this vague question that could have many different meanings: "Can you help clean?" Instead, you want to say, "I would really appreciate it if you could clean the downstairs bathroom." Even if you suggest something other than what they're offering, let them help you. Accepting help isn't a sign of weakness, inadequacy, or incompetence on your part. The opposite is true — it's intelligent to accept help.

Sometimes you'll have friends come by to help, but they'll end up being anything but helpful. These people usually fall into two categories. One group includes those who sit around expecting you to take care of them, as opposed to the other way around. The other group includes those people who are truly trying to help, but instead are actually making your life more chaotic. Remember that you don't have to protect their feelings. Don't worry about offending them or about what they might think. I don't mean that you should blast them or go out of your way to make them feel bad, I'm just saying that it's your well-being that should be on the front burner.

Structuring Your Day

Moms with PPD often have the sensation that they're in a time warp — perceptions of time are definitely altered. When I had PPD, everything seemed to slow way down. It was like moving through sludge (I'd say molasses, but it wasn't that sweet). A minute would feel like an hour. I remember being so sure that my husband was on his way home (he usually came home at 5 p.m.), only to realize with dismay that the clock said 10:30 a.m.

If you've worked outside the home, chances are you've had some kind of schedule: You got up at a certain time, got to work by a particular time, and so on. As much as you may have disliked the schedule, it did provide you with something very important — structure. One of the biggest adjustments to staying at home after having a baby, even if for only a few weeks, is the lack of structure. Suddenly your structure flies out the window and throws your life upside down. Whether you're in bed, out of bed, dressed, or in your nightgown make no sense anymore. Without the reference point of going to work outside the home, everything is topsy-turvy.

Because it provides you with a guide, having some kind of structure will help you move more easily through your day. I'm not talking about making a rigid schedule where every fifteen minutes is spoken for. Instead, I suggest that you just create an easy plan that you can follow.

Making lists

One of the best ways to build structure into your day is by using lists. If you dislike lists, bear with me for just a moment. You may have this dislike because of the way you or someone else used lists in the past. Just listen to my suggestions and see if any of them are useful to you. If you're already a list-maker, or at least used to be, hear me out because my way may be an even easier way for you to use them (at least for right now). With my system, you make two different lists: the master list and the daily list.

You can pull items off your master list and transfer them onto your daily list, but be careful. If you're dealing with a major project, such as cleaning your garage, break down that task into a few smaller ones and put the smaller ones on your daily list until the whole garage is done. If you put "clean garage" on your daily list, you'll be too overwhelmed and won't go near your list.

The master list

To use my list-making system, begin by making a master list. This master list includes everything you need or want to do, from the tiniest chore (writing a thank-you note) to the most massive overhaul (landscaping the backyard). Think of this list as the brain dump list. Every time you think of something that needs to be completed, write it here. You'll find that as you write down the things that have been buzzing around your mind, your head can begin to clear.

Keep this list where you'll always be able to find it, but not right in your face — such as on the refrigerator. Here's why: If this long list is posted in a place where you see it frequently, it will drain your energy. You'll always be thinking, "Ugh! Look how much I have left to do!" So, keep it in a kitchen or desk drawer, or another place that's easily accessible, but tucked away.

The daily list

Each day, preferably when you have some support, make the second list, called the daily to-do list, for the following day. This list provides you with a structure, but you're allowed to do these tasks in any order that you want. Many moms make this list before going to bed, because the likelihood of having a partner there at that time is greater (and having a partner around can help you concentrate better). If you don't have that support, make this list during your baby's nap time so you can focus a little.

Only put three or four items on this daily list. Three of them can be tasks, and at least one of them needs to be something for you. Using this system allows you to literally put yourself on your own to-do list so that you're not forgotten. You should schedule three or four larger chunks of time throughout the week during which you can take care of yourself. If you're extremely depressed right now, the following list may be all you can handle (and everything listed, even though some are for you, may feel like chores):

1. Get up (task).

2. Feed the baby (task).

3. Take a shower (for me).

4. Eat breakfast (for me).

If you're more functional and you'll automatically do these basic items, you don't need to list them. At this point, your list may look more like this:

1. Go food shopping (task).

2. Dust office cabinets (task).

3. Walk the dog (task).

4. Read my book for a half hour (for me).

Here's the rule: After making your daily list, take a look at it and see how you feel. It should feel totally workable and not overwhelming. So, if you find that your shoulders start rising up by your earlobes and you're thinking, "I *think* I might be able to get this done," you have your first signal that the four items you've listed are feeling like too much for one day. Adjust it until it feels so simple that you know you can get it done.

Don't wait until tomorrow to make tomorrow's daily list. If you wait until the day is upon you, and you're feeling down, you won't be motivated to make a list. You need to wake up and already have that structure in place. Then you have a plan to follow no matter how tough the PPD is that day.

Setting yourself up for success

You can plan the best you can with the structure of the daily list, but some things may pop up (as they often do). For example, suppose your baby is particularly fussy that day or you receive a phone call about an insurance paper that needs to be turned in right away. Adjust your list accordingly. Sometimes you can just trade one task for another. Other times a task on your list needs to wait until tomorrow's list — and that's okay because you did the best you could.

Compare these two moms who are suffering from PPD — Anne and Jenny. Anne doesn't make a daily list. She only uses a master list. Jenny uses both. At the end of a particularly productive day, each had accomplished the exact same four items. However, their outlooks are quite different. Anne looks at her master list and says, "I only did four things on my list! Look how much I still need to do." She may feel dejected, unproductive, and defeated.

Jenny, on the other hand, crossed off each item she put on her daily list as she completed it. At the end of her day, she looked at her crossed off list and exclaimed, "Wow! Look what I did. I completed every single task I set out for myself today. I feel proud that I actually got everything done."

Each of these women accomplished exactly the same items, yet one feels bad about herself and the other one feels good. The key is to keep your expectations manageable so you set yourself up for success — not failure.

Knowing It's Okay to Lighten Your Load

You may have already been great at setting boundaries and limiting your activities before the PPD. Even so, you may have noticed that trying to take on the same number of tasks is not only difficult when you have a baby, but almost impossible when you have PPD. It can be frustrating when you know you were always able to handle certain things, such as balancing the bank accounts or organizing a birthday party, and those functions are now, to say the least, challenging. You haven't lost IQ points. This is just what PPD does.

It's not only okay to move some of these usual tasks off your to-do list whenever possible, it actually helps your recovery if you do. As you feel better, you start doing these tasks again, but for now, get them off your plate.

Deciding whether to take it on

When the PTA president calls you and compliments you with, "You're the best person to do this. You're so good at it. Can I count on you to come through?" you have to remember to take several steps before saying yes or no. If you're thinking that because you *can* take charge of the parent-teacher party at your kid's school, that somehow you ought to, beware — this thinking is a trap. Follow these steps to avoid taking on projects you shouldn't:

1. **Always buy yourself time.**

   No matter how sure you are that you want to accept, never do so on the spot! You may end up regretting your decision, and it's a lot more difficult to get yourself out of a commitment than it is to turn it down at the beginning.

   Answer the PTA president or other person wanting you to participate, with this: "Thank you for thinking of me and for your kind words. I'll need to think about it and get back to you." If they're persistent, just keep repeating that sentence. Don't let them wear you down until you say yes. Stick to your boundaries, and get some distance from the request so you can evaluate the proposition objectively.

2. **Ask yourself the correct question, not the wrong one.**

   For example, the wrong question is "*Can* I do what this person is asking?" Your decisions shouldn't be based on whether you're *able* to do the task, but rather, if it's *right* for you to do it. So, the correct question is, "Is it healthy for me and my family if I take on this task?" The answer to the first (wrong) question is usually yes. But, the answer to the second (correct) question is often, absolutely not. Just be sure to listen to your gut feeling regarding the answer to the correct question.

Spending quality time with your kid(s)

Even though you do need to take ultimate care of yourself right now, remember to put time in your calendar to spend special time with each of your children. Many times moms with PPD are feeling guilty (so what else is new?) about not spending enough time with their kids. Even if you're feeling so low that you can't leave the house — or in some cases, your bed — make a time for each child to have Mom all to herself. When your 4-year-old knows that every Wednesday afternoon, for instance, you'll read him a book and play a game, he won't be vying for your time as much when you're with the baby. Similarly, Dad should make sure that he sets up special time with each of the children as well. Not only is it good for dad, and good for the other child or children, but this helps to take more of the pressure and demand off the new mom.

Slacking for the good of your health

You may have been taught that slacking on your chores is irresponsible, but right now, slacking is exactly what you need. You need to save your energy for the important things, like spending quality time with your family. So, here are some tips to get you started:

✔ **Let the laundry pile up.** The concept of "getting your house done" is a myth. A house is never "done" — it's always a work in progress. It's you who decides when it's "done" for the day. Just like the house is never done, the laundry — especially when you have a baby in the house — is constantly a work in progress. If you've put two loads of laundry on your daily list (see the section "Making lists" earlier in the chapter) and they're complete, you're done. If other tasks take priority for the next few days, let the laundry wait. No one ever died from lack of a clean undershirt.

If you can delegate your laundry duties to someone else, either lay or professional, do it (unless you get satisfaction from doing laundry, which some do).

✔ **Allow the dust to settle.** If you're in charge of at least half of the housework, it's okay to let the dust build a bit before you wipe it off. Unless the dust is really impeding someone's health, let it go for a while. If other chores take precedence, put dusting on the list for the end of the week or next week. So what if your great aunt runs her finger over your mantle with a white glove to examine its cleanliness. If she wants to clean your house, make sure to accept!

If you can hire a person to clean your house twice a month, now is the time to do so. If someone wants to buy you a gift, tell them you want a housekeeper.

✔ **Order take-out.** Putting dinner on the table doesn't always have to involve cooking. You may typically enjoy cooking, but right now with your lack of appetite and a master to-do list a mile long, cooking can feel like one more grueling task.

Many happy couples divide the nights that each is responsible for providing dinner. And here's the deal. The agreement needs to state that any way food is provided on the person's night is okay — barbecue, stove-top cooking, frozen dinners, or takeout. If you need to do a couple of weeks at a time with straight takeout, so be it. Pick whichever restaurant has the healthiest food and you'll probably feel better about it.

You won't be responsible for single-handedly destroying the environment if you use paper plates and plastic utensils for a few weeks.

Chapter 13

Coping with Your Feelings

. . . .

In This Chapter

▶ Preparing yourself for the ups and downs of PPD

▶ Releasing stress the healthy way

▶ Understanding how to boost your self-esteem

▶ Controlling your control issues

▶ Knowing how to respond to others when you're upset

. . . .

As you've probably figured out by now, having a baby wreaks havoc on your hormones. And, as it turns out, these hormones cause postpartum depression (PPD) to feel very different from other depressions. When people suffer from depression at other times — not after pregnancy — they're constantly down in the dumps. PPD doesn't feel like that. You're probably up and down and all around, like a rollercoaster. At 8 a.m. you may feel anxious, at 10 a.m. you feel okay, at 2 p.m. you may be feeling depressed, and then at 5 p.m. who knows what emotions may be swirling around your head.

Unfortunately, these ups and downs are part of the PPD ride. However, you can survive the ride by using the coping skills in this chapter. Here, I explain the importance of your mindset in your recovery. I give you specific methods for coping with your wide array of feelings, and I discuss the positive aspects of being honest about your emotions. By the end of this chapter, you can expect to know how to boost your self-esteem, let go of perfectionism, and handle your feelings when other people are judgmental or negative about your situation.

Learning to Ride the Waves

Your expectations regarding your recovery are extremely important. In other words, the way you psychologically prepare yourself for this bumpy ride can affect how it goes. The healthiest mindset is to understand that you can only control so much. For example, you can arm yourself with good information and set up your support system and environment. But, after those elements are in place, you then have to roll with the waves. Just as you couldn't completely control the experiences of labor and delivery, you also can't control your moods.

If you're determined to try and control your moods and you've convinced yourself that you can will away your negative thoughts, I guarantee you that you're setting yourself up for a hard ride — you may even need an extra seat belt. The more you try to stay in control, the more out of control, disappointed, and frustrated you will become.

Having this mindset can also set you up for negative self-talk, which will make you more depressed. After all, if you feel you've let yourself down and have failed (because you're never in total control the way you want to be), you probably won't be compassionate with yourself — and it's compassion that you need the very most.

Facing Your Feelings Head On

Feeling certain emotions, such as anger, frustration, sadness, fear, and disappointment, is obviously quite uncomfortable for most people. However, ignoring these feelings, as many people want and try to do, usually makes the situation worse. For example, if your mild anxiety isn't given proper attention, it can grow worse and worse until your stress is released in ways that you may regret. If you try to push away or bury your feelings, you may find yourself snapping at your partner or handling your toddler too roughly.

Instead of bottling up your feelings, make sure you have an outlet to release them. When I used to have difficulty releasing stress, I would pencil-in a date with myself. During my solo date, I would rent a movie that was sure to make me cry. Some of my favorites were *Ghost* (I'd close my eyes for the 30 seconds of gore), *An Officer and A Gentleman, When Harry Met Sally, The Way We Were,* and *South Pacific.* Crying like a baby is always a great release for stress!

Throwing a party for yourself! A pity party, that is

You know you should be happy about having a new baby to coddle and coo at. And everyone's assuming that you're delighted with your "bundle of joy." But, you're not. So, you judge yourself for crying and freaking out at the littlest things. You're probably asking yourself "Others have it so much worse — what's the matter with me?"

Life would be much more pleasant if you could just skip over these "poor me" instances and go directly to feeling happy about all those things you know you should be grateful for. But unfortunately, that's not how it works. You need to accept all your emotions, not just the upbeat ones, in order to be psychologically healthy. You may think that allowing yourself to wallow in your negative thoughts will keep you stuck down in the dumps forever. Quite the contrary! The only way you can emerge from your sadness and begin to experience more of what you've been looking forward to is to give the negative emotions an escape route, much like releasing steam from a pressure cooker.

As a release, I recommend that you throw a full-blown pity party. For those of you who were taught never to feel sorry for yourself (you know who you are), this assignment may be tough, but you need it more than anyone.

To get started, carve out some time — between a half hour to an hour — where you're completely alone (and where no one can hear you — the party may get loud!). During this time, follow the upcoming steps that I outline to help you get your feelings out in the open:

1. **Let out all the negative feelings.**

   The specific negative feelings will be different for each woman. But, here are a few examples:

   - I'm angry that my mother-in-law burst into the delivery room.
   - I'm hurt that my sister decided at the last minute not to be my labor coach.
   - I'm scared that my baby isn't eating enough.
   - I'm frustrated that my doctor didn't warn me about PPD.
   - I'm worried about how long this depression will last.
   - I'm disappointed and sad that my partner doesn't understanding what I'm going through.

   Use the method of your choice to vent. Shouting to the sky, writing, and recording your thoughts on tape are the old standbys. But remember: No censoring! Be as honest as you can, and don't worry about saying things such as "Why me?" or "It's not fair!"

2. **After about 30 to 45 minutes of venting, wind down.**

   To wind down, say something like, "Okay, so I was dealt what I was dealt. It could have been worse. I'm going to move on." Then remind yourself of at least ten specific things you're grateful for.

3. **State (or write, or draw, or whatever) positive truths with oomph (wimpy isn't effective).**

Here are a few ideas to get you started:

- This time in my life is really difficult, and I'm taking positive steps to recover!

- My baby loves me!

- I'm a good mother!

- This depression is temporary and I'll get myself back!

- I'm looking forward to feeling happy again!

You may need to throw yourself another pity party in the future, which is fine. If you want to throw another that same week, go ahead. Or, if you don't need another one for a few months, that's okay too. Whatever you need is what is right. Don't deny yourself, because as silly as it sounds, this release will boost your recovery. You'll find that each time you empty your heart of negative emotions, you have so much more room for the positive ones to enter in.

Releasing your perfect pictures

Perfect pictures are those dangerous little expectations of perfection which are, by definition, unattainable. You may expect perfection from yourself or from others around you, or you may be convinced (whether real or imagined) that others expect perfection from you. Or, you may even have a combination of all of the above. The discussion here is mainly about the self-imposed perfection.

Realistic expectations are necessary for health. You don't expect your child to learn how to walk overnight, right? He's going to take it one baby step at a time. And sometimes he'll fall flat on his face. But, you wouldn't tell him he's a failure. You'd tell him how great he did and how proud you are of him for trying. So you should do the same for yourself.

You may be struggling with perfect pictures that you're not consciously aware of yet. Check yourself — see if you believe any of the following statements:

- ✔ There is such a thing as a perfect mother, and I can picture her.

- ✔ A stay-at-home mom should have a clean, orderly house when someone visits.

- ✔ There is such a thing as a perfect child.

- ✔ I need to make the "right" decision every time.

- ✔ There's only one right way to accomplish a task.

If you read any one (or more) of the previous statements and felt as if it were true (even though you know better rationally), this discussion will help you. You can start by releasing the perfect pictures that have begun to overwhelm you with this new job of being a mother. Parenting in general requires flexibility in just about every area. This realization can be one of the biggest parts of the learning curve for new moms.

A major myth of motherhood is that this job is instinctual. I mean, women have been having babies since the beginning of time, right? If everyone else is doing it, how difficult can it be to take care of a baby? You know darn well how difficult! And a lot of the tasks expected of you have nothing to do with instinct. This job needs to be learned just like any other. Even knowing what to do with those two watermelons hanging from your chest needs to be learned!

After you've identified your perfect pictures, it's important (and healthy) for you to toss them out. To do so, you have to consciously change your way of thinking. Simply pat yourself on the back for catching it, acknowledge the false statement or belief, and flip it around so you're telling yourself the truth.

Letting your worries float away

One of the most common symptoms of PPD is anxiety. Not every woman with PPD feels it, but most do. And some women mainly have postpartum anxiety and don't feel much depression. If you do indeed have anxiety, this section can help you keep it under control.

Understanding your anxiety

You may be the worrywart who has always worried about worrying. Or maybe you're the one who always let things roll off her back, but now you don't recognize yourself at all. Or maybe you used to worry more than your partner or your friends and family, but it never felt as intense as it does now. My purpose here is to provide you with tools to alleviate your worry. As your mind relaxes, it will in turn, help your body relax (your heart rate and breathing may comfortably slow down, for instance), and vice versa.

Anxiety is caused by the following factors:

✔ **Physiological factors:** With PPD, *serotonin,* an important brain chemical, is often low, and so by raising serotonin, you can greatly reduce your anxiety. Specific nutrients (refer to Chapter 12) can help enhance serotonin production. Also, medications are available that can help increase the amount of serotonin that can be used in the brain. Also, cortisol levels are often high in moms with PPD, which leads to anxiety and depression. You can usually treat these high levels naturally by using the suggestions I provide in Chapter 12.

✔ **Psychological factors:** Perfect pictures and myths of motherhood can cause anxiety because they make you think that you can never measure up. The great news is that this can be alleviated by using the techniques to help release perfect pictures (see the section "Releasing your perfect pictures" earlier in this chapter) and to reform your negative self-talk (refer to Chapter 4).

Another cause of psychological anxiety stems from how you were raised. For example, if a parent showed you that life had to be handled by worrying all the time, or that love equals worry, this way of thinking is probably engrained in you. But, don't worry! Thoughts are reversible.

✔ **Environmental factors:** There are many different situations I could mention here, because for each woman, the factors will be different. Stressors and changes in your life, such as moving, death, money problems, relationship issues, job changes, sleep deprivation, and so on, can all be factors here. I'm sure you've recognized that at least a couple of those listed apply to you.

For instance, if you just moved to a new community and are missing your friends and family, chances are you're feeling lonely and isolated. "Will I ever make new friends?" is a thought that could make you worry. Other common examples are when a baby has health issues or when a partner travels a lot or has long hours at work. No matter what the environmental factor is, you're sure to find an antidote. Your therapist can help you work out a plan that suits you.

Relieving your anxiety

When you're anxious, no matter what it's caused by, nothing is more annoying than someone saying to you, "Just relax!" If you could have willed yourself out of worry, you would have done it long ago. No one would ever choose to feel this way.

During the height of my PPD, I remember my friend telling me to listen to her favorite relaxation tape while lying on the floor and breathing deeply. This exercise was futile and frustrating because I was unable to sit still, let alone lie on the floor and breathe! If you're able to use a good relaxation tape, that's great, and I encourage it. But, if you try and it doesn't work, don't worry more about yourself because you can't do it quite yet.

Here are just a few simple suggestions that can help you relieve your anxiety:

✔ **Get as much off your plate as possible.** For example, don't sign up for extracurricular activities that require a lot of your time and attention. This just isn't the time to take on Room Mother for your eldest child's class.

For those activities that you must keep in your life, write down the daily tasks so you aren't trying to keep them in your head (refer to Chapter 12 for more on how to keep lists super simple).

✔ **Be kind to yourself.** Putting yourself down only creates more stress and anxiety and sets you up on a never-ending and ugly downward spiral.

✔ **Do gentle aerobic exercise such as walking or swimming.** Exercising two or three times a week can lower your depression and boost your mood. You'll also feel better about yourself when you're doing something active to help yourself recover.

If you're prone to panic attacks, however, make sure to build up your exercise program slowly. Prolonged exercise when your muscles aren't conditioned can increase lactic acid, which in turn can cause panic (lactic acid is also what makes you sore).

✔ **Eat healthfully.** Increasing your intake of specific nutrients can help alleviate your anxiety by increasing serotonin, dopamine, and other brain chemicals that affect mood (check out Chapter 12 for more details on how to eat healthfully).

✔ **Stay off the Internet.** Information on the Web, as it is on the news, is often very negative. And negative information just doesn't help your worries. In an anxious state of mind, you'll find that you'll be attracted to, and tend to obsess over, negativity. Also, because Web information isn't filtered, you're often becoming unnecessarily anxious about misinformation anyway.

✔ **Do whatever activities work for you.** If an activity increases your level of anxiety, stop. If you find something that helps calm or relax you, do it. Just trust your intuition about what's right for you now, and treat yourself with respect and patience.

Dealing with depression after your anxiety subsides

When your anxiety thankfully subsides, you may become aware of some underlying depression. For example, sometimes my clients become concerned that even though they're enjoying relief from the old anxiety, they're now feeling depressed. Even though you should mention these feelings to your doctor or therapist, you typically have nothing to be concerned about. What's happening is that you're getting better.

It may appear that this depression rears its head suddenly, but really the depression isn't new — it was there all along. You just weren't aware of it, because the anxiety was the most prevalent and bothersome symptom — the one that got your full attention. Now that the anxiety is calming down, you feel the depression. So, despite what you initially thought, you aren't getting worse. On the contrary, this change is a sign that you're recovering.

One woman's journey down recovery lane

Tami Muser was a client of mine. She has been a crusader for mothers with PPD ever since her own recovery from the illness, and she's now the coordinator for the Bay Area Postpartum Depression Stress Line. Here's her story, in her own words:

"My baby is a week old. We waited five long years to start a family. Most of my friends are on baby number two by now. My husband and I favored waiting in order to work on our home and our awesome marriage. So, why do I feel like the walls are closing in? I wish I could turn my head off.

Waiting in that paper gown for the doctor to come in was killing me. Panic was rising. I called to the nurse, crying that I just wanted the door left open so I didn't feel so alone. Did other moms feel alone? I wanted this baby so bad. I can't believe it feels this awful now that he's here. My OB came in and I told him I didn't want to live another day. No, I wouldn't actually *take* my life, but I didn't want to be alive. I wasn't sure which was worse. I just felt *stuck* in this shell of a body. My house felt like a box. The nurse held my hand and I secretly wished she could come home with me so the silence wouldn't scream at me. I never realized how loud silence was.

My OB said to go down the hall to psychiatry and make an appointment. 'Oh sure. Like I'll do that.' No thanks, I'd rather go home to the silence. Maybe I should have left a radio on. . . .

Pulling into the garage, I felt like I'd died at that appointment. I went for answers and came home desperate. Maybe if I left the car running and the garage door down? Shoot, the phone is ringing! Great, and now the baby is crying. I prayed they'd left a message. I called our voice-mail from the garage phone afraid to go inside my box — I mean my house.

I slumped to the floor of my garage sobbing as I heard the voice of Dr. Shoshana Bennett telling me I'd found the right place and that she could definitely help me with this disorder called PPD. Thank God it had a name! I felt better just knowing I actually had 'something.'

We hired a nanny. Call her what you want, I just want someone by my side all day until the Prozac kicks in and does its job. Other women in Dr. Bennett's support group said medication gave them their life back. I hoped it would for me too. The nanny goes everywhere with me. Showers can be lonely, so she's sweet enough to sit in my room until I turn the water off. I'm so grateful my husband gets it. Other women in the support group said their husbands tell them to get it together. That would kill me. Dr. Bennett assured my husband that I would go back to the woman I was before and that PPD doesn't last forever. I hang on to those words because every second feels like forever with PPD."

Boosting Your Self-Esteem

PPD is a thief. It's sneaky and can quickly steal away your good feelings about yourself — in other words, it steals your self-esteem. If you've previously enjoyed a healthy outlook on your self-worth in your job, at home, and with your friends and family, you may be wondering where that confident woman went. And if you've never felt really solid about yourself before, chances are those negative feelings toward yourself are now greatly exaggerated.

One client recently told me that she has always struggled with feeling slightly less competent than her colleagues, even though her production and ratings were higher than theirs. No one at work would have guessed that she had been feeling bad about herself. Now with PPD, my client's minor self-esteem issue has exploded to the point where she even has a difficult time maintaining eye contact with others at work, doubting that she even deserves the job.

Assessing your self-esteem

Low self-esteem is quite different from understanding that you're not perfect. For example, being able to take an honest look at yourself and realistically assess your strengths and weaknesses is healthy and can help you grow. A strong sense of self is important for all aspects of your life, including as a mom. The key to having a healthy self-esteem is to become aware of your strengths, and at the same time to accept yourself as a worthy individual in spite of your weaknesses. So, taking a look at what you can strengthen in yourself and following through without judgment is, in and of itself, a strength. If you can feel good about your ability to be honest and grow from it, chances are your self-esteem is in pretty good shape. If, on the other hand, you take a look and start criticizing yourself, this is an indication of low self-esteem.

I bet I know what you're saying to yourself right now: "But, how do I know for sure if I've crossed the line to low self-esteem?" To help you out, I've put together the following checklist to help you determine where you fall on the self-esteem continuum. Put a check by any statement that you know is *completely* true. If you start thinking too much and come up with, "Well, it's sometimes true or mostly true," that's not clear and strong enough to earn self-esteem points. You need to be sure that the statement is true to check it. Otherwise, leave it blank. This isn't a test you can fail. I put it here to help you take an honest look so that you can get some necessary information if you need to grow. Here are the statements:

- ☐ I'm a happy person.
- ☐ I like being with others.
- ☐ I'm easily honest and open when I'm wrong.
- ☐ I'm valued.
- ☐ I'm confident about my opinions.
- ☐ People like me for who I really am.

☐ If I feel something, I'm honest about it.

☐ I like myself.

☐ As long as I approve of myself, that's enough.

☐ I know inside when I've done a good job.

☐ I have a right to be just as happy as the next person.

☐ I'm good at praising myself.

☐ My opinion counts.

☐ I can stick up for myself.

☐ I can accept criticism without feeling bad about myself.

☐ I deserve respect just like anyone else.

☐ I'm worthy of love.

☐ I accept myself even though I'm not perfect.

☐ I'm a good person.

☐ I'm useful to others.

Now that you've gone through the statements, tally up the number of checkmarks you have. The more checks you have, the better you are in the self-esteem department. If you have 18 to 20 checks, your self-esteem is in great shape. If you have 15 to 17 checks, it's high but needs work. A score of 13 to 15 checkmarks is moderate and 11 to 12 is low. If you have less than 10 checkmarks, your self-esteem is extremely low. Remember, feeling bad about receiving a low score, is just another indication of low self-esteem. In a few weeks, I suggest you retake this quiz to see if your score has changed for the better.

Improving your self-esteem

If feeling bad about yourself is mainly due to your PPD, your self-esteem will naturally rise as you recover. On the other hand, if your self-esteem has always left something to be desired, this is an excellent time to start shedding the old negative thoughts.

Here are some tips that will get you on the road to recovery:

> ✔ **Do what's right for you, not what's right for everybody else.** If going back to work outside the home feels like the right step for you and your family, do it. If bottle feeding the baby works best for your family, go ahead. Whatever decision is at hand, you have to know how to trust your gut.

PPD can make you doubt yourself, so trusting your gut isn't always easy to do. When the doubt about whether you made the right decision creeps in, remind yourself that you made a good decision and that you'll be able to handle whatever happens from it.

✔ **Practice those skills you need help with, and don't put yourself down in the process.** Instead, congratulate yourself for trying. Everyone is better at some things than they are at others. The only way to improve those skills you're not so good at is to practice and be patient with yourself. Beating yourself up only lowers your self-esteem and feeds the depression. It also models unhealthy patterns to your kids, and they'll likely grow up doing the same thing.

✔ **Respect your needs and wants and take care of them.** If you don't respect your needs and wants, others won't either. Write down what you need daily (and nightly!), as well as your longer term goals as you recover.

Remember, these needs and wants are personal and will differ from person to person. If, for example, you need to have privacy in the bathroom, make sure you get that privacy (as long as everyone's safe). And, if you're hungry, make sure you finish your lunch, even if a fussing (or even screaming) baby needs to wait two extra minutes.

✔ **Set realistic goals so that you'll be successful.** Challenges are fine and good, but until you recover, you need to make sure your goals fit with what's reasonable for you right now.

✔ **Concentrate on your strengths.** In other words, concentrate on what you can do, not what you can't. Accept that the PPD will limit you in some ways for the time being, but also remember that you can indeed accomplish a lot. As you recover, the limitations will start disappearing.

✔ **Set yourself up for success and then acknowledge yourself when you accomplish the task.** If you're extremely depressed, just getting out of bed in the morning can be challenging. So, set it as a goal, and when you actually do it, check it off your list and let yourself feel good about it.

✔ **Speak positively to yourself.** Catch yourself when you're judging or doubting yourself, congratulate yourself for catching it, and then change the thought to something positive.

✔ **Put your negative feelings on a shelf long enough to deal only with what's in front of you at the moment.** For example, if a family member says something judgmental to you, you may think, "My relationship with her is over." Then you may feel depressed about it. In a case like this, remind yourself that it was just one silly comment she made and that your relationship probably hasn't ended. If you jump from a little comment someone made (no matter how icky the comment was) to a catastrophe like, "it's all over," that's the lack of perspective from depression or anxiety talking. Ask yourself what reasonable steps you can take to get your perspective back.

✔ **Allow yourself to solve problems you can handle.** For instance, don't take on major decisions that aren't necessary at this time in your life. Only do what you can, and feel good about your efforts. However, some major decisions will be right in your face, so to speak, so I know they can't all be avoided. But, if you can delay the decision to move, change jobs, or to have another baby, that helps. It's better to wait until you're less stressed and overwhelmed, and you're thinking more clearly. It often helps my clients (and their partners) to actually choose and circle a date on the calendar a few months out. On this date, they allow themselves to start making decisions about whatever they've been healthfully delaying.

Knowing What You Can and Can't Control

Control is a huge issue for people in general. But mothers in particular are prone to the kind of control that eventually makes them feel like they're in a prison with no key. PPD, on top of this kind of control, exaggerates this feeling. This happens for many reasons, including the fact that moms with PPD are feeling so out of control that it's a way to compensate and get the control back. Unfortunately, though, it doesn't work that way. I know I certainly tried doing it this way and it just brought more dysfunction to me and my family.

Coming to terms with the truth

As you probably know by now, accepting what you're in control of and what you're not in control of is essential. For example, you can take some actions that help or hinder the outcome of any situation, but the bottom line is that you don't always have final say. And if you don't have final say, that situation is out of your control. Here's a short list of situations you're not in control of:

✔ Getting pregnant

✔ Staying pregnant (miscarriage)

✔ How you feel during pregnancy

✔ How the labor goes

✔ How the delivery goes

✔ The temperament of your baby

✔ Your biochemical reactions to pregnancy and delivery

Criticizing yourself for not having been in control of any of the previous situations is rather inappropriate. No one is in control of these things. No matter how hard you concentrate, you couldn't change your estrogen or serotonin level. Nor could you change the strength of a labor contraction.

Even though certain events are out of your control, you are, in fact, in control of what you choose to do with any of these events. For instance, if you're having a difficult time getting pregnant, you have choices about what to do next. If you're feeling sick while pregnant, you can search out some treatments. If you have a spirited child, you can read a book on the topic, talk to an expert, or join a parent group with others who are living with the same thing. Just remember that PPD wasn't within your control, but now that you know what you're dealing with, you have a lot of options on how to cope.

Relinquishing the reins to your partner

It's exhausting to feel like the world is on your shoulders and everything regarding your baby is your responsibility. When the baby first comes home, some moms report that they like the feeling that they're the cruise directors, orchestrating what needs to happen when. However, that role is a trap, and it usually begins to breed resentment. What these moms often don't realize is that they helped to create the situation that caused this resentment and that they need to take responsibility for fixing the environment.

Often clients say to me, "Why doesn't my partner just take over and do baby care and house chores without my asking?" Other than reminding her that he can't read her mind, I'll ask her how she reacts when her partner does actually do house chores and baby care. She usually responds, "He doesn't do them right, so I have to do them over again. If I can do it better, I may as well do it myself."

Who would want to step up and do a task if it's going to be judged as wrong or inadequate? After a while, anyone would stop trying. If you truly want to feel more like you have a full partner and less like it's all on you, you need to change your mindset and behavior. Following are some guidelines that can help you change your attitude and give up some control. I refer to partner here, but these suggestions apply to any close support person who's in charge frequently (or could be!):

 ✔ **Be willing to give up some of the control.** Other people are quite capable of taking care of the baby. You'll always be Mom and you'll never be replaced. By allowing yourself some help, you'll only be relieved of the self-imposed burden of feeling alone with this huge responsibility.

Sometimes this need to control comes on when nursing ends because many women believe that what sets them apart from other caretakers is their ability to breastfeed. If this applies to you, please remember that your breasts don't make you Mom. You'll always be special as Mom no matter how you're feeding your baby.

✔ **When your partner does a baby or house task, accept it the way it was done and leave it alone.** Give your partner a compliment whenever possible and appropriate. Good ol' positive feedback — the more you pay off a behavior, the more frequently it will occur.

✔ **If it's too difficult for you to see your partner take care of the baby in a different way than you do, leave the room or the house so you don't see it.** Your partner will have a different way of doing most every task, but that doesn't make his way wrong — it's just different.

✔ **When you hear the baby cry when your partner is on duty, don't swoop in and take over.** If you do, you just undermine your partner's efforts, feelings of competence, confidence, and the relationship between your partner and the baby. This situation isn't good for any member of the family, including you.

I used to leave a few pages of written notes with my husband even if I was leaving the house for just a half hour. The notes would have copious instructions about how to feed, diaper, clean, and hold our baby, plus details about where to find certain items in the house. I could barely get out of the door when I'd remember something else and come back in to add it to the list. I found out years later that Henry would throw out my notes, because he knew very well how to take care of his child.

Responding to Others Honestly (But Appropriately!)

Moms with PPD are especially vulnerable to giving their power away. This happens when she isn't feeling secure and thinks that someone else has the "right" answer, or does something a "better" way than she does. In this section, I outline how you can keep your power by appropriately answering inappropriate questions from others or responding to comments that are out of line. I also show you what to do if you feel like you're about to lose it and say or do something that you'll regret.

Taking a timeout when you feel snippy

As you've maybe already witnessed, when you're stressed to the max some ugly things can come flying out of your mouth — and, well, I probably shouldn't repeat them here. And sometimes depression manifests itself more as anger than sadness. So, if you're already feeling crummy about yourself, it surely won't help if you lose your temper with a big or little person who doesn't deserve it. I mean c'mon, if you yell at your toddler or snap at your partner, you just feel bad.

Even when you set up your wellness plan just right, and you're doing everything you should, you'll still hit those difficult points. At those times, it may feel like you don't have any control at all regarding what you do or say. The truth is that you have more control than you think.

Consider "timeout," the disciplinary technique used on children. Believe it or not, when you hit one of those rough times in your PPD and you just lose it, you can gain control by using the same technique.

The adult version of timeout is mostly like the child version: You simply time yourself out and physically leave the room. Or you can have your partner respectfully and privately suggest to you that you need a time out (perhaps whisper it into your ear or have a signal like wiggling an ear). If you have a toddler, preschooler, or older child, tell him that Mommy said something she shouldn't have and that she needs to sit by herself, think about what she said, and calm down. Place your child somewhere safe. If you need to apologize to anyone, you can either do it before or after your time out.

To make your timeout go as smoothly as possible, designate a place where you can go to be alone. Tell your kids that you're not allowed to have any company during this time. The rule is that no one can talk to you during your timeout, because you need to collect yourself (is this not suddenly feeling like a punishment?). When my children were very little, I used the stairs for my timeout spot. They took this time very seriously, just like when I timed them out.

If you're getting regular breaks, hopefully you won't need to time yourself out on a daily basis. Remember that timeout loses its value if used too much. And, if you're tempted to purposely act out to get yourself put in timeout, you now have a clue that you need a few more scheduled breaks!

Dealing with comments that put you on the defensive

Why is it that women feel obligated to answer personal questions just because they're asked? For some reason, women in general often feel rude when ignoring other people's questions or comments, no matter how inappropriate they are.

But, remember, unless you're mandated in court to do so, you never have to answer any question with the complete and unadulterated truth. Give yourself permission to answer in a way that suits the occasion. Sometimes that may mean totally ignoring the comment. Not every comment needs a response, you know.

There are better ways and worse ways of dealing with unwanted questions and comments. Especially with depression, it's easy to let ignorant comments affect your head, so beware. If you're vulnerable to criticism and have low self-esteem, as is common with PPD, you may feel put down, chastised, shamed, and guilt-tripped whenever people make inappropriate comments. Use these times as opportunities to strengthen your affirmations of the truth, and you'll continually get better and more confident.

Following are a few scenarios that you may encounter. Along with the inappropriate comment, I go into details about what you may be feeling and what you should and shouldn't say when faced with the situation. After reading through these few examples, you'll get the idea and will be able to apply the concepts to any topic.

> **Inappropriate comment #1:** "You're supposed to be happy — what's wrong with you?"
>
> **Possible feeling:** That person just threw a myth of motherhood at you, either by accident or on purpose (though it really doesn't matter whether he or she meant to or not). Remember that new moms are in bootie camp and are usually not feeling very happy, even without PPD. If you're not careful with how you handle this comment, you could experience shame, and you may doubt your worth as a mom until you get your bearings straight.
>
> **DO NOT say:** "Oh, REALLY? Thanks for telling me. Now I'll be happy." Sarcasm gets you nowhere.
>
> **DO say:** nothing and walk away. If the person who said this comment to you is your partner or someone else in your close circle, he or she will need to be educated by this book or in a consultation with a professional so that you get the support you need. If the comment was made by someone else, it probably won't be worth the effort.
>
> **DO say:** "This mommy stuff is harder than it's made out to be. I'm told by the experts that the good times come in time."

DO say: "I'm looking forward to feeling happy. I'm getting there." This works as an affirmation for you, as well as giving the other person a clear message that the judgment doesn't work.

Inappropriate comment #2: "You should be breastfeeding."

Possible feeling: This judgmental individual is trying to make you feel guilty. If unfortunately it starts working, remind yourself in firm statements that you're an excellent mom who made and will continue to make great decisions for your baby. Tell yourself that you're doing the very best that you can and that you feel proud about your decisions.

DO NOT say: "It's none of your business how I'm feeding my baby!" (even though it's technically the truth).

DO NOT say: "I know" and go into apologetic explanations. You have nothing to apologize for. Based on your individual situation, you either couldn't breastfeed or it was the healthiest choice for you and your family not to. Feel good about taking excellent care of yourself — a happy mom is the best gift you can give your child.

DO say: nothing and walk away. Remember, not all comments deserve a response.

DO say: "I can't. I'm suffering from a life-threatening disorder" (yes, depression is life-threatening). That usually backs the person way off. After all, your disorder may be contagious!

Inappropriate comment #3: "I always put socks on my babies when they were little — you should put warmer clothes on your child."

Possible feeling: This person is usually female. She may or may not be judging you as a mother. Give her the benefit of the doubt, because she may be trying to help. But, of course, it really doesn't matter what the intent was anyway, because how you choose to feel about that comment is what's important.

DO NOT say: "That was in the ancient days when you had no heat in your apartment!" Becoming defensive simply hands the other person your power. And, remember, you want to hold on to your power. So, stay cool, calm, and collected.

DO NOT say: "You're always so critical! Leave me alone!" Your statement and feeling may both be real, but responding this way isn't good for you. Even though, on some level it would be satisfying to blurt this out, you'd end up feeling lousy and it would hurt your relationship with that person.

DO say: "That's great you found a way that worked for you and your babies. It sounds like you were a really good mom." This is an important one to remember. Notice that I ignored the "you should" part of the person's comment. That part just wasn't worth responding to. This is because usually when a person speaks about the way she parents or parented, she just needs some validation of her own. Don't take it personally. After she gets the validation she craves, usually the criticism stops immediately.

Forcing Yourself to Laugh

This section may be the most bizarre for you, but stay with me, because it's an important one. Why? Because humor is very healing and can help you with parenting in general. Unfortunately, keeping your sense of humor can be really challenging with PPD. When PPD tries to steal away your power so that you feel weak and helpless, however, humor can bring it back. The irony is that the more serious you feel, the more you need humor. And the more you need it, the more difficult it is to access. So, here's a quick and dirty way to get some of the world's best medicine.

Just as you can write positive affirmations on 3 x 5 cards and tape them all over your house, you can also write reminders to laugh on those same cards or on different ones. Some of my clients use a particular color or symbol to remind themselves to laugh, even when they're in no such mood.

When you really don't want to laugh — when everything is looking pretty darn awful — that's when you really need to laugh the most. Force it. That's right — force the laughs with some oomph (give them at least a medium amount of air). You don't have to feel happy, just force a few laughs no matter how stiff or awkward they may sound. Make sure to fake smile a bit while you're forcing your laugh. I'm not kidding! It has been found that endorphins — chemicals in the brain that help make you happy — are released when your eyes and mouth are in the position of a smile.

I warned you — my advice sounds weird, but it's amazing how well it works. Here's what will happen: Nine times out of ten, (for some of you, ten times out of ten) your laughing will sound so odd that the ridiculousness of it will make you break out into a real giggle. It works. Try it. Nothing can change energy and help you feel your strength faster than a laugh.

Chapter 14

Finding Somebod(ies) to Lean On

In This Chapter

▶ Reaching out to others

▶ Creating and using your support team

▶ Talking to people about your PPD

▶ Avoiding the myth that you should be autonomous

Social isolation is a top risk factor for postpartum depression (PPD), and sometimes, believe it or not, this isolation is brought on by the woman herself. A woman may think that independence where she feels the need to do everything herself is healthy, but it really isn't. If you suffer from PPD, being by yourself perpetuates your condition and may even make it worse. If you spend countless hours home alone with your child or children, you're headed toward even greater suffering than if you were completely alone without kids.

Reaching out to others breaks through your isolation because it's a courageous and healing act. It helps you see just how much support you actually have. Seeing the amount of support around you is important because one of the cruelest parts of PPD is that those who suffer from it tend to see themselves as having little or no support. Because they feel so alone, they fail to take advantage of the help that's actually available to them. By reaching out into your world, you'll not only gather the support and contact that you need to feel better, but you'll also find that your anchors of support are closer and more numerous than you originally thought.

This chapter helps you determine who your backers and cheerleaders (and related organizations and support groups) are, how you can best tell them what's going on with you, and how to ask for and receive the support that you need. By reaching out to the loved ones around you, you'll most certainly find that the universe really does help those who help themselves.

If you're new in the community, without friends or family in the area, or aren't close to them at all, you may be wondering whether this chapter applies to you. You bet it does. And you need to read it twice. Just because you haven't met those support people yet doesn't mean they're not there waiting for you.

Emerging from under the Sheets

Contrary to popular belief, when a baby is brought into a home, he isn't the only one who needs love, attention, and nurturing. The mother does too! Many cultures across the globe even build in special ways of taking care of new mothers because the people of these cultures understand that the moms are quite vulnerable physically, nutritionally, and emotionally. Sometimes in these cultures, many generations of the same family live together, so there's always someone to watch over the children or help out with daily tasks. The new mother doesn't feel guilty or weak that she's getting help because these customs are expected.

Naturally, no matter what part of the world she's from, a new mother feels the pressure of taking care of the new life she and her partner have created. Just as her baby may be screaming, she may hear a voice in her own head screaming "Who's going to take care of me?" Please know that this reaction is normal. Because nurturing you, the new mother, is just as important as your nurturing your new baby is, (and because in our culture the mom's needs aren't taken care of automatically), you'll have to find ways to reach out and make sure that you're taken care of.

The more you may be suffering from PPD, the more unhappy, anxious, tired, and depressed you may feel — and the more important it is that you find ways to make sure that you receive the nurturing you need. If your tendency is to withdraw and tough it out, you have to find a way to overcome this tendency.

Accepting the fact that you need a support circle

Some bleak philosophies (such as existentialism) emphasize that people are born alone, die alone, and that for many, most of the time in-between is fundamentally spent alone. Taking that thought a bit further, some observers of human nature believe that people are all inherently self-interested and downright selfish.

But, while some people cling to these negative thoughts, I truly believe this isn't the case. From my years of experience as a therapist and as a survivor of PPD, I'm here to point out that not only are human beings social animals, but in most circumstances they actually enjoy helping and taking care of each other. When given the opportunity, most people willingly help others, especially when those people who need the help are close to them.

Consider, for example, the many stories of how people pulled together after major disasters, such as the terrorist attacks on September 11, 2001. Or, think about the thousands of people who gave time and money to help those who lost everything during Hurricane Katrina. Even during simple power outages, reclusive homeowners find themselves transformed into caring neighbors, sharing everything from flashlights and water to blankets and warm places to sleep.

It's true that people need to do some things alone, such as riding a unicycle or playing solitaire. But, on the other hand, there are many other things that people are far better off not doing alone if it can be avoided — and facing PPD is hands-down one of them. Contrary to what you may have gathered over time from modern-day society, the plain truth is that getting help when you need it is a sign of both strength and intelligence.

Ideally, your support circle will comprise your primary partner, family members, friends, and other close support people who are ready and willing to hear you out, accept your situation, and then pitch in and make a difference. If you don't already have this kind of support available, you may have to quickly extend your network or be prepared to bring in paid support (for example, a nanny or regular babysitter) or support that you trade for (such as a babysitting co-op). In any circumstance, you need others to help you get through this bumpy ride. You need people who can grab the wheel when you don't have the strength to drive.

Deciding whom to tell

The more support you have as you go through your encounter with PPD, the faster and more complete your recovery will be. Does that mean you need to inform everyone you meet about your personal encounter with PPD? Of course not. You may want to skip the guy on the elevator or the lady with the big umbrella at the bus stop. But, in addition to your primary partner and close family members (if you have these), there are most certainly a few other people in your life who should know about your situation so that they can offer their help and support.

In addition to those who you're close to and who you'll naturally want to inform, you have to consider the individuals who you frequently encounter as part of day-to-day living (the person you share a cubicle with or the nice mom of your oldest child's best friend). Pretending that you feel fine when you don't takes a tremendous amount of energy and can be both psychologically and physically exhausting. Instead of wasting your energy acting, you'll probably find it easier and more productive to clue in the people you frequently see or spend time with. And if some of these individuals aren't "safe people," you probably shouldn't be around them so frequently.

The strength of your relationship with a particular individual, how vulnerable you're feeling, and the individual's safety level all determine how much energy you want to invest in educating him or her. For instance, if you feel sensitive about your PPD, you may not want to share what's going on with a casual work buddy. If that casual work buddy asks "How's the new mom doing?" you can say something like "This mommy stuff is more difficult than I expected, but I'm moving in the right direction. How are you doing?" Asking about the other person helps take the focus off of you and put it onto him or her. You may want to come up with a few of these pat answers so that you can elegantly respond to some of the innocent inquiries that you may receive. You don't have to lie — just be general and move on to another topic.

On the other hand, if you want to educate everyone around you and you aren't feeling particularly vulnerable, feel free to let loose! There's certainly nothing wrong with doing that. Spread the word! You may be surprised with how much genuine compassion emerges and how much assistance you're offered.

Diversifying Your Support Team

As you consider whom in your life to open up to — and exactly how to do that — you may find it useful to begin by taking a step back and considering the broad range of people and relationships that are already in your life. No doubt a great diversity exists among these people and relationships.

For instance, one person may be great at shopping for you or vacuuming your carpet, but lacking in the emotional department. Another person may be your patient walking buddy who helps you get dressed and out of the house, but she may be a bad babysitter or terrible at housework.

By making educated guesses as to who will be emotionally receptive and who will be able to offer the kind of support you need, you will have taken an important step both toward conserving and maximizing your available energy and toward getting the help you need and deserve.

Your partner

Except in the most unusual of circumstances, you need to fully and completely inform your partner of what's going on with you. And you can't be afraid of asking for what you need whenever you need it (assuming that you know what you need, which sometimes you won't).

Sometimes a depressed mother may feel too inhibited to tell her partner about her suffering. The fear of disapproval or rejection can loom very large in the heart and mind of someone who's already feeling inferior. Feeling like "damaged goods," some PPD sufferers may even fear that their partners will throw up their hands, say that this isn't what they signed up for, and then simply leave.

If you have good reason to believe that your partner will have a highly negative reaction — perhaps you opened up the discussion and he quickly shut down or reacted in a hostile or judgmental way — you may want to first open up to a different family member or a close friend. With the support of this other individual, you may gain the strength and comfort to have the necessary discussion with your partner (perhaps with this third person present). Or, you can have this other trusted friend or close family member talk to your partner when you aren't present, acting as a kind of go-between. Your therapist can also be of great help in educating your partner.

There isn't a right or a wrong way to talk to your partner. Just believe in yourself and assess the situation as realistically as you can (remembering that you'll likely have a more negative assessment of the situation than is actually called for), and then find some way to move forward.

As odd as it sounds, don't thank your partner for helping you, because doing so implies that taking care of the baby and house is actually all your job and your responsibility, and your partner is simply helping you with *your* job. Remember that these responsibilities are your partner's as well (after all, he lives in the house too, right?). Instead, you may want to say something like, "I love the way you take care of our baby. I can tell from how she looks at you that she's bonding with you and adores you." Similarly, you may say, "Thanks for cleaning the house — it looks great." In turn, your partner should be thanking you and complimenting you on baby care and house tasks. That's how happy couples live: Every member feels valued — not taken for granted.

Home sweet home: The core of your support

Members of your own birth family can be among your best or worst support people, depending on your individual relationship with them. At best, if you have members of your own birth family close by — those who you grew up with and who you can totally relax with and be yourself around — you're in luck. Their presence can be an amazing comfort. With such a close family member, you won't feel as if you have to pretend or act like you're fine.

Even family members who truly mean well can sometimes be bossy or judgmental. Or, they may even presumptuously try to take over your house and your care. Be clear with such family members about exactly what you want and need. If you're fortunate enough to have lots of family around, try designating a family member (or your partner) to help coordinate who should do what. Having a go-to person makes it so people aren't stepping on each other's toes — this just isn't the time for a family feud.

Extending the innermost circle

After you feel safe and secure in your innermost circle — your partner, your family, and perhaps one or two of your closest friends — you want to extend that innermost circle and bring others into the loop — for example, friends and neighbors. It's important to remember that the timing and extent to which you inform others (and perhaps ask for their help) is totally up to you. In other words, there aren't any rules about what's right or wrong here.

Friends

When you're extending your innermost circle, pick one or two friends who you implicitly trust and share your PPD experience with them. Let them know generally (or specifically, if you wish) what feelings and other symptoms you've been dealing with and how they can help you. Answer their questions the best you can because the more they know, the better they can help. But, unless you want to, you don't need to disclose anything that wouldn't help them help you (for instance, the names of your medications or your partner's first reaction to PPD).

Many of my clients have told me that going through PPD showed them who their real friends were. You may find that the person you thought was your friend is unable to give, and instead she only takes. You may reflect on all your close times with her to discover, much to your surprise, that those were nearly all times when you were giving to her. Disappointing as it may be, you're better off shedding that person and moving on to spend time with your other real friends (or the new ones you've recently made). Give and take is important with true friendship, and right now you need someone who's around for you to lean on.

After you've pinpointed a true friend, you may want to ask her to call you or come over on a regular basis to check in, to encourage you to take a walk, or to do some other activity together. Don't be worried about imposing on your friends or burning them out. By asking for help in your time of need, you're giving them permission to ask you for the same when they need it. That's the way real friendship works.

Missing Mom: Coping with past losses

Moms who have lost their own moms (or those they were closest with) can feel an extra pang of loneliness when they first have a baby. Especially if you've lost your own mother, or don't have one who is available or supportive, you might be grieving for that loss especially intensely right now. This feeling of loss happens whether the loss is from death or from other causes, such as alienation and ostracism or simply great physical distance. Whether your own mom is deceased, on another continent, or simply completely out of your life, it just makes things that much more difficult (which gives you yet another reason to cut yourself a break and find some local, real-time nurturing and assistance). It's perfectly normal and understandable that when you become a mother, you'd want your own to mother to be mothering you. If you have strong feelings about this issue, it may be particularly helpful to discuss it with a therapist.

If you've been neglecting any of your friends because of your PPD (perhaps a friend sent you nine e-mails and left three phone messages and you still haven't called back) this may be a good time to get back to her. Even if you just call or send an e-mail saying, "I've been out of it for a while, but now I'm beginning to come back down to Earth," your friend will appreciate that you took the time and effort to reach out to her.

If you have a number of friends who you want to clue in but you simply don't have enough energy to contact all of them, pick someone who's particularly close to you to make the contacts for you. Have that person give the rest of your friends a brief description of what's going on in your life right now, and have him or her note that as soon as you can, you'll be making individual contact. And it never hurts to explicitly express your love and caring, even through an intermediary.

Neighbors

What about the neighbor down the street who approaches you and asks if she can help you out in any way? You may find, to your surprise, that people who barely know you are making genuine offers of help and assistance. If you aren't good at accepting help from people you don't know too well — get over it now! Start taking them up on their offers to buy groceries, drive you to an appointment, or bring you dinner (or whatever else feels appropriate). Often such strangers genuinely want to help and are expecting absolutely nothing in return. So, do a nice thing for them, and accept their offers. You, your child, and everyone in your world will benefit from your gracious acceptance of such unbidden help.

Increasing the circumference to outside communities

After padding your innermost circle with a few extra supporters, you're probably ready to extend your circle even farther. At this point, then, it's time to bring in people from work and other outside communities, including religious groups, support groups, and professional caregivers.

The same general principles that apply to your innermost circle members also apply to these new supporters. Be true to yourself by trusting your intuition, and bring in only those people whom you trust or otherwise want to be closer to. If it's someone who can offer you a type of assistance that no one else can, you may want to bring them into the loop sooner rather than later. But, never feel as if you're obligated to inform anyone: It's your life, and your condition, and only you get to make the call of who you do or don't want to trust and communicate with.

Co-workers

Friendly people who you work with now or have worked with in the past can be a big help, but they're not necessarily friends. They may truly be good friends, and that's great. But, I'm including this section because hundreds of women have been surprised (the bad way) by co-workers who they wrongly thought they could trust. Many women have set themselves up only to be let down when they expect work "friendships" to continue outside of the work setting. You may think that because you've shared so many intimate details of your life with these people that they're truly your friends, but this isn't always the case. So, be cautious, and until you have a secure feeling about a workmate, play it safe.

Keep in mind that because the relationship you have with co-workers is a professional one, you must be careful about what you share regarding your mental and emotional health. If you disclose too much, it can sometimes backfire and get ugly. Trust your gut. If you're not totally sure that a co-worker is a safe person to share with, don't do it.

Religious communities

When I say religious communities, I mean not only the obvious religious groups, but also all the spiritual groups that you may be part of. If any of these groups throw absurd or ignorant comments at you, such as "If your relationship with God was stronger you wouldn't be depressed," you should leave the group — fast. You don't want to affiliate with a group that truly believes these absurdities, and you really don't want to be part of a group that treats distressed members so disrespectfully.

When they're working as they're meant to, religious communities can be an excellent source of comfort and support. Often they're organized so that, for instance, members will bring a new mother dinner on a particular night.

Group support

Groups are a great way to get the emotional support you need, and they're easily accessible — new groups are popping up more and more around the country (and the world) as awareness and training in the field of PPD increase. If you're severely depressed or anxious, check with your therapist to make sure you're ready to pop into a group. I say this because sometimes a woman needs a few (or a few more) individual therapy sessions before she's ready to take advantage of a group. The exception may be the therapy group, if this group is set up to handle this level of illness.

You can take advantage of the following three types of PPD groups:

- ✔ **Self-help groups:** What sets self-help groups apart from the other categories is that these groups don't have a designated leader. If you and your friend walk around the neighborhood listening to each other and supporting one another, guess what? You got it — it's a self-help group.

  However, these groups may be arranged more formally, too, with a set time and day each week. I began running self-help groups out of my living room as I was still recovering from my second bout of PPD. The groups soon became support groups, with me as the facilitator.

- ✔ **Support groups:** As opposed to a self-help group, a support group does have an appointed facilitator who acts as a resource person and who helps keep the group running smoothly. However, this leader isn't required to have particular credentials in medicine, training, or otherwise. Even if credentials aren't required, the group truly benefits if the leader has some training in the specific skills of facilitating groups. The leader should also have expertise with PPD.

  You can contact me if you want training and materials regarding how to set up and run a successful PPD support group. This training provides tools about how to keep the group members safe emotionally, how to decide when to refer to professionals, and how to make sure each member has time to receive support. The training also gives you ground rules for the participants and ideas for marketing and advertising.

- ✔ **Therapy groups:** These groups are run by a licensed psychotherapist (usually a psychologist or a marriage and family therapist). The therapist may allow only private clients or he or she may open the group up to others in the community.

  Unlike the other groups, in this one, the therapist is the authority and the participants are receiving actual therapy within the group. The therapist may work individually with women during the meeting time, or he or she may work with the women at the same time as a group. The therapist, in this case, isn't a participant of the group, but instead is present in a professional capacity.

All of the groups I list here have benefits. But, the support group model is my favorite because it's a wonderful mix between the self-help and the therapy groups. Support groups are especially helpful to women because the facilitator isn't regarded as the one who has all the answers. But yet she helps participants feel safe by setting ground rules, clarifying when necessary, and making sure each person who wants a turn gets one. Even as a psychologist, I never ran therapy groups — just support groups. I wanted the groups to feel like women helping each other figure out their own answers. My role was important, but often quiet.

Typical new mom's groups, depending on the leader, can be one of the worst places for you to be right now. I remember taking the strong suggestions of my OB and therapist (a very ignorant psychologist) and going to a new mother's group. I walked in already feeling like a terrible mom and thinking that something was very wrong with me. I was suicidal and saying to myself, "I hate this mom stuff — I can't do it, and my family would be better off without me." The other moms in the group expressed that their worst problems were such things as how to remove formula stains from a baby's T-shirt! I left the one and only group I attended feeling more alienated than ever, and I was convinced that all the negative feelings I had about myself were correct. Depending on how depressed you are, you may be able to join a regular group to discuss all the normal new mom stuff, and leave the depression and other tough feelings for your PPD group.

Contact Postpartum Support International (see the appendix for contact info) to see whether an appropriate group is listed in your area. Keep your ear to the ground, and ask around at health centers, therapy centers, and venues that are oriented to supporting new mothers. Hopefully as you were leaving the hospital you were given a pamphlet with PPD support information. If not, call the hospital and inquire.

Online chat rooms

Online chat rooms can be wonderful or horrible depending on a variety of factors. For example, it can be a blessing to have the convenience of finding other moms who have PPD without having to leave your house (no one will ever know about your sweatpants and wild-looking hair!). On the other hand, if you're anxious or you tend to obsess, hearing about other moms' worries can make your condition worse.

Another blessing of online chat rooms is the anonymity factor. These venues provide a comfortable environment for you to openly share, without worrying what others might think. If this idea appeals to you, a good one to try is www.ppdsupportpage.com.

Being on the Internet in general can be anxiety producing because you never know what information may present itself or how accurate it is. Let your gut and inner wisdom guide you. If you start feeling more anxious during or after being online, decrease your online time or disengage entirely.

Professionals

Professional support includes basically any person who's paid to be your expert help. As you can imagine, with a definition like that, many kinds of professional support are available. One obvious possibility is a therapist, who can help you stabilize your mental and emotional state. On a more physical level, a lactation consultant can be helpful if you need one. And don't forget a housekeeper, who can unburden you and your partner so that you can have more time alone, together, or with your baby.

Using a birth doula, another helpful professional, can potentially cut the rate and severity of postpartum depression. Studies show that moms who are supported by a doula during labor and delivery are less depressed, less anxious, and have higher self-esteem and self-confidence postpartum than those moms who don't use a doula.

Professionals who can care for your baby may include a nanny or a postpartum doula. Most nannies are paid to care for your baby, but sometimes they'll watch older children as well. Postpartum doulas are trained in baby care, but they also know how to take care of the mother's needs. She can be an extra pair of hands for you — she'll sometimes do light housework, shop, fix you food, and be someone you can talk to and lean on.

Good nannies and doulas are worth their weight in gold. If much of your stress can be alleviated by one of these professionals coming to your home a few hours a week, consider the expenditure an investment in your new family. If you have any savings, this is a good time to dip in. The key is to have great support, whether this is a hired professional or not. You can contact Doulas of North America (DONA) to find a doula in your area (call 1-88-788-DONA or visit www.dona.org). When you're interviewing a doula, ask her about her expertise with PPD.

It's good for babies to experience other loving caregivers (besides you and your partner). I don't mean a different person every day, but a few consistent and caring adults that the baby can bond with. Having taught early childhood education for years, I can tell you that separation anxiety is often less for these babies, because they know that Mom or Dad is coming back and that in the meantime they'll be safe in someone else's hands. As a teacher looking at an incoming kindergarten class, I could always tell which kids had never been away from their mothers and which had. The ones who had experienced aunts, uncles, nannies, doulas, grandparents, or other wonderful caregivers on a regular basis adjusted more quickly and had fewer and less intense separation problems.

Explaining Your Depression to Others

After you've reached a clear awareness of your situation and you've created your safe innermost circle of support (see the previous section "Diversifying Your Support Team"), you're ready to let others know about your PPD. However, you may find that merely telling them about your PPD isn't enough. Instead, depending on exactly whom you're talking to, you may have to explain it to them (or have someone else explain it to them), slowly and patiently, using a variety of different methods, until they really "get" it.

Adapting your info according to the listener

As you'll likely discover, each person you encounter may have a very different image of what PPD is all about. So, you must be prepared to change both what you communicate and how you communicate it, depending on whom you're talking to. Not only will different people have different levels of compassion, intelligence, and openness, but they'll have different predispositions toward the whole idea of PPD being a real condition that takes courage and intelligence to overcome.

Virtually everyone who hears the word *depression* has a different picture in mind of what depression is, how it's caused, and what, if anything, can be done about it. Many people still have in their heads the stereotypical picture of a crying woman in her fuzzy slippers and bathrobe, who's completely unable to function. Even though this can be the way PPD manifests itself for some, it may not describe you — instead, you may be one of those women who pulls herself together everyday only to crumble behind the facade. So, using the word *depression,* or the term *postpartum depression,* may not be enough to convey what's going on with you. Show your listener the appendix of this book so he or she can read about PPD or watch a film on the topic.

What reaction to expect from the people you tell

When you tell people about your PPD, you're likely to get a range of reactions — from good to bad to ugly. If you're fortunate, among your closest loved ones and friends will be one or more individuals who quickly come to understand what you're talking about. These individuals may have experienced PPD or other forms of depression themselves, or they may be otherwise well-informed about depression generally or PPD specifically. Just a few words may be enough for such individuals, and in some cases these supporting people may rapidly and empathetically respond with physical nurturing and offers of assistance.

More typically, however, you find that most people don't have a good understanding of depression, let alone PPD. As you convey your situation, you may be met with blank stares and glazed eyes, or even worse, with hidden or outright judgment. When you encounter such people, it's critical to remember that their reaction is their problem, not yours. Do your best not to let their reaction affect you, and you'll be that much farther ahead of the game.

Getting past a poor reaction

If you receive an upsetting judgmental reaction from someone who's close to you or who you thought would understand, cut yourself a break. For example, if in mid-sentence you realize you've picked the wrong person to share your situation with, change course and deflect the conversation to another topic. You can say, "Thank you very much for wanting to know what's going on with me. When I'm able to put it into words, I'll get back to you."

It's common to initially feel bad if something like this happens, but the quicker your recovery time from the conversation, the better it is for you. No one deserves uncompassionate responses from others, but sometimes it happens, and when it does, the best you can do is just accept it and move on.

You're under no obligation to explain your situation to anyone, including people who want to know and who have politely or aggressively made direct inquiries to you. (Note, however, that leaving your primary partner and close family members in the dark is probably not a wise idea for the long run. See the section "Diversifying Your Support Team" earlier in the chapter for details on talking to these important people.)

Getting personal with other adults

Consider the other adults in your life (not the primary ones, such as your partner and your family). If they're people you're close to, should you just bring up your PPD out of the blue? The answer is: It depends. Really, there isn't a right or a wrong way to divulge your situation. If you think somebody should know — and by *should* I mean that somebody could be part of your support team or network — go ahead, take a chance, and bring it up. Waiting isn't a good strategy when you know that someone may be able to help you if you can just get through that first awkward conversation.

If you have PPD, you're no doubt feeling inferior, and you may be wary of other people's reactions. On the one hand, you desperately want others to know (so that they can help you and so that you feel less alone with what you're facing). But, on the other hand, you may be worried about a possible negative reaction. In fact, you're probably *projecting* (as psychologists call it) like crazy. In other words, you're expecting to see the worst possible reactions from others. That is, you're expecting to see just what you fear the most, since that's how you're viewing your own PPD.

Given your fears, projections, and the real possibility that you may get a negative reaction, it's understandable that you just want to hold back and not bring it up at all. In this situation, though, it's very important to remind yourself that you really don't know how the other person is going to feel or react.

If you find that you're blocked from communicating by fear (of rejection, judgment, and so on), consider working with one of the affirmations in Chapter 11 of this book. Another tactic is to visualize the entire conversation ahead of time. Make some quiet time for yourself, sit or lie down, and then visualize, in your mind's eye and ear, how the conversation will go. See and hear yourself bringing up your PPD; see and hear the other person listening carefully, attentively, and openly; and then see and hear them offering you the kind of love, attention, and assistance that you need and deserve.

If you want, you can write out the exact words that you want to use ahead of time. For example, you might say the following:

> *Thanks for taking the time to sit down with me and have this conversation. I want you to know that I'm suffering from PPD, postpartum depression. This condition is a result of my brain chemicals being out of whack, and my serotonin being too low, following my pregnancy and delivery. This is a very fixable and treatable disorder, and I'm already getting good help for myself. So, right now I am having a difficult time processing information, and I may seem a bit moody to you. In truth, I'm not my usual self right now. I may cry easily, or get angry, or suddenly become sullen and withdrawn. What I really want you to know is that this isn't the "real me." And I want to assure you that I'll be 100 percent well in time. I'm hoping you can understand and support me as I get through this.*

No matter the response you receive, just remember that you have done a brave thing by taking a step to explain your condition to someone else, regardless of whatever limitations that person has in being able to process the information. If you can, have compassion for that person. Just because the circumstances, upbringing, and programming of this other person have rendered him or her incapable of compassionately and openly responding to you, you have done your best here, and you should be very proud of yourself. Also, as you become more confident, the less another person's reaction will matter to you.

Giving the gist to older kids

As tempting as it may be to try and hide your depression from your own children (or other close youngsters) as a way of avoiding potential discomfort, be aware that they'll know something's not right with you. It's always better to be open and honest with kids — they see and sense much more than grown-ups usually give them credit for. However, you do have to communicate at a level they can understand.

By letting kids know that something is up with you, they'll typically feel a lot more comfortable, and you may even be surprised at just how much compassion and assistance children are capable of giving to someone in need. So, take the time to sit down with the children you're around the most.

Follow these steps to make talking to children about PPD as easy as possible:

1. **Ask them if they've noticed whether you've been acting a bit unusual lately, perhaps crying more or getting mad more than they're used to.**

   Make sure that you listen to the children's responses carefully (both their words and their body language) because in the very act of paying close attention, you validate their experience and let them know that you still love and care for them regardless of how strange some of your recent behaviors may seem.

2. **Tell them your side of the story:**

   - Remind the children that you love them very much, and that you love your new baby very much as well.

   - Tell them that you've been feeling unwell lately, but that it's not their fault or anybody else's fault.

     Use words that children can identify with. For example, it may be easier for them to understand "Mommy feels sad (or grumpy or worried)" instead of "Mommy is depressed and anxious."

   - Explain that you've been taking good care of yourself, and that you'll get better as fast as you can.

     Make sure the children know that it's not their responsibility to cure you. But, let them know what they can do if they want to help you out (for example, they can give the baby a bottle, draw you a picture, make you laugh, and so on).

   - Let them know that even though you'll probably still have some more bad times, that you'll get better and better until you're completely healthy again.

   - If you've stopped doing any activities with them — such as taking them to the park or the beach — reassure them that you're looking forward to resuming that activity as soon as you can.

     By showing your children that you're looking forward to feeling better and you're getting help, you're modeling an important lesson: When life throws you a curve, you can do something about it and make it right again.

   - As you finish the conversation, remind them that you love them very much.

If you have a difficult time talking to your children without crying, don't worry. It's okay to show your feelings (tears or not) to them or any other children you're close to. As long as you can handle their reaction to your tears with honesty and they have non-depressed adults around them too, they'll be fine.

Finding a Healthy Balance between Support and Self-Sufficiency

A pervasive myth says that the following is true: You're better off being a rugged individualist and relying only on yourself than taking advantage of the assistance of others, regardless of how freely it's offered. But, it's absolutely critical to understand that at the beginning of your PPD recovery, it's simply impossible to lean on outside help too much.

 Telling a depressed person that they're relying too heavily on others is like telling someone who has a broken leg that they shouldn't keep using their crutches because they may become too dependent on them. Just as using crutches aids and speeds the recovery process of a broken leg, relying on your network of support helps you get through your PPD that much faster and more effectively.

In fact, at the very beginning, just get used to the fact that others may be doing practically everything for you — baby care and housework included. As soon as you can, of course, it's good to start participating in the day-to-day aspects of your life. But, at the beginning, it's simply fine and dandy to graciously accept help. Eventually, as you feel better, the support person will fade into the background as you take over more and more of the necessary activities.

The bottom line here is that you shouldn't worry about becoming overly dependent on your support system. Just because you have to take on the tasks again in two months when your mother goes back home or your partner resumes full-time work, doesn't mean that you should take it on now. Take full advantage of the help you have now and you'll recover more quickly and get back on your feet sooner than you think.

Chapter 15

Helping Your Partner Help You

. . . .

In This Chapter

▶ Keeping your partner involved

▶ Staying positive even when your rope is short

▶ Knowing how to communicate with your partner

▶ Dividing tasks with a business meeting

▶ Nurturing your relationship with your partner

. . . .

More than anything, what you need when you travel through the dark tunnel of postpartum depression (PPD) is support — someone to shine a flashlight so you can see what lies ahead (and more clearly see the real you through the darkness) and someone to hold your hand and walk through the unknown with you. And no one is more qualified to serve as that steady source of assurance than your partner — after all, he probably knows you best.

While you're wading through the dimly lit passageway, though, you must remember that for your partner to go through it at your side, he must do just that. In other words, even though the sludge on your side of the tunnel is undeniably deeper and tougher to move through, your partner is still walking through it too. Before both you and your partner understand that what you're facing is PPD, your partner may be confused, impatient, angry, annoyed, scared, or sad (or all of the above). This lack of understanding and the subsequent reaction may cause you to feel even worse about yourself, especially if you've been blaming yourself. Your partner may be saying things that reinforce the negative thoughts you've already been thinking and feeling. You may feel responsible for your partner's feelings, and you may think that you've let your partner down. Before you know it, you may think that this whole ordeal is your fault and that you deserve your partner's negativity. You may also be afraid that your partner will leave you. After all, your partner wasn't expecting to have to take care of you and the baby at the same time, at least not like this, right?

I can assure you that many couples make it through this dark time together, and when you focus on making the recovery a team effort, your heart will feel that much lighter as you walk through the shadows. Above all, the more your partner knows about what to expect from you and your illness, the more support you'll get. Because the success of your relationship (and the support you need) may potentially be hanging in the balance, this chapter discusses how to accept and nourish a broad range of relationship aspects. The advice given here is rooted in real-world experience (both my own and that of the many clients I've assisted over the years). This chapter can help you get what you need from your partner during this rough time, and it can also help you to understand what you can do to help your partner as well.

Understanding Your Partner's Role in the Battle

Given how debilitating PPD can be, it's crucial that you recognize the effects that your condition has not only on you, but on your partner as well. While PPD may be *your* demon, it's likely to have a tremendous impact on your partner as well. In fact, your partner may be going through a completely different hellish experience of his own. Like yours, your partner's experience wasn't expected and isn't understood (especially at first). You, your baby, and your partner (and any other children or adults you live with) constitute a system, and with PPD, everyone in the system is impacted.

You shouldn't feel guilty about these systemic effects, but you should recognize them so that they can be most effectively dealt with. You need to get your partner on board as soon as possible because your partner is in a better position than anyone else to help you on an ongoing and in-depth basis. It's an obvious point, but studies have confirmed that good partner support improves your recovery, while poor partner support usually extends and intensifies your condition.

In addition to a tremendous amount of confusion, many difficult emotions are likely to be felt not only by you, but by your partner — especially before anyone has figured out that PPD is in the picture. Your partner may very well be thinking, "Hey, we finally have our wonderful baby, so what's the problem? Isn't this what we wanted? What's wrong with her? Why doesn't she just buck up?" To you, this type of annoyance, confusion, and judgment may look and feel much like anger, thereby intensifying any preexisting guilt or shame that you may have. In this situation, what your partner really needs — and what you need your partner to have so that he can best help you — is information and education.

Often, however, because you're the one with PPD, you won't be in the best position to give your partner such education and information. You'll be just as (or even more) confused and disoriented than your partner, and especially in the beginning, you're unlikely to know what's happening. Chapter 16 will be very helpful to your partner.

Typically, especially in the physical and emotional realm (but also in the realm of ordinary household chores and tasks), the partner is the one who gets the short end of the stick. If you happen to have anything left over at the end of the day— energy for cuddling or general affection — that's what the partner gets. And that's all the partner gets — the leftovers. It's far too easy for you as the new mom (especially one with PPD) to put your relationship with your partner on the back burner. After all, your partner is an adult, is expected to not incessantly demand real-time attention as your baby often will, and therefore is supposed to just accept the neglect and lack of attention and comfort. This way of thinking is a mistake and leads to sadness in both of you, plus an array of other negative feelings and consequences.

Thus, partners are often left with the feeling that they're last on the list of priorities and simply don't count for much. The resulting resentment and lack of intimacy can lead to a large and debilitating disconnect, which can also lead to divorce. Sadly, the divorce rate in the U.S. is about one out of every two marriages, and many of those divorces happen within the first year of a baby entering the picture. I believe that *untreated* PPD plays a big role in these divorce statistics. Postpartum partners develop depressive symptoms as well, especially when the moms have PPD, so be sure to keep that point in mind when seeking treatment (Chapter 2 has detailed information about when and why partners get PPD).

Dealing with Your Partner When You Want to Be Left Alone

With PPD, it's difficult enough just taking care of yourself, let alone a baby (and the rest of the household). So, it comes as no surprise that you may feel completely drained when it comes to the prospect of physically, emotionally, and energetically nurturing your partner. New moms often say that they're "all touched out" by the end of the day. The amount of lifting, cuddling, rocking, feeding, changing, burping, and carrying that's required can leave a new mom craving an *absence* of touch. Even without the effects of PPD thrown into the mix, being a new mom can make it tough to have any spunk left to share with your partner.

Wanting and needing to be by yourself is fine. For instance, you may need some space to emotionally or physically regroup, you may be overstimulated, or you may be about to emotionally boil over. The need to be alone comes up for all new moms, but it's especially prevalent with new moms suffering from PPD. As part of taking care of yourself, you should be clear and direct with your partner when the need arises for you to have some alone time — without turning into Mrs. Hyde, that is. Don't expect your partner to interpret your behavior and simply know when you want to be alone.

Confusion is likely when, out of the blue, you may really want your partner to be physically near you — working in the same room, sitting on the couch together, or holding you. Acknowledge to your partner (without apologizing for it) how confusing it must be for him to live with a person who suddenly wants alone time, and then swings back to wanting together time. Keeping your humor about it can help both of you ride the waves.

As much as humanly possible, don't let yourself become "all touched out." Save some of the good stuff for your partner by not giving it all away to your kids. You have more of a choice than you think. If that means not picking your child up for the umpteenth time or having your 5-year-old sit next to you instead of on your lap, do it. The most important relationship in the house (other than the one you have with yourself) is with your partner, so some physical affection needs to be reserved for the end of the day — not necessarily sex — to nurture this relationship. If you're wondering what planet I live on, let me tell you that what I'm suggesting (strongly) is quite possible, and new moms — even those with PPD — make these changes all the time. You don't need to be one of the Stepford wives, and sometimes you'll have more to give than others, but at least you won't be cringing when your partner touches your arm or tries to kiss you at the end of the day.

Kindly explaining your need for solace

Ultimately, as in so many other aspects of a relationship, the key to success is clear and conscious communication. Let your partner know ahead of time that you'll want to be by yourself at certain times, and that it's important that he not take your solitude personally. It's crucial that you communicate that your wanting to be alone isn't a rejection. Try saying, "I'll need to be alone at times. It's not you, it's the PPD."

When you can't warn your honey in advance, the very best way to communicate your need to be alone, whether that means going into another room or leaving the house for a while — is to be direct (without being rude, of course). Controlling your tone of voice and your body language — not easy, but possible — will save you tons of wasted energy later on if your partner feels slighted or hurt. Take the time and energy in the present moment to muster a pleasant tone, no matter how overwhelmed, sad, or anxious you feel, and politely and matter-of-factly state your needs: "I'm ready to burst.

I've had a rough day emotionally, the baby has been crying incessantly, and I can't find my purse. I'll be in the bedroom for a while. Thanks for taking charge." Also, stick in an "I love you" or "We're fine; it's just me" (or anything else that will quell your partner's concern).

If using words when you think you're going to explode with emotion is too difficult, think of a signal — maybe even a humorous one — that will alert your partner that you need to be alone. For many couples, a code word can serve as an effective break signal because it's simpler than finding the right words, especially if you're filled with emotion. If it's set up ahead of time, any word that's decided between you (one of my clients picked "rhubarb") can trigger both a knowing smile and an open door for you to take your walk. Another of my clients decided on "red" as her code word (and color), and she and her husband had fun communicating at a birthday party when she picked up a red plate and waved it in the air. He didn't worry as he watched her walk outside, and he had a hug for her when she came back in.

Here's how you *shouldn't* go about signaling that you need a break (this is my own ineffective strategy when I was unknowingly struggling with PPD): Every day after work my husband would peek through the living room window with an apprehensive look on his face — he was checking to see how many of his family members were crying. If just one of us was crying, it was usually me — not the baby. As soon as he got one foot in the front door, I'd toss him the baby, storm out of the house, jump into the car parked in the driveway, and then sob for about 20 minutes. Even though that was my way of taking a break, I don't suggest you try it.

Instead, you may want to try this set of steps when your partner gets home:

1. **Greet your partner at the door.**

2. **Give your partner 15 minutes to use the bathroom, change clothes, and regroup.**

3. **Let your partner know that you need a break right now and gently (and as lovingly as possible) hand your partner the baby.**

4. **Calmly leave the house and take your break.**

5. **Come back at the agreed time and thank your partner.**

Keeping your cool

Anger and short-tempers are high on the list of PPD-induced experiences. It's imperative for your own mental health, as well as the mental health of your partner and your children, that you remove yourself from the room (swiftly, if need be) if you think you're about to blow a fuse. When you feel your stress level rising and you want to release, remember that your partner isn't a verbal punching bag. When you feel angry, you can easily justify yelling or otherwise heaping emotional junk onto your partner. But, if you unload your stress onto your partner, feelings will be hurt, apologies will be required, and you'll end up feeling guilty about what flew out of your mouth. Instead, the healthy way to handle your stress is to simply leave the room — not in a huff, but just as calmly as you can possibly pull off. Going for a walk can be an effective way to let steam out without directing it at your partner.

Keep in mind that your partner actually is on your side (whether you believe it or not), which means that you'll be far better off doing whatever it takes to cultivate his support (instead of alienating him during stressful times).

Minding your partner's need for space

Just as you sometimes want and need some space, your partner most definitely feels the same way. Remember, your partner is affected both by having a new baby to care for, and by your having PPD.

If possible, try to arrange for scheduled times when someone else can come over to keep you company while your partner goes for a walk or does something relaxing alone. Ideally, you'll have someone on call for those unexpected times when your partner says, "You know, I just need to be alone right now." If you don't have someone who can be there in a jiffy, when these times occur, have your partner agree that he'll just take a walk around the block or be gone for only a certain amount of time. Having a certain time to look forward to makes sure that your feelings of being abandoned for hours on end — or permanently — don't kick in and exacerbate your condition.

Communicating Effectively on a Regular Basis

When you feel lousy (as you likely do if you need this book), it's difficult to communicate kindly and effectively. But, because your partner's support is so important to your recovery, it's crucial that you find ways of communicating effectively, regardless of how bad you feel. The first step to communicating well is knowing that doing so takes some work, so consider yourself already on the way.

In my own case, I hadn't received any professional help and I didn't have this book or any other materials to rely on, so I had no good guidance on how to communicate my experiences. So, the very fact that you're reading this book means that you're much better situated than I ever was in terms of knowing what you have to do and finding a way to do it.

An important part of communication is receiving feedback, so there's a continuous back and forth loop about what's working and not working, suggestions of ideas to try, and feelings to process. This section outlines specifically how partners can enjoy this kind of healthy sharing.

Listening, not just hearing

Women often hear their partners differently from what their partners intend to communicate, and with their hormones in upheaval, women are especially sensitive and can easily misread a partner's questions or statements. Consider a common example. A mom with PPD finally sets a time to take a break to go see a friend. As she's walking out the door, her partner, holding the baby, says to her, "When will you be back?" Her reaction? Yelling, complete with tears, "Why are you guilt-tripping me? This is the first time I've taken a break in two months and you're asking me when I'll be back? I do this all day, every day, and now you can't even be with the baby for a couple of hours? This is your child too!" Her partner, dumbfounded, hurt, and standing in shock for a second gets defensive — after all he was just attacked — and then a bad argument ensues.

Now, if your partner is truly a jerk, all bets are off. But I encourage you to give your partner the benefit of the doubt and assume that your partner was simply requesting a bit of information (when you'll be home). If this scenario describes what tends to happen in your home, next time try to smile and simply answer, "I'll be home at (fill in the blank). Have a great time. See you later." That will be that, and everyone will have a good afternoon.

Scheduling regular debriefing sessions

Also important in achieving effective communication is making sure that you set aside time to regularly sit down and talk with your partner in a calm and uninterrupted setting. (Notice that I say talk *with,* not talk *to.* Communication has to be a two-way street, or it just won't work.) I recommend that in addition to the time you set aside for your weekly business meeting (which I discuss later in this chapter) you set aside 20 minutes each evening to talk with your partner. During this time, don't discuss finances, chores, or childrearing opinions — handle those heavy issues at your business meetings whenever possible. Rather, use this "debriefing time" to connect with your partner.

Of course, sometimes things come up that you feel you just have to talk about with your partner right now, or at the very first opportunity that arises — instead of waiting until your regularly designated time. Unless a real-time physical emergency is involved (your 3-year-old gets his head stuck in the dog-food dish, you need your partner to pick up dinner because the baby projectile-vomited into the casserole you prepared, or a co-worker accidentally put your car keys through the shredder), do your best to resist this urge to bring up serious issues outside of your debriefing time. Forcing an immediate discussion about something that you have strong opinions on rarely helps or produces the result you want — it usually just makes things worse.

You may have to work this time in around the baby's schedule, or you may have to call in someone else to watch the baby for you. Generally speaking, though, it's easier if the baby isn't present because you and your partner can give each other full and undivided attention. But, if that's not practical, wait until the baby is asleep or happily and safely playing on her own.

Telling your partner what you need (without making him guess or making him wrong)

One of the most frustrating aspects of PPD is articulating how you feel. Finding words for the confused and intense web of emotions affecting you can be challenging, and that's putting it mildly. So, to keep the lines of communication open, whenever you do actually have a clue as to what it is that you want or need (or feel), make sure to tell your partner as quickly and clearly as possible.

For example, if your partner asks you how you are, take the time to really check inside yourself and answer as accurately as you can. I encourage using percents as a way to communicate, because this type of system is quick and easy. Because you're giving a numerical answer (for example, maybe you'd say, "I feel like I'm at about a 35 percent right now), you won't have to search for the right words, and your partner won't have to struggle to make sense of them.

If you can't tell your partner what you need (because you don't exactly know either), and your partner therefore isn't always doing the "right" things to help you, a serious rift can begin to develop in your relationship. Because you're not spelling out what you need, your partner is probably trying to guess. Often your partner will start doing tasks or taking care of items that he himself would like someone to do for him if he were in your situation.

For example, one particular client recently told me in frustration that her husband came home and immediately started vacuuming. I asked her what the problem was, and she exclaimed, "I had called him earlier to tell him I was having a bad day!" Now, "having a bad day" to my client meant she needed some emotional comforting. Her caring husband assumed that she needed a house chore done for her (that's what he would've wanted done had he been feeling unwell). I told her that because she never communicated her specific need, she shouldn't assume he knew. She went home, thanked him for doing what he thought she needed, and told him that what she'll want next time is a hug and a chat.

In any case, remember that when you feel frustrated you're allowed to feel that way, but it's not your partner's fault — so don't dump the blame on him (or yourself, for that matter).

Maintaining sensitivity in your speech

Even though it sometimes seems that you aren't in control of what you say, you are. You're responsible for what you say and how you say it. I'm the first person to understand that it isn't easy, but I want you to be empowered quickly and take charge, because your recovery will go more smoothly and more quickly. To help guide your conversations with your partner, keep in mind the following range of facts and recommendations about PPD — many of which I explain in detail throughout this book:

✔ **Don't place blame.** Even though you may be feeling bad, it's not your fault, your partner's fault, or the baby's fault. Often people think that if someone feels bad, someone did something wrong. Not true. Sometimes a person just feels lousy, plain and simple.

If there's a specific problem or incident in question, bring it up in as neutral a way as possible (that is, if you really want to do something to prevent its recurrence in the future rather than just laying the blame). Talk about it in a calm tone, as much as humanly possible. If your partner feels attacked, he'll get defensive, won't listen as well (because he'll be busy trying to defend himself), and the bottom line is, your communication won't be very effective.

✔ **Give yourself time to heal.** Remind your partner that you'll get better over time and that eventually you'll return to your "old self" (or maybe even transform into a "better self"). In the meantime, help your partner remember not to take your moods personally.

✔ **Wait until you're calm to talk.** If you're too riled up, you're overly emotional, or you're just feeling really rotten, don't bring up serious issues until the situation has cooled and you're feeling more calm and neutral. As a general rule, don't try to discuss something if the very thought of it makes smoke come out of your ears.

✔ **Don't lash out.** Do whatever it takes to avoid lashing out at your partner — no matter how angry you may feel. Lashing out is simply not effective, and it makes getting what you need or want in the future much less likely. If there's a serious, ongoing issue between you and your partner, consider couples' counseling.

✔ **Share the love.** Let your partner know that you love him. Tell him that you appreciate all the support you've received already and look forward to that which you'll receive in the future.

These guiding points may seem like a lot to remember, and many of these suggestions are easier said than done. (Do as I say, not as I did!) But, if you can follow these recommendations and suggestions, you'll spare yourself a lot of extra pain and vastly cut down on the amount of time it takes to repair your relationship with your partner. In time you'll create the kind of family life that you had always hoped for.

If you feel as if an issue is just too hot too handle, you're far better off discussing it with a therapist or some other trusted neutral third party (such as a member of the clergy or a family friend who understands the nature of PPD).

Seeing a Therapist Together: Benefiting from an Extra Set of Brains

In addition to talking things through with your partner on your own, seeing your therapist together can be an effective way to communicate and to hone your communication and coping skills. What I'm suggesting here isn't couples therapy but simply your partner accompanying you to your therapist for some practical tips that can help you both. Speaking with a knowledgeable therapist, you'll have a safe forum to bring up whatever tough feelings you each have regarding the PPD. A therapist can address any reactions your partner may have to information regarding your illness and your recovery. Also, you can discuss expectations of child care, household tasks, and other chores with a mediator there to help you. Sometimes one or two sessions together will be all you need. As many couples have found, a great deal of deep and long-term healing can occur in this environment.

When one of my clients brings her partner along, I offer practical advice about how the partner can handle some of the common situations that arise in their home. As the new mom is listening to our discussion, I ask her for feedback. I keep her in the discussion because I want to know whether the mom thinks the information I'm giving the partner is helpful, accurate, and on target. The new mother usually feels relieved to know that her partner is receiving good support and that practical issues are being addressed.

I've found that my clients often like to speak with me by themselves the first time so they can dump their guts out and not feel like they need to censor what they say about their partner or about their thoughts (as you probably know, thoughts can get quite dark when you're depressed). Both getting reassurance about your recovery and feeling that you have a solid plan of action make including your partner in a therapy session easier.

When your partner needs to talk to someone alone

Like new moms suffering from PPD, partners often need to talk through their feelings about their own PPD experiences — instead of simply bottling them up. Even though talking to you is important, your partner may need to find another outlet to discuss what's going through his head.

Often, the partner will have the correct intuition that some things just shouldn't be said in front of a new mom suffering from PPD. Not only will she tend to rapidly fall into increasing guilt or shame, but it simply won't help her to hear certain things from her partner. For example, she may not be able to handle money worries, the fact that it makes her partner really mad when she acts in certain ways, or that she has unfairly slacked off on her share of household chores. Like moms, partners need to be able to vent without being censored, and to do so they need to find the appropriate outlets.

What I say to the partner can be therapeutic, but it isn't really therapy. The information I give, along with the opportunity to ask questions and express concerns, is usually very helpful for the partner, but that's about as far as I go. If actual therapy is needed, I refer the partner to another therapist, possibly one who specializes in dads. If I have permission from the mom and her partner, I'll be in touch with that therapist to help give some context and get the therapist up to speed on the situation.

Sometimes the partner will want to use me as an outlet — to speak to me alone and vent so that he doesn't hurt the mom's feelings. As long as I have my client's permission to speak with the partner, this can be very effective. (Sometimes even multiple family members, including children, call for a session without the mom being present, which can be helpful for everyone involved.)

What if a partner wants to speak to someone, but doesn't want to see a therapist? In some areas of the country support groups exist especially for dads and other support people. Some of these groups, which may focus on PPD in the house, are in the real world and some are online.

Another option is for the partner to talk with friends, a workout buddy, or members of the partner's own birth family. There's a real danger, however, in the partner confiding in individuals who may be ignorant about or downright prejudicial against PPD. If a partner confides in an individual like this, the situation may worsen because the partner's anger and lack of understanding is reinforced. For example, when my husband talked to his friends and mother (who was a mother of five and a postpartum nurse for many years), all he heard were reinforcements about my incompetence, which just made him more frustrated with me. Even if the partner's support people are good-hearted and positive in spirit, they may simply not be capable of providing any useful advice.

If your partner resists joining you, make sure you reassure your partner that he's not attending therapy nore will he be blamed for your PPD. He's just joining you to be a support to you. And if anything about your behavior is bugging him, he'll have a chance to ask his questions and vent his concerns. That brief explanation is usually all it takes to get a partner on board.

Getting Support when Friends and Family Make You Feel Worse

If you have certain family members who you'd never choose to spend time with — or even know — if you weren't related to them, or if you have family members or friends who you love, but who are unhelpful or even downright toxic during your time of need, listen up. This section is for you.

If you're in this situation, your partner can be quite useful. For example, he can slip into the protective role and act as the following:

- **The go-between or buffer between you and your unhelpful friends and family:** If any of these folks want to pass a message to you, make sure it goes to your partner first. If the message is harmless, your partner can choose to pass it along to you.

  If the nature of the message is even the slightest bit in question, have your partner agree to put it in the circular file (the trash can) and spare you and your feelings entirely. Partners often feel virtuous when they assume protective roles, so this kind of agreement can serve both of you quite well.

- **The bearer of news:** If you have a piece of news or an update that you want your troublesome friends or family to know, but you don't want to be the bearer of the news, your partner can spread the word. This news can be anything, including, "If you're sending baby gifts, please send them in the form of money," or, "We're moving out of state and will be in touch when we can." Informing the ones who bug you — no details necessary — can help you be less bugged in the long run.

- **Your personal superhero:** If a family member insists on speaking with you directly — and goes so far as to show up at the door, send a zillion e-mails, or leave tons of voice-mail messages — you can send in the superhero. Have your partner speak to the family member directly and tell him or her to back off until you're ready and willing to initiate contact.

  If the family member is so insensitive that he or she isn't taking strong hints or gentle directions, tell your partner not to worry too much about hurting feelings. Your partner should be direct and say something such as, "I guess I haven't been clear enough, so I apologize. I'll be clearer now. Don't try to contact [the new mom's name] again. When she's ready, she'll contact you."

  Some of my clients' partners have had to turn some of these types — the ones who don't take no for an answer — away at the door. Do whatever it takes. If someone gets offended, remember that this person wasn't at all considerate of your feelings. They're usually not hurt, anyway — just annoyed at not getting their way!

You need a strong support team, so don't hide from too many people (take a look at Chapter 14 for tips on gathering your supports). Reserve the suggestions in this section for the toxic ones — you know who they are. They're the people who make you feel worse when you're around them and their "help" is never really helpful. I call them "energy vampires." They can suck the life juices right out of you!

Sharing Responsibilities

Running a household is like running a small business. From laundry to money matters, many chores need to be done, especially with a new baby in the house. In my experience, having regular "board meetings" to nail down the details, work out "personnel" issues, deal with finances, and work out logistics is tremendously helpful. The more business-like and unemotional you can keep this part of your life, the more smoothly your business will run.

Having a business meeting

The main purpose of a household business meeting is to discuss logistics for family members, household tasks, and other mundane matters (basically, everything you aren't allowed to talk about on a date). For instance, every Sunday afternoon (or whenever works well for both of your schedules), you and your partner can schedule your business meeting and discuss the following items:

✔ Who's on duty with the baby during the week and when

✔ When each of you gets a break

✔ Who's in charge of each household task

✔ How you're handling money matters

✔ How you're handling various child-rearing issues that crop up

When both of you know the plan, your week will likely go much more smoothly. Even though the weekly business meeting can also be a time when you hash out weightier issues, such as differences in opinion about childrearing and how money is spent, it's probably best to set up a separate meeting — possibly with a therapist or other neutral third-party. This separate meeting allows you to discuss such heavy-duty discussions rationally and calmly.

Whatever wasn't right about your relationship originally will probably be magnified and exaggerated both by the presence of the new baby and by the PPD. These business meetings, then, can serve as a wonderful opportunity to rearrange business matters that weren't healthy or balanced to begin with.

Splitting household chores for now and always

These days, as opposed to a couple of generations ago, couples are arranging the division of cooking, cleaning, outside chores, childcare, and other home-related tasks much more evenly. Not that the split is ever exactly 50/50 — that goal is unattainable and therefore unreasonable. The way to go about splitting tasks is whichever split makes sense at any particular time in a couple's life. If at any time, one partner isn't functioning at his or her best, the other should be able to pick up the slack and take care of business. There's always this kind of give and take and balance and harmony in healthy homes.

Sometimes a new mom with PPD is afraid that after she starts recovering, her partner will want to cut back on the amount of household chores that he's been covering. To make sure that the new mom won't have an incentive against completely recovering, it's necessary to come to agreements about splitting chores that both parties feel good about continuing indefinitely.

Problems arise when there's rigidity of roles, and there's either little willing-ness to be flexible or just a lack of practice. Sometimes a partner may react negatively to taking on household chores that he feels aren't "manly" or other-wise appropriate for him. (This can be worse with partners of certain ethnic and national origins.) But, the partner needs to be willing to accept the situa-tion because so much work is involved with a new baby and with having a family — horizons and competence have to be expanded. Likewise, a woman needs to be comfortable filling her partner's roles at times.

If worse comes to worse and your partner is inflexible, you may need to move in with a close support person during this time. And as you recover, you and your partner should get some serious counseling. Unfortunately, the same kind of rigid person who refuses to do "women's work" often won't go to counseling. If this is your situation, you have some choices to make, and I strongly recommend that you discuss them with your therapist so you have the support you need. If all else fails, another option is to hire someone to do the cleaning, laundry, gardening, and so forth. Any competent housekeeper can do the cleaning, and any competent gardener can handle the grounds. If you need help with child care, now is the time to ask relatives to pitch in or to hire a nanny or doula if you can manage it.

Handling money matters

Money is often a heavy topic for couples — one that's highlighted and intensified by the coming of a new baby. It can be an especially sensitive subject if your role has changed from a professional working outside the home to a part- or full-time caretaker of the baby. In this case, much of your identity may have been associated with earning your own money. PPD alone often assaults your self-esteem, so not earning your own money can have a further devastating effect on your self-worth until you come to terms with the immense value of your job (and if you calculated how much money you'd pay to hire people to do everything you do, it would cost thousands upon thousands of greenbacks).

If you find that you may be trying to self-treat your PPD with excess spending, mention this behavior to a therapist. If you're going on actual spending sprees, running up credit cards, and putting your family in serious debt, please see a therapist or psychiatrist as soon as possible. This behavior may be a sign of postpartum bipolar disorder (see Chapter 3 for more on this disorder).

After conducting couples sessions for many years, interviewing financial advisors, and attending classes led by wise and insightful teachers, I've gathered some information that all couples, especially when major role changes are occurring, find useful regarding handling finances. Even though this section could easily be expanded into an entire book, here are just two key points to keep in mind:

- **You aren't a second-class citizen.** Don't let anyone get this idea stuck in his or her head — you, your partner, your friends, or your family. This is especially important to remember if you're now staying home to raise your child and your paychecks have stopped.

  If you're happy with your new full-time or part-time home role but your partner, on the other hand, wants you to work outside the home to make money, you may want to consider either a bit of couples counseling to hash things out, a meeting with a financial counselor, or a combination of both.

- **Except for "fun money," your partner's money is your money, and vice-versa.** The happiest couples share a joint checking account, but they also have separate checking accounts (in addition to the main family account).

  The separate account is used for whatever each partner wants (barring illegality or health-impairing addictions). But, neither partner should judge, criticize, or veto the other. Each partner should receive *exactly the same amount* of money in his or her account each month or pay period. If your partner wants to save enough money for yet another widescreen TV, that can't be any of your business, even if you think it's ludicrous. And the same goes for you and your shoe fetish.

Watering Your Relationship and Letting It Grow

Many times, couples with a new baby find it challenging to dig up the time and energy to nurture their relationship. And, as a new mom with PPD, you're suffering from a significant illness, which makes it far too easy for your relationship to get lost in the chaos. Keep in mind your partner's perspective as well: Your partner thought you were both just gaining a baby, but now your partner has, in his mind, lost at least part of his lover and partner. At the same time, you're likely feeling especially dependent on your partner. You can probably see why neither one of you may feel as if you have a balanced relationship at this point.

"Nurturing your relationship" doesn't mean just being together in the same room. And, unfortunately, due to your new baby and your PPD, this kind of "spending time together" may be the only kind of together time you're having. Maybe your partner has taken a leave from work to spend time with you and the baby. Even though this is good family time, the focus of this time isn't on the two of you.

Make it a point to talk *with* each other — really talk and really listen — for at least twenty minutes every evening. But, force yourself to talk about things other than your PPD (for instance, normal couple things, such as what cute faces the baby made today), whenever possible. Reach back in time to your common interests and whatever it was that originally drew you two together, or talk about movies, politics, sports, the garden, or whatever else you're both interested in. The longer you work at this, the more skilled you'll become, and the easier it will get.

Continuing the dating stage

Twice a month, you and your partner need time alone without the baby. Even though going out to a restaurant with the baby gives you a change of scenery, it's just not the same as being out on a date because you're still parents on duty, not lovers. Your dates should be set on a regular basis — for example, every other Thursday night or Saturday morning. Just make sure your date time is consistent so you can each count on the time together and won't be wondering when you'll ever see each other again. Here are some ground rules for your dates:

✔ **Get dressed up.** It doesn't matter where you're going — just wear something that you wouldn't dream of wearing while holding your baby. Something silk, perhaps? Dressing up is important because you want date time to be set apart from the rest of your day in as many ways as possible.

✔ **Limit kid-oriented discussion.** The two of you should agree to only discuss your child — the happy, cute stuff as well as the challenges — for the first ten minutes. After that, the subject is off-limits, because dates are for connecting with each other as partners. After all, you're more than the mother of your partner's kids, and he's more than the father of yours. (And don't fall into the trap of calling the babysitter on the cell-phone every time your anxiety about the baby happens to get above your comfort level.)

When you're just starting to date again or leave the baby with others, allow yourself one call to reassure yourself that everyone's fine. If you happen to call when your baby is fussy and you hear her in the back-ground, though, you likely won't feel calm — it may raise your anxiety instead. So, if it were up to me, your cellphone would be turned off (the sitter can always call the restaurant), but keep it on if you must. Remember, the babysitter knows how to reach you and will if need be.

✔ **Fluff up the conversation.** After the first ten minutes of kid talk, the rest of the date should be as fluffy as possible. Talk about light and fun stuff like your next vacation. Or reminisce about why you were first attracted to each other. And remember that dates should never be business meet-ings (see the "Sharing Responsibilities" section earlier in the chapter for details).

If you experience some awkwardness, allow yourselves to giggle — even your discomfort can be intimate. Such awkwardness merely indicates that you need a whole lot more dates! You're just getting to know each other again.

Enjoying Mars and Venus: Sex (for him) and intimacy (for you)

Sex may be the last thing on your mind right now, for all kinds of reasons. These reasons, to name just a few, include decreased serotonin levels, med-ication side effects, sleep deprivation, general fatigue, baby care stresses, possible low thyroid, and physical healing. Between your hormonal shifts, your altered brain chemistry, and your overall depressed state, it's no wonder your libido is low. And, you may feel all "touched out" because you-know-who is sucking on various parts of your body all day long.

Nonetheless, sex is an important topic, both for you to read about here and to discuss with your partner.

Acknowledging the importance of "the deed"

If you're having difficulty rekindling your sexual fire, you may want to consider the reasons why sex is so important in the first place. Don't think of sex as your "duty," and don't think that you're doing your partner a "favor" by having sex. This thinking only breeds resentment.

Instead, remember that sex is just as much for you as it is for your partner. Here are some reasons why sex is so important to your relationship, especially now:

- ✔ Sex is a part of who you are, and that part of you has probably been missing for quite some time now. You want to get that part back as soon as you can.

- ✔ Sex is also a way to allow your partner to express his love to you, and vice versa.

- ✔ Generally speaking, your primary relationship is the only relationship you have where you *can* be sexual — it sets your relationship with your partner apart from all other relationships. Sex is designed to bring about increasing closeness and intimacy on multiple levels.

It's important that you not wait too long to get your sexual self back. Only you know what "too long" means, but don't necessarily wait until you feel completely comfortable, either emotionally or physically. Feeling 100 percent comfy may take a while (obviously you need the go-ahead from your doctor). And, if you wait too long, it may be much more difficult to find a way to be together and start things up again. So, stretch your boundaries and get your groove on as soon as you can.

Try adopting a start-without-me-and-I'll-catch-up approach if you're waiting for your desire to kick in. Often, with a little stimulation in the right places, a woman can start revving her engines and then join her partner's enthusiasm. Also, talk with your partner about not wanting pressure to "perform" with enthusiasm all the time. Your desire level may be at various points each time you have sex — with or without PPD — and your partner needs to learn to be okay with that.

Communicating about a low libido

Talking to your partner about your low libido may be difficult, but as a starting point, reassure him that you're looking forward to feeling interested in sex again (and emphasize this fact often). Let him know, however, that for right now, you prefer cuddling and nonsexual touching, both of which are very healing. Sometimes you may not even want these, especially if you're nursing. If this is the case, you'll have to do an even better job of communicating to your partner that you aren't personally rejecting him. Let him know that you're still attracted to him, and that the problem is just your low libido.

As you're communicating about your ailing libido, make sure you put yourself in your partner's shoes (if not his underwear). Right now he may be feeling much like a second-class citizen — he may feel that you have little energy left for him both with respect to affection generally and sex in particular. But, even if you're not up for sex, your partner doesn't have to feel like he's absolutely last on your list. If you can't enjoy hanging-from-the-chandelier-sex right now, you can provide just a little bit of touching and affection — even a small effort goes a long way.

In some situations, the tables may be turned and your partner may be the one showing a lack of interest in sex. His flagging libido could be due to a variety of reasons, such as experiencing the extra financial stress of supporting a baby, having difficulty continuing to regard you as a lover and not just the mother of his child, and sleep deprivation.

As an example, sometimes, some men are pretty freaked out if they're present in the delivery room and witness the birth. He may have seen your body parts in a way that he never has before, and it may now be difficult for him to regard you as a sexual being rather than as the mother of his child.

What's most important is that you openly discuss the topic so that you both can avoid unnecessary hurt feelings and misperceptions. In some cases, if he's having a lasting difficulty in being sexual with you, the situation may require a therapist's intervention to set things straight.

Ready, set, go (slowly, lovingly, and creatively)

When you're ready to have sex (and your doctor has given you the okay), things may feel pretty strange for a while. Your body may feel different and unfamiliar to you, with physical sensations registering in different or unusual ways. Similarly, you may feel quite different to him — especially during intercourse if you delivered vaginally and this was your first baby. Take the time to slowly and thoroughly explore your body together as you discover what feels good and what doesn't. And remember that things may continue to change as you heal, as your lubrication level increases, and as you recover from your PPD.

Especially at first, try not to focus on orgasm — yours or your partner's. Outside of its procreative function, sex is first and foremost a way to be intimate with one another. You can be as athletically or intensely sexual as you want, but if it doesn't bring you closer together, it really isn't good sex, no matter how momentarily pleasurable and good it may feel. Ultimately, it's the closeness and intimacy accompanying good sex that helps you (and your partner) feel much better about your overall relationship. You are wife, mother, and now, once again, lover.

Even though it's not uncommon for a new mom just beginning to have sex again to worry that she'll let her partner down, or that she won't perform the way she once did, try not to pressure yourself. And, if you're afraid of getting pregnant again (nothing lowers libido in a hot second faster than that thought), make sure that you've discussed whether birth control is an option for you, and if so, which method(s) you'll use.

Oddly enough, if you really take your time, and go about reinitiating sex in a nice and gentle manner, you may find yourself experiencing greater levels of intimacy than ever before. The various obstacles that you encounter can lead to a kind of creativity that pleasantly surprises you or even turns you both on.

You do have, of course, many ways to be intimate and even overtly sexual that don't involve intercourse. Don't forget about the passionate kissing you used to enjoy. Be creative and try new things, such as an entire body massage with scented oil or caressing each other with an ostrich feather. Make your nude time an opportunity to get out of the old rut and experiment a bit with the person you love.

Showing love to your partner even when you feel empty

So, you're feeling terribly low, depressed, and empty. And then your partner — the love of your life — walks into the room after a long day. What are you going to do? Well, if you've read the rest of this chapter, the answer should be clear: You aren't going to vent, you aren't going to lash out, and you aren't going to let your partner get caught in the cross-fire if your mood is rotten. Greet him with a hug, kiss, and "I'm glad you're home." You can still be real and talk about the hard parts, albeit with great civility (even if you also experience a release of tears at the same time).

Positive reinforcement is always a good idea. Even though you may not feel like putting on a smile or being charming at the moment, if you're kind and positive, you'll get more of what you want in the long run. Act as if there's no one on the whole planet whose presence would make you happier. And say thank you and show your gratitude as often as you can remember to.

Chapter 16

Helping the One You Love: A Chapter for Family, Friends, and Partners

Maybe you think your loved one hasn't been acting like herself for a while now and you've been encouraging her to seek professional help. Or maybe you're annoyed or angry with her for not responding to motherhood the way you or someone you know did or the way you think she ought to. Maybe you didn't even believe that depression was an illness at all until now. And, finally, maybe you're curious: You're really happy with the new baby, so why isn't she? After all, she's the new mother — she should be the happiest of all. You may be asking yourself, "What's wrong with her? Doesn't she realize what a great blessing has come into her life?"

Lucky as she may be to have her new bundle of joy, a mom with a new baby may, in fact, realize the nature of that great blessing but may be completely and helplessly void of joy due to depression. But with the help of another blessing in her life — that is, you, her loved one — she can be set on the road to recovery much faster. The fact that you've picked up this book is a good sign for the new mom because even if this is the only chapter that you look at, you'll get a good idea about what she's likely feeling and thinking. And as you gain clarity about what she's experiencing, you're bound to be better motivated and equipped to help her get the support she needs.

In this chapter, I show you the best ways to support a woman who's suffering from postpartum depression (PPD). I show you everything from knowing how to react to the diagnosis and how to handle the ups and downs, to staying kind throughout the ordeal (even if you *are* close to ripping your hair out).

In American culture and in other cultures as well, when a woman is quickly active again after delivery — maybe going to the gym, making meals, fitting into her pre-pregnancy clothes, and so on — she's often complimented for her ability to adjust to motherhood. Sometimes she really is just adjusting well. But, sometimes it's more than that. For instance, if at one or two weeks postpartum her house is immaculate, you may want to ask the new mom who's cleaning her house. If she says she is, the new mom may not be sleeping (she may have insomnia so she's cleaning instead) and may need some help. In other words, never assume from how it looks on the outside that she's doing well on the inside.

Reacting in a Healthy, Helpful Way

If you're reading this book, odds are that the time will come when you and your loved one have a one-on-one discussion (or maybe you already have) in which she clues you in on what she's facing. Remember and heed this fact as you communicate with her: Everything you say and do will have an impact on her, whether she's present or not. So, do your best to let good thoughts, encouraging actions, and respect and love be your guide. Before you even consider handling the details of working through this illness with her, think ahead so that you can determine how to best react to her and her PPD diagnosis. If you're totally in the dark and you're not quite sure how to react, don't worry, the following sections give you some tips.

Showing your understanding and unconditional support

It's critical for you to realize that your outward reaction to your loved one's PPD diagnosis is important because it can affect both how she feels about herself and her ability to move firmly onto the path of recovery. Remember that she may be feeling ashamed and therefore worried about and vulnerable to possible judgment from those people she's closest to.

You may feel the urge to offer your opinion, to go into judgment, or to criticize her, yourself, or the doctor who gave her the diagnosis. Hold all that in and wait until you understand more. Any sort of negative judgment on your part will only aggravate and exacerbate the bad feelings she already has about herself. Instead, simply say something like, "Interesting. It's good to know this condition has a name. Thank you for telling me. As you learn more, I'd love to hear about it." And give her lots of reassurance that she'll get through this time just fine — support and reassurance is what she craves and needs.

Stay calm and be open to her sharing. Encourage her to talk, but don't push her to do so. The more you listen in this way, the safer she'll feel with you — and the safer she feels, the more open she'll be. But, if she chooses not to share much, don't take it personally. Her unwillingness to open up to you doesn't mean you're doing something wrong. She simply may be a private person in general, or just not ready to open up to anyone yet.

Acknowledging your difficult feelings

Your acknowledgment of any possible difficult feelings about depression in general or PPD in particular is hands down the most helpful thing you can do for your loved one. I don't mean you necessarily need to talk about those feelings directly to the new mom — in fact, I don't think that's a good idea at all (unless it makes for an interesting discussion after you've worked those feelings through). You need to acknowledge them to yourself and be completely honest. If you're struggling with accepting depression as an illness, for instance, you must accept it before you can be of real emotional support to the mom who's suffering. Reading a few more sections of this book would be helpful to you. Also, consult a therapist for yourself if, for instance, you have some depression issues that are being inflamed due to the new mom's PPD.

Keeping your lips sealed

You have to watch what you say about your loved one around other friends and family members. I can almost guarantee that anything negative you say — any knee-jerk reactions or judgments — will inevitably get back to her and make things even worse (this goes for all forms of communication, including e-mails). If you want her to get well as soon as possible, do whatever you have to do to keep your criticism to yourself (and your foot out of your mouth).

Information about your loved one's PPD is private information and should be treated discreetly until she's ready for others to know. Even if you're sharing the information with others as a way to be caring and supportive, get her permission first (if possible) and be careful who you share with — you don't want to undermine her trust in you. Sometimes she'll want you to spread the word for her, but that, of course, is a different story. (Chapter 14 shows my tips for those moms who want loved ones to relay their messages.)

Getting Information if Depression Is Foreign to You

It's easy to deny that depression exists if you've never been depressed your-self. Perhaps you're from a family that doesn't "believe in" depression. Or maybe you've always been told to "snap out of it" when you're feeling blue.

The truth is that depressed people can't just "snap out of it" any more than you can snap out of the flu. If this is your first encounter with depression, you're likely to be frustrated, confused, perhaps scared, and somewhere between mostly and completely unprepared. So, here I give you some of the basics on what a mom is going through when she's suffering from PPD.

For example, given the nature of PPD, try to regularly remind yourself that the new mom will probably be constantly experiencing a mixture of many confusing thoughts and feelings:

- ✔ She may be relieved that she has a diagnosis, but she may also be embarrassed about that diagnosis.

- ✔ She may be feeling weak or inadequate because she can't cope with her daily life, yet grateful that she has you and others helping her.

- ✔ She may be glad deep down that she has a baby, but she may also be afraid of taking care of it.

All of these conflicting emotions will often bombard her at the very same moment. PPD is known for tossing moods hither and thither, so your loved one probably doesn't know how she'll feel at any given time. Just remember, you don't need to figure out every mood she's having. You're helping her just by showing patience with her ever-changing moods.

In order to be the best support you can be, you really need a good under-standing of what your loved one is going through, and you should always try to put yourself in her shoes — not literally, of course, but enough so that her needs and the reasoning behind them are clear to you at any given moment. Give the new mom a break and familiarize yourself with the nature of PPD. You can refer other chapters or to the resources section at the back of this book for more information.

Sometimes making an appointment with a knowledgeable professional can be helpful for gathering information. Often the professional can give just the information that's needed by a loved one trying to help. I believe that the more support and information the woman's loved ones get (including psycho-logical counseling or help from a support group for themselves), the better off the new mom is. In fact, I love it when family and friends call me to receive their own support, education about the disorder, or information about what will be helpful to the mom. When this happens, I immediately know that the woman whose loved ones are calling has people around her who care and who are doing whatever it takes to help her recover. I provide them with specific do's and don'ts about helping her, and I explain what her reactions and comments probably mean so that they aren't in the dark and guessing.

As PPD becomes less foreign to you, you'll be able to remain more grounded and centered in the face of what the new mom is going through, and you'll be more able to serve her as a valuable resource and ally.

ANECDOTE

Seeing but not comprehending: A sister's outlook

From my sister, Karen Gelender:

"What I remember most clearly about my sister Shoshana's early motherhood are actual conversations we had during her first pregnancy. During one interaction, she explained that because she was on the best diet and was doing all the best exercises, her labor was definitely going to be natural and easy. She was also convinced that she was going to just go on with her regular life after the baby's birth, insisting that not much would need to change. (She mentioned a friend who had effortlessly taken her infant camping.) I remember warning her that things with babies don't always turn out exactly as planned. But not wanting to undermine her confidence and optimism, I didn't press the point.

I was present in the delivery room for Shoshana's difficult labor and for the miraculous birth of my gorgeous niece. I also observed that my sister's reactions to her newborn were very different than my own had been. However, I misinterpreted her early detachment as a kind of shocked reaction to things not going as perfectly as she thought they would. I thought that she'd soon adjust.

As weeks turned into months, however, I was puzzled to observe that my sister didn't seem to be 'in love' with her baby daughter as I was with mine. She didn't appear to be excited as Elana reached milestones. Sometimes, I found myself enthusiastically pointing out to my sister how beautiful, smart, strong, and sweet her baby was. Her responses usually ranged from mild agreement to slight surprise.

I had never heard of postpartum depression. I wish I had. I felt sad because my sister was missing out on some marvelous moments, but I tried not to be judgmental. Were we just different kinds of mothers?

When our mother and sister came to visit, they stayed in Shoshana's home. They told me that things were 'really bad' with Elana and her mother and they claimed to have witnessed a coldness toward Elana that I had never seen. Even after their reports, I continued to see my sister's parenting style as simply different from mine. In retrospect, I feel very guilty that I hadn't recognized that something awful was eating away at my sister.

I wish I had persevered more. I wish I had gotten more involved. I wish I had seen what was really going on. I tried to be a support for little Elana, but I regret that I wasn't a source of support for my sister during this incredibly painful time. I just didn't know about postpartum depression. I had no idea what I was seeing, and I had no idea what to do about it. I must mention, though, that seeing the relationship between my sister and her daughter now, after years of effort, is a magnificent thing to behold.

Thickening Your Skin: Not Taking Things Personally

Unless you happen to be a saint, odds are that you'll be defensive from time to time when you're around your depressed loved one. The closer you are to her, the more likely it is that you may react negatively to her behavior. Because it's your friend or loved one who's suffering from PPD, it's far too easy to assume that what she says, doesn't say, does, or doesn't do, somehow has something to do with you. However, take the negativity with a grain of salt, and by all means, don't take it personally. And, read on because the following sections give you tips on how to best deal with your depressed loved one.

The negative actions or reactions aren't about you!

You may be the suffering woman's nearest and dearest, but you absolutely must keep this point in mind at all times: Her PPD is about her, not you. For instance, if she acts antisocial — which is very likely — remember that she isn't trying to attack you, make you unhappy, or push you away. It's the PPD — not the way she feels about you — that's making her withdraw socially.

So, don't be offended if she doesn't answer your phone calls or e-mails, gets irritated at the littlest things, or forgets your birthday. Instead of taking her strange behaviors as insults, remind yourself that you're important to her, and that she's probably just so overwhelmed that even the tiniest of tasks are now difficult for her.

It's important that you not react negatively to her lack of communication. If you write ten e-mails or make five phone calls criticizing her for not returning your communication, you'll only worsen her depression, because she's no doubt already worried and feeling guilty that your feelings (and the feelings of others) are being hurt. So, reassure her that you aren't judging her and that you stand behind her 100 percent. You can say something like, "I know you're having a really tough time right now. I love you, and I want you to know I'm here for you. When you're up to it, give me a buzz. I'll be here when you're ready."

You aren't the trigger (or the fixer) of your loved one's PPD

Friends and family members (especially partners) often tell me that they feel responsible for the new mom's PPD, that somehow they should've been able to protect her from it — or at least fix it after it happens. For her sake, not just your own, you need to know that you didn't cause her PPD and you can't take it away. This situation isn't like a broken hinge on a door. In a half hour you can't just find the tools, fix the door, and that's that.

It doesn't help that some women often outwardly blame their friends and family for their PPD. Just remember, in general, people are rational beings, so they try to make sense of the irrational way their minds are behaving with PPD. It's easy to blame the ones closest to them, which makes it difficult for you not to take on the blame. But, it's imperative — for her and for you — that you not take it on.

However, if you've been unsupportive in the past for whatever reason, you may have contributed to her depression — but you still didn't cause it. And even if this were the case, by reading this book and following the suggestions I've outlined, you're demonstrating an active and positive change in your attitude and behavior.

Always keep these two important truths in mind:

- ✔ **No one is responsible for causing PPD.** Many friends and family members tend to believe that if they had done something differently — been a better friend or partner or insisted that she eat differently or exercise more or less during her pregnancy — the PPD wouldn't have happened.

  A husband recently told me, "I must not be doing something right. Maybe I caused her depression. She's not happy with me." If you feel this way, keep in mind that, even though sometimes you may need to change some things about your behavior toward her, you didn't cause this. Much of what she's undergoing is biochemical, and your job is simply to support her as she recovers. Recriminations about what went on in the past aren't going to make a bit of difference in helping her recover. In fact, they can actually get in the way.

- ✔ **You can't make her depression go away.** Her recovery is an ongoing process (see Part III for treatment options), and your ongoing support during this process is critical. So, if you feel the "fix it" response arising, simply channel that desire and energy into your willingness and ability to provide whatever kind of support she needs — watching the baby, cooking, being around to listen, and so on.

Caring for Yourself . . .

To be the best supporters they can be, many of those people closest to a new mom suffering from PPD need some support of their own. Especially if you're the main — or one of the main — support people, make sure to get whatever help you need for yourself. Calling the mom's therapist and asking for a referral is my top suggestion. Or sometimes just being able to speak openly to a close friend is enough. If you don't, however, you won't be able to support the new mom as fully as possible. Remember, even if she always has been before, the new mom obviously can't be your support person right now. Instead, all her energy needs to be directed toward healing herself.

. . . *to benefit her*

Ultimately, the new mom needs to know that you, a major pillar of support, are getting support for yourself and aren't being debilitated by your constant caring for her. Unless she knows you're well and being taken care of, she'll be concerned that she's burning you out, that you're getting sick of her and the situation, and that you're thinking of leaving for good. You know that you wouldn't ever get sick of her and leave, and you may assume that she would never think that you would, but in her current state of feeling weak, dependent, and unworthy, she needs your reassurance. So, follow these guidelines:

- ✔ **Communicate the truth to her.** Tell her what you're doing for yourself to make sure that you don't burn out or fall apart.

- ✔ **Be honest and tell her if you do need a break from helping her.** By being honest, she'll then know for sure that she can trust you and she won't have to guess if you're okay.

  If your main job, for instance, is to be on duty every afternoon for two hours, and you need a couple of days off, line someone else up for those days so that you can get your break (just make sure that she's comfortable with the person you choose).

- ✔ **Reassure her that you'll see her through this illness, just like she would see you through one that you were having.**

When you're visiting her in person, make sure that she doesn't end up taking care of you — especially if in the past she typically had the role of care taker. For example, if she tries to serve you, insist that she sit down and let you do the work.

. . . *to benefit you*

It's a commonly recognized phenomenon that when partners don't get the appropriate help for themselves while holding down the fort, they often get depressed too — either during the PPD or as the moms get better. For example, my colleagues and I have noticed that when partners take on the stress of their jobs, take care of their partners and children when they get home, and finish much or all of the household chores without allowing some relaxing and recharging time for themselves, they can fall apart during or later.

It's easy to avoid this trap — just take time for yourself and get the proper support, including professional support, if you're under severe stress. Men, especially, aren't used to being given permission to talk about feelings or to get help, and some men think it's wimpy and weak to accept help. So, if you're one these men, get over it. Do your family a huge favor and get the help you need now.

As a key source of support for your loved one, now's the time to cash in some chips with old friends to ensure that you're being lifted up as well. Let them know what's going on and that you need their support to help you through this so you can give the new mom everything she needs. A simple discussion will help, especially if you're new to depression in general. As you talk to people you trust and unload your feelings, you'll find that taking care of everything becomes easier and that you have more energy to help the new mom through her challenges.

Only share information about the new mom that others need to know in order to help you. For instance, to understand your frustration, your support people may need to know generally how unpredictable her moods are, but they probably won't need detailed information about what medication she's taking and at what dose. Be respectful and present what's going on with her in an enlightened, nonjudgmental, and noncritical way.

Keeping Kindness in Your Countenance

If you know someone who's struggling with PPD, it's important that you acknowledge the effects of this illness, both emotional and physical. You're likely to see your loved one endure a substantial drop in energy, frequent aches and pains, and the inability to cope with simple physical tasks, such as getting a bowl of cereal (let alone addressing the needs of a newborn). How, then, do you act around that person without crushing the eggshells you're walking on? The following sections show you how.

Continually caring even when you're frustrated

According to general principles of law, if you see someone in an emergency — you aren't obligated to save them. But after you do get involved, you're obligated to see the rescue through all the way to the end. The same applies to seeing your loved one through her PPD: If you're her partner or a close family member, you've committed (even if not verbally) to being her ultimate support; if you're her friend and you decide to get involved, be prepared to see her through to recovery, regardless of how long it may take or how frustrating it may become.

Even though you love this suffering woman and always want to be there to support her, the effort of trying to figure out what she needs can make you go crazy, because much of the time she doesn't know what she needs either — she just knows she feels awful.

If you're her partner, you face that helpless feeling day in and day out. So, it may help your frustration, sadness, or worry if you accompany her to one of her therapy or doctor's appointments so you have a chance to ask questions, vent concerns, and stay informed as to what she needs.

If you're a friend of a woman with PPD, you're in a unique position — you can help her in ways that are beyond even what her partner can do. For one, if she needs to vent or wants suggestions about how to handle her home life, you may be able to lend an objective ear. You also may know more of her friends than her partner does, so organizing a meal "help wagon" or a team of babysitters for a couple of weeks could be extremely constructive.

Suppose you get tired or frustrated as the days, weeks, or sometimes months of supporting her go on (you should assume that at some point you'll feel as if you've reached your limit). In addition to calling on your own support systems (see the "Caring for Yourself . . ." section earlier in this chapter), remember that her "best" will keep getting better as time goes on.

When she dips, instead of expressing your frustration or otherwise negatively coming down on her, reassure her that you understand that she's coping the best she can right now (see Chapter 11 for more info on dips). Every time you don't react negatively, but instead turn it around and express your unconditional support, you make her full recovery that much easier. Make a point to do something nice for her at the very moment when you feel like giving up. It will change your mindset back to the positive, and will help her at the same time.

Holding closely the virtue of patience

The flip side of not becoming frustrated is knowing how to cultivate patience. Living with PPD is a difficult situation, and you're not going to be perfect in your deliverance of support, just like the new mom won't always be perfect in the way she receives your support. So, having patience can help you both make it through to recovery.

If you tend to react quickly to things when they don't turn out the way you expect them to, try to focus on the positive in whatever situation you find yourself. And if you tend to speak too quickly when you're angry and later regret what you've said, practice counting to ten before you speak. Deep breathing can work wonders as well. Taking ten deep breaths when you're stressed can have a surprisingly positive effect on your mental outlook under almost any circumstances (it sounds simplistic, but it really works). In addition to those two suggestions, here are a few more:

> ✔ Let her know (nicely) that you need a break and go outside or into another room.
>
> ✔ Take the baby for a walk.
>
> ✔ Direct your energy toward a task you've been wanting to tackle.
>
> ✔ Repeat to yourself, "We'll get through this. The PPD is temporary and she's recovering. I'm doing a great job supporting her."

It's especially important that you have patience with respect to the mom's willingness to share what's going on with her. She's probably embarrassed and confused, among the many other emotions she's feeling, and she may not feel like talking much with anyone. Respect this and have patience, but don't take it personally. Simply accepting your support may be a big step for her already.

Radiating optimism and hope

A mom with PPD may be lacking or incapable of generating something that you, as supporting loved one, can endlessly provide: A positive attitude that radiates optimism and hope. Like yawning, a positive attitude is usually catchy. Clinical depression and anxiety, however, tend to filter out the contagious aspect for anything positive, so don't be too disappointed if she doesn't immediately "catch" your mood.

There's a fine balance between being positive and being over-the-top happy, and it can get confusing for both of you. If you're too exuberant and cheerful, you may actually annoy the depressed mom. So, just be positive and upbeat, and understand that for the most part, even if you can't see the positive rub off, she appreciates being around your uplifting mood. If she reacts negatively, on the other hand, you've probably crossed the line. You don't need to change your behavior — don't squelch your enthusiasm for life — just understand that she may need to distance herself for the moment. The truth is that she's probably envious and wants so much to enjoy life again like you do.

Even if you don't feel particularly happy or optimistic on any given day or you feel bummed out that your friend or family member has PPD, it's still your job to act as positively as possible. Think of it as part of your long-term caring commitment to your friend, family member, or partner.

For instance, personal growth seminars, books, and CDs often teach people to pretend or to "fake it until you make it." The same applies in your experience with PPD: Regardless of how you feel on a particular day before spending time with the new mom, make up your mind ahead of time that you're going to be positive. As your attitude has a positive effect on the new mom, you'll likely begin to feel better as well.

You're allowed to have a bad day. Simply make sure you check your anxiety at the front door. Do tell her about your day — she knows you well enough to know when you're having a difficult time — but do it without spilling the worry onto her. It's a delicate balance between sharing information and spewing anxiety and negativity. On the other hand, don't try to protect her, thinking that her depression will worsen if you tell her what's happening. Her imagination about what's going on is usually worse than the reality anyhow. Just make sure that if you have an anxiety-producing situation that you get outside support (and tell the suffering mom that you're getting it for yourself). Most importantly, don't expect the guidance from her, or she'll take on the worry.

Putting Your Love into Action

You care deeply about the mom with PPD, and now you're thinking positively about her recovery and feeling good about your role. But that's not enough. There are a few more specific points that, when put into action, can make the remaining recovery time and your ongoing relationship even stronger.

No matter what your relation is to a PPD sufferer, you need to keep two important principles in mind as you walk with her to recovery:

- **Support her choices.** What she craves hearing from you is that you'll support whatever actions she feels she needs to take (within reason) in order to recover.

- **If you're attacked unfairly, stand up for yourself.** PPD often shows itself with short tempers and anger. If you're being pounced on irrationally or unfairly, you'll be doing yourself, your relationship, and the new mom a favor by calmly but firmly standing up for yourself.

  Don't yell back at her or be critical. Just say something like, "I don't think I deserved that. When you can talk to me with respect, I'll be glad to listen." Or, "I'm sorry you're having a difficult time. The PPD is not your fault or mine. If you know what you need right now, tell me and I'll help you." Walk out of the room, if necessary, letting her know that when she calms down, you'll be glad to talk.

Listening without trying to fix her (or her problems)

If you haven't already, give up the "fix-it quick" mentality — she's not broken and she can't be "fixed" with the flip of a switch. As a support person, you have to develop your ability to listen to her without offering advice, or otherwise trying to fix her. If she asks for advice, feel free to give it to her (if you can). But, remember, often a great deal of healing happens in the simple act of her talking and you listening. Allow yourself to believe (because it's true) that you're accomplishing a great deal just by sitting there and listening. On the deepest level, she just wants to know that you're tuned in to her, that you're there to support her without any judgment on your part, and that you love her.

When you do get together, invite her to talk, if she's open to it. Let her choose the topic, and don't offer your opinions or suggestions unless she asks for them. Sometimes she may want you to do the talking, however, so ask her if she prefers to talk about her PPD experience or would rather be distracted from it.

Moms with PPD get sick and tired of what's going on in their heads, and they sometimes feel they can't escape from their thoughts. So, offer her a distraction if she wants one, and talk about normal adult stuff that has nothing to do with PPD, her situation, babies, or mommyhood.

Providing the partner support she needs

If you're the depressed new mom's partner, you obviously play a special role that no one else can. In particular, the following types of support are those that only you can provide:

- ✔ **Back her up in her decision making.** If she needs to see various practitioners, take medication, join a PPD support group, stop breastfeeding, or whatever else, she needs to know you're behind her 100 percent. You can certainly participate in the decision-making process, but the decisions themselves should ultimately be hers.

  It can be helpful for you to accompany her to a therapy or doctor's appointment so you can ask any questions you may have regarding her treatment. As a therapist, I find the partner's attendance useful and I encourage it at least once. My client is always relieved to know that her partner is getting support and now understands more about her situation and the illness.

- ✔ **Show her you're a willing caretaker of your house and child.** She may think that all the housework and childcare is her job. New mothers, especially stay-at-home moms, often think this way. With PPD, she takes on an extra layer of guilt if she can't do it all.

  Start out by setting her straight and telling her that it's your home and child too, and that she can rely on you to do your part. By sharing the duties, you'll end up bonding much more with your child, and your marriage will be strengthened as well. Everyone wins (and you get a cleaner house, too).

- ✔ **Don't mention how much her care costs.** She's already feeling guilty about what she's costing the family, both emotionally and financially.

You're talking about your partner's mental health — without it, nothing else matters. During PPD recovery couples use up savings and take out loans — consider it an investment in launching your new family in a healthy way. Be open to doing (and spending) whatever it takes to get her the right, specialized help, not just whoever is covered by the insurance plan.

✔ **Take over for half the night.** Like everyone else, a new mom needs at least five to six straight hours of sleep per night (it's not enough, but this many hours at least allows for a sleep cycle).

Let her know that you recognize that she's working hard too, and that you know she needs her sleep. (Take a look at Chapter 11, which shows you an in-depth discussion on how splitting the night can work, even if she's nursing and you need to leave the house early for work.) Reassure her that you, too, should have bags under your eyes. You may both be tired, but at least you'll be a matched set!

✔ **Practice the work/life balance.** You've probably read your employee handbook at work about your company's work/life balance program. Well, now's the time to make it work for you. Tell your manager what's going on at home, that you need to leave work every evening on time, and that you can't take extended business trips for the foreseeable future.

You may see this practice as career suicide, but it isn't. Many of my clients' spouses and partners have taken parental leave, and have made the effort to be at home on time every night during this difficult period. Federal law provides husbands job-protected time off from work following the birth of a baby or to care for a seriously ill spouse. If you're a domestic partner, it depends on the state in which you live whether or not you'll be covered.

If necessary, go ahead and move off the corporate fast track to help your partner recover. Your physical presence to her is more important than the next promotion, and years from now, when you look back on your life, you'll never regret having chosen family over work. I hear over and over from my clients that they don't care about the big house (with the big mortgage). They just want their partners at home. So, if you're thinking that it's for her and your kids that you're working long hours, traveling, and so forth, you may want to ask her what she thinks — you may be surprised.

✔ **Maintain intimacy.** As you and your partner walk the road to recovery, it's important to maintain intimacy, even if it's (for now) void of any sexual activity. You may be rolling your eyes with the thought of "just cuddling." After all, what's the point of cuddling if it doesn't lead to anything? But for her, just being close to you and being held by you is comforting and healing. She may also have some physical healing to do following the birth process. Just remember not to take her lack of interest in sex personally. This isn't a rejection of you — it's mainly about hormones, brain chemicals, and life changes.

If you're the one returning from work at the end of the day, make sure you greet her first, before you greet any other member of the family (including furry, four-legged ones). The relationship with her is the most important one and without it, no other little person would be there (see Chapter 15 for these and other sex and intimacy issues).

Lending a helping hand

Ultimately, talk is cheap. In other words, it's the physical actions you take to support the new mom that will get noticed — they'll signal to her how much you care for her. Few things are appreciated more than a helping hand. Of course, you don't want to overcommit yourself, but you do want to do whatever is reasonably within your limits and capacities to make her life easier right now.

The kinds of help that you can and should offer differ depending on your relationship with the new mom, but in any case your actions make a tremendous difference to her and her recovery. Here are just some of the many actions that you can take:

✔ **Be proactive.** Don't wait for a mom with PPD to ask for your help — you may find yourself waiting for a very long time. Remember that she's probably feeling inadequate, embarrassed, or ashamed, and that asking for help in such a state can be difficult. Instead, call her and ask if you can do something for her. Ask her what she wants you to do. If she has a difficult time telling you or even knowing what she wants, ask her partner, if she has one, for suggestions.

✔ **Baby-sit.** Take care of her baby for a couple of hours, or come over and be on duty with the baby while she naps, goes out, or talks with you. If she has an older child, invite that child over to your house, or offer to drive him or her to school. If you have children, consider having your kids play with hers at your house or at the park.

✔ **Organize her support network.** As part of her social circle, you may know more of her friends and social acquaintances than her family members do. You're therefore in a perfect spot to pull these friends and acquaintances together and create a support squad for her. You can organize who's bringing dinner when, who's driving her older children to school or daycare, who's calling her on what day to check in with her, who's coming over to keep her company. If you aren't good at organizing this kind of schedule, you can figure out which one of her friends is good at it, and you can delegate.

✔ **Give her gifts (for herself, not the baby).** Gifts for the mom (such as a massage) or for the couple (such as money for dinner out and babysitting) can be much more helpful than more gifts for the baby. It's the mother who needs the extra nurturing right now — typically, the baby will already be getting tons of attention, clothes, and toys.

Here are some gift suggestions (some not requiring money) that you can give or pass on to others:

- Babysitting (or paying for a babysitter)
- Watching the older kids
- Cooking
- Bringing food
- Shopping
- Taking over at night
- Cleaning
- Doing other chores
- Hiring (and paying for) a housekeeper

If you're bringing a gift in addition to your smiling face and heartfelt energy, make sure not to bring her anything that ultimately causes her more work. For example, don't bring flowers or other plants that need watering (unless of course she has specifically requested these items). I remember giving away all of my plants — and even my pets — after I came home from the hospital. I could barely take care of myself and my baby, let alone the so-called calming bonsai tree. Just the thought of other living things being dependent on me for their lives — even if they sat in potting soil near my sink — made my anxiety shoot out through the top of my head. It was just way too much to handle.

Encouraging healthy habits

Someone who's depressed and overwhelmed may very well fall prey to preexisting or new bad habits. At the same time, many of their good habits — such as eating well and exercising — may fall away partially or entirely. This cruel irony is important to consider because right now those good habits are necessary and the bad habits are harmful.

Take exercise as an example. If you know her "real" self loves taking walks, offer to be her exercise buddy. If she resists, ask her if it would help if you came over and helped her get ready (for example, depending on her level of functioning, she may need anything from you coming over to prod her a bit to you actually helping her physically get dressed). She just might say yes. If she says that she really isn't up to walking yet, don't bug her. Just remember that you reserve the right to ask her again in a few days or weeks.

The same thing goes for all activities. If you think it may be something that she'd enjoy, encourage her to do it. Sometimes it just takes a little nudge for her to decide to muster the energy it takes for her to do the activity. Just make sure you stay on the inviting and encouraging side of the line and don't cross over into anything that's annoying and nagging. If she says it's too much for her right now, respect that.

Regarding her nutrition, which is a vital part of balancing brain chemistry (see Chapter 12), be consistent and inviting, not judgmental or pushy. Follow these guidelines to help her with healthy eating habits:

- ✔ If you bring food over, make sure it's as healthful as possible. For example, bring turkey, chicken, nuts, or cut up veggies or fruit. Bringing sugary foods will not help her — they'll only make her blood sugar levels spike and crash, which won't help her PPD.

- ✔ While you're with her, make sure that you model for her what it's like to drink plenty of water.

- ✔ If you're having a meal out together, order wisely and go light on (or avoid) things like white bread, fried food, caffeine, sugar, and alcohol. If she's taking an antidepressant or antianxiety medication, she should avoid alcohol. Caffeine should also be avoided, especially if she has any anxiety or insomnia. You aren't her police officer, but it would be easier for her to resist these things if you're ordering more healthfully for yourself.

- ✔ Even when you aren't with her, consider stepping up the healthfulness of your own lifestyle as a way of strengthening yourself so you can provide her (and yourself) with more energy and support. The mom with PPD can use this difficult time as an opportunity for growth — and so can you.

Referring her to helpful resources

Another way of lending a hand is for you to do the research and other leg-work necessary for the new mom to access the spectrum of resources that are available to help her. There are written resources, such as this book, and electronic sources, such as the Internet, which can be a vast gold mine of resources, especially concerning alternative and complementary health options (see Chapter 9). The Internet, by the way, is only for your use — not hers. Anxiety can easily be worsened by the Internet, so you can filter the information and share only what's positive and helpful. Be willing to check out these resources and make the calls for her (even book the appointments for her, if she wants you to).

In addition, you can help the new mom by finding appropriate support groups and professional assistance for her. The woman herself may be so depressed or overwhelmed that she isn't capable of seeking out and making a determination with respect to groups, therapists, or doctors. You can make the initial inquiries for her, and then help her make decisions as to which support options to go with. As a therapist, I have received hundreds of calls just like this from wonderful friends and family members of women with PPD. I smile to myself when I get these calls, because I know the woman will recover much better with this kind of a support system paving the way. To help out even further, you can drive the new mom to her appointment or you can watch her children while she's at the appointment.

When PPD Escalates: Recognizing the Warning Signs of Suicide

If your loved one starts exhibiting any of the behaviors listed below, stay with her or make sure someone is watching her at *every second* — including in the bathroom — until she's seen by a doctor (which should happen immediately) and becomes more stable (which may take days or weeks). Most of these signs are warning behaviors of suicide, and the last two bullets may also indicate psychosis (see Chapter 3):

✔ Saying things like, "I'm a burden to my family and they'd be better off without me."

✔ Putting herself in dangerous situations.

✔ Talking about or showing interest in death quite often.

✔ Avoiding all social contact.

✔ Feeling hopeless most of the time.

✔ Talking about strange things that don't make rational sense.

✔ Talking about hurting herself or the baby.

If you feel she or the baby is in imminent danger, call 911 or another emergency number even if she doesn't want you to. Having her mad at you (but your family safe) is much better than the alternative.

Practicing Sensitivity: Knowing What's Okay and Not Okay to Say

Given the nature of PPD, what you say and don't say to your friend, family member, or partner, can make a huge difference in your interactions with her. If you're really there to help, you need to vigilantly practice sensitivity and cultivate a strong internal sense of what is and isn't okay to say out loud.

As a starting point, try putting yourself in her shoes — imagine that you feel depressed, overwhelmed, and anxious and that you have a new baby to care for — and then decide whether what you're about to say will likely help the situation or make it worse. Practicing self-censorship is highly advisable when talking to a woman suffering from PPD.

Most importantly, don't approach her directly until you can do it with no judgment. She'll probably be sensitive to your comments, so even an implied criticism could damage your long-term relationship and otherwise set her recovery back.

Leaving constructive criticism by the wayside

Most new moms, depressed or not, tend to be sensitive to criticism. So, when you add in PPD, new moms are often even more sensitive, which means you need to be particularly careful that you say only positive things to her. Praise her as often as you can, and keep criticism to yourself, even if you feel it's justified. Consider the following sets of statements as an example of staying positive with the new mom:

> **DO say:** "I love the way you hold your baby — just like a pro."
>
> **DO NOT say:** "The way I always held my baby was like this."

As a general rule, unless a new mom (with or without PPD) asks for suggestions, don't offer any. And even if she does ask for suggestions, you can offer them without putting her method down. Remember that with PPD, she will often doubt her worthiness as a mother and even as a person. She has enough dragging her down, so you should try to build her up whenever possible.

Lauding her efforts

PPD isn't a disorder that you somehow contract by wandering around the house with nothing to do. Being extra busy can sometimes distract the mom from feeling her depression, but it certainly won't help her avoid the reality of her condition for very long. Acknowledge her for what she has been able to do, however little it may seem to you, and soon enough she'll be able to do more. Check out the following set of statements that show you how to best acknowledge a mother's efforts:

> **DO say:** "This is a lot to deal with, and you're doing such a good job."

> **DO NOT say:** "I never had time to be depressed."

Keeping her stress under wraps

PPD may make a new mom feel like she's all alone and having to face an impossible burden by herself. Using the word "we" can help alleviate that feeling and give her the strength to go on. For example, consider these do's and don'ts:

> **DO say:** "We'll get through this together."

> **DO NOT say:** "I can't take this much longer."

Steering clear of mentioning her shortfalls

Reminding your loved one that PPD is temporary can be very healing. Hopelessness is caused by losing the faith that the suffering will eventually end. However, be careful when you talk about bringing a new mom's "old self" back. For example, consider these two statements:

> **DO say:** "I know you miss the old you. I miss her too, but I know you'll get yourself back."

> **DO NOT say:** "Boy, I liked the old you a lot better. When is she coming back?"

The previous "do not say" statement refers to her "old self" in a critical way that puts the burden on her to somehow bring herself back — like somehow she's in control of the PPD. Using this statement also increases her worry that you'll get sick of her and leave because she's a burden and is unlovable. Instead, by simply affirming that she'll be back to her old self at some point soon, the new mom will feel relief and hope.

ANECDOTE

PPD from a dad's-eye view

The following excerpt of my first bout with PPD was written by Henry, my husband of 25 years. Keep in mind that our first baby, Elana, was born in 1983, long before PPD was recognized in this country. It was about a year after our son Aaron was born in 1987 that PPD started to be officially recognized in the United States. Henry writes:

"My wife was gone. I could see it in her eyes the instant our daughter was born. She was holding her and smiling for the camera, but the smile was fake. I could tell. Her smile, the real one, didn't come back for over two years. During that time, the happiest in my life, my wife suffered from a disease with no name. We knew something was wrong, but we didn't know what it was, what to do, or what to say.

Everything we did was wrong. Her obstetrician told her to take a cruise and buy a new dress. My mother, a mother of five and a postpartum nurse for over 30 years, said Shosh wasn't ready to be a mother. I came from a 'just snap out of it' family, where you took control of your own sadness. That approach didn't work here.

Every night I came home from work, I was greeted with a smiling baby and a wife in tears. She handed me the baby and left the house. The house was a disaster: No food, clutter everywhere, dirty laundry on the floor, and dishes piled up in the sink. It was chaos. On weekends, when I suggested family outings, she grudgingly went along, but I knew she didn't enjoy them.

I thought that if we acted like a normal family, she'd just snap out of it. Boy was I wrong. Family gatherings were abysmal. My wife was a good actress, and smiled her way through, but I knew it was just for show. Driving home, I just got more tears, more 'I hate this Mom stuff,' and more despair about losing the life she once had and hating the life she had now. I knew telling her to shut up wasn't the right thing to say, but that's what came to mind.

I loved my new life as a dad — it was hard work, but the best work ever. I tried not to let my wife's misery affect me, but I'm not as good an actor as my wife. I couldn't keep it bottled up any longer. I finally had to tell someone what was really going on at home. I confided in a trusted colleague at work and an old friend. Neither had ever heard of such a thing, but I felt better talking it out and getting their sympathy and support. Unfortunately, it didn't end the misery at home.

I focused my attention on my daughter, giving her the eye contact, hugs, and love she needed. I wasn't going to let my wife's behavior affect her. My wife would eventually come around — or so I hoped.

A miracle finally happened. My wife recovered and began enjoying life again, and she finally enjoyed being a mother. Only after the birth of our second child and another year of pain did we learn what she was suffering from. It was a real illness that had a name and a treatment."

Remember also that she may be doubtful of her worth as a person, a woman, and a mother. The more you compliment her mothering, the more secure she'll feel about herself. Even if she's not physically able to do much of the childcare, you can always find ways to compliment her. For example, if she's hospitalized, and she has expressed concern about who's taking care of the children, her concern shows that she's a good mom, so you can truthfully tell her that she is. Take a look at these statements:

DO say: "You're such a good mom."

DO NOT say: "Once the PPD is over, you'll be a great mom."

The person who said the previous "do not say" statement probably meant well, but he or she has inadvertently implied that the woman isn't a good mother now.

Making her sure of your loyalty

A mom with PPD may be feeling like "damaged goods," wondering if you regret being her friend or marrying her. To reassure her, make sure you tell her often that you love her, just as she is. And avoid statements that try and force her to get better (which is impossible and only increases pressure and stress):

DO say: "I love you."

DO NOT say: "I'll probably feel a lot better about our relationship when you get better."

By showing up physically to help, and then verbally reaffirming that you're committed to helping the mom as much as you can, you're telling her how important she is and how much you love her. Give her a reminder that even though you can't fix the illness, you can give her hugs and reassurance, and you can share the physical responsibilities of caring for the home and the children. For example:

DO say: "I can't take the PPD away, but I'm here, and I'll do everything I can to help."

DO NOT say: "No matter what I do, it's always wrong. I give up."

Part V
Moving Beyond PPD

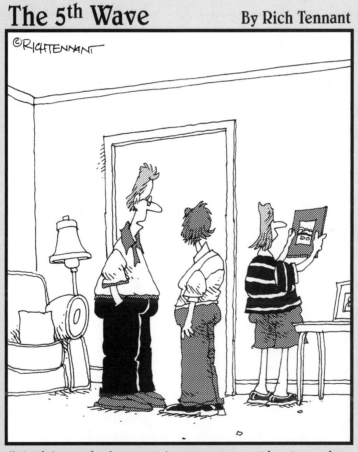

The 5th Wave By Rich Tennant

"I think she's getting better. She bought three 'Life is Good' T-shirts yesterday."

In this part . . .

This part discusses what it will be like when you're most or all of the way through your treatment and feeling substantially better. Believe it or not, you may end up with a better you. You may feel more fully integrated and able to take care of yourself than you did before you had your baby and got hit with postpartum depression (PPD). I also discuss the various considerations that go into the decision to have another baby if you've previously experienced PPD.

Chapter 17

Delight at the End of the Tunnel: Emerging with a New Sense of Self

In This Chapter

▶ Examining the progress you've made

▶ Handling your life and the activities in it

▶ Moving on while taking the experience with you

*N*ear the beginning of this book I promise you that there will be a time when you'll be done with your postpartum depression (PPD) and will finally see that proverbial light at the end of the tunnel. If you've followed most or all of the suggested guidelines throughout this book and have persevered through a treatment plan, not only are you alive and breathing, but you're probably doing very well. You're probably fully on the road to being even better than ever before.

PPD isn't an easy road to travel (to say the least!), but you hardly had a choice in the matter. It's the same kind of choice as that of a woman in active labor who turns to her doctor and birth team and nonchalantly says, "I've decided not to go through with this after all. I've changed my mind and I'm going home." So, if you've made it through all the obstacles and have done what was necessary, you need to take a breather and congratulate yourself. But, don't forget to also shore up any loose ends and make sure that your forward progress continues.

Just like getting through your PPD is primarily your responsibility, the responsibility for creating your post-PPD world the way you want it rests mainly on you. That's not to say that you can't still ask for help at this stage (you should) or that every moment will be wonderful. But having been through the ringer, you still need to stay aware of your progress, your environment, and any challenges or obstacles that come your way.

To that end, this chapter takes a look back at some of what you've endured (if you're at this stage of recovery), and it also focuses on the here and now as well as the coming days. By spending some time thinking about where you've been, where you are now, and where you're headed, you're far more likely to avoid any setbacks or regressions. In fact, you may instead find yourself in a better place than you would have once thought possible.

Looking Back: Build Yourself Up, Buttercup

Just in case you haven't had the time to notice just how good you're feeling, it might be useful to review a little bit of what you've been through and how you came through it. Although the tendency to push the unpleasant memories into the past is completely understandable, it's really not a good idea. You don't want to simply lock up those memories and throw away the key. By seeing and honoring the past, it becomes possible both to fully understand it — to see the puzzle pieces and put them together — and to fully take advantage of it. You don't have to like what happened, but by acknowledging that it did happen and accepting how it happened, you put yourself in a much stronger place to go forward. Similarly, there's a great deal of value to be had in acknowledging what you've been through and where you are now.

Remembering the past: The healing gift that lasts

The best way to become grateful and joyous for where you are now is to remember where you were back when it wasn't great. Remembering the past, however, does *not* mean focusing on and reliving all the negative details — it simply means to generally and briefly review how you used to think, and then quickly come back to the present and revel in the difference of how you think today. Just allow yourself to review your past perspective about your self, your life, and the illness you were pushing through. Sometimes you simply leaf through a journal (don't immerse yourself in it — just pick a paragraph or two every few pages) or speak to a loved a one who reminds you of your successful journey. But the majority of your time is in celebrating now and marking this time as the triumph that it is.

There tend to be two kinds of survivors when it comes to PPD:

- ✔ **Those who try to push their past PPD into a dark closet and shut the door on it forever.** Many women, having made it most or all of the way through their PPD, simply want to forget that it ever happened to them. For these women, the attitude is "It's over and it's done. I never want to think about it again. I'm moving on." (Interestingly, these are the same women who tend to end therapy too early and cut off support systems before they really need to or should.)

- ✔ **Those who make it through the full recovery plan and who are willing to fully remember, embrace, and learn from the past.** I urge you to join this second group. If you try to push your memories down, they'll likely pop right back up when you least expect it.

Based on my own personal experience, and on the experience of hundreds of my clients, I can assure you that you want to remember what you endured in your bout with PPD. Consider just a few reasons why:

- ✔ It reminds you how strong you are.

- ✔ It helps you continue the healthy steps you started in your recovery, such as sleeping, good nutrition, and taking breaks.

- ✔ It awakens you to what helped shape who you are today (as all important experiences do). In order to benefit from the PPD and find some meaning in it — and take all you learned with you into the future — you need to remember what happened.

If you're clear about what happened to you, and what you did to face the intense adversity that dominated your life, you'll not only be more able to enjoy the fruits of your labor (pun intended), but you'll also emerge stronger and more able to enjoy the silver linings that now cover your life. As you face the past, you may find that you gain an even deeper level of understanding, strength, gratitude, and self-compassion. You're probably better at taking care of yourself than you were before. You're probably more able to let go of little things and let them roll off your back. You've probably grown an extra antenna, a heightened sensitivity that enables you to recognize when another woman is depressed, even if no one else can tell. Some women at this point report a sense of "waking up," as if they've come out of a dream or a coma.

One woman I know felt that when she finally faced what she had been through, a great deal changed. She said "It seemed to me that I became aware of my surroundings for the first time in ages. I looked up at my dresser and suddenly became aware that it was covered with an inch of dust. I guess I knew that on some level, but it didn't even register since I was dealing with the PPD."

Every feeling you experience is relative. You know what *hot* is only because you've experienced *cold.* You understand *happy* only because you've felt *sad.* After you've been through PPD, you're more able to enjoy the little pleasures and to stop and smell the roses much more keenly than many who never experienced PPD. To this day, when I feel a complaint coming on, I catch myself and remember that I have so much to be grateful for, reminding myself how productive I can be now, how I can enjoy my children, how sunny the sky looks, and more. I know this can sound a bit sappy to some, but if you've been through PPD, it's difficult to take even one good day for granted, and I know you know exactly what I mean.

Consider German philosopher Friedrich Nietzsche's famous quote: "In life's school of wards, that which does not kill me makes me stronger." It's true that you're stronger for having recovered from PPD, and if you allow yourself to remember how exactly you recovered, you'll be able to take maximum advantage of all your experiences as you move forward in your life.

Congratulating yourself for pressing on the journey of healing

Take some time to pat yourself on the back. It was a long, hard road — one that sometimes seemed impossibly difficult. It took your strength, your courage, and your ability to keep believing in yourself. It also took willingness on your part to discard old beliefs and myths about motherhood and to ignore or brush aside the unkind and uninformed judgments of others. Despite the many challenges that you faced, you were able to push through them, putting one foot in front of the other. You did what it took, and look where it got you — to a much better place than you thought possible.

Understanding the need to celebrate your triumph

In order to recover, you probably had to let go of numerous habits and tendencies that weren't healthy. For instance, if you were too hard on yourself, you had to learn to be kinder in your self-talk. If you held double standards about certain things ("It's okay if almost everyone else is out of shape, but, regardless of my PPD, it's not okay that I'm out of shape."), you had to let go of those as well. If you and your partner had an unhealthy arrangement with respect to splitting chores and household tasks, you've probably already worked it out. And, hopefully, you've learned to say "no" to people when you mean it and to ask for help when you need it.

All of these positive changes took a great deal of inner strength, and it's important that you allow yourself to acknowledge and even revel in that strength. By doing so, not only are you more likely to keep the old crud from coming back in and taking over your life, but you can also keep your transformational momentum going strong. It's not just about recovering or a temporary fix. It's about lifestyle changes. You want to be healthy enough not just to emerge from the quicksand, but to emerge from it as your own person, the deserving queen of your own hard-earned reality.

Because you already find yourself extremely grateful to have made it most or all of the way through the PPD tunnel, you may think that a special emphasis on celebration is unnecessary. Just as survivors of other traumatic events or life-threatening illnesses are wholly changed and have an ever-present sense of gratitude, some women who come through PPD never again take for granted a good day with their babies. Even so, you should still find the time to cheer for yourself, and let your accomplishment really sink in.

You may even want to take this to the next level and throw a little post-PPD celebration party with your partner, family, and friends. You don't have to make it a big deal with dozens of people, balloons, and a three-tiered cake (unless you want to), but instead, have an intimate gathering with those who supported you and those who can help you affirm your strength, courage, and newfound wisdom. Rites of passage are important and should be acknowledged.

Meditating on your progress

Just to make sure that your moment of glory doesn't slip away, take a few minutes and arrange for some alone time, light a candle (if you're a candle person), and then sit down in a cozy spot to read the following paragraphs. If you have a tape recorder, you may want to record the paragraphs and then play the recording for yourself after you're all settled in and relaxed — following an imaginary journey is somehow much easier when your eyes are closed!

> *You've arranged some free time in a relaxed setting, so now you can take this short mental and emotional voyage. Feel your body as it rests against the chair, couch, bed, or floor. Once you are ready, relaxed, and comfortable, take a deep breath, let it out with a sigh, and if possible, allow yourself to become even more comfortable.*

> *Now allow your mind to drift back to when you first knew you were going to be a mother. Picture yourself remembering the feelings, whatever they were, that you had then. Now fast-forward to when you first held your baby, and then see yourself at home with your baby. Watch yourself experience that, like you're watching a movie on a screen. Were you already depressed or anxious, did it sneak up on you, or did it hit later all at once?*

Allow yourself to watch this screen and scan the struggles you had — with your baby, your partner, family members, friends, or with yourself. Remember how difficult it was, especially when you knew very little or perhaps nothing about PPD.

Picture yourself in the middle of the depression and give that woman lots of compassion. Let her know that it will be okay and that she will recover. If tears are ready to come, allow the release. These are healing tears. If you have no tears, that's fine too.

Now, shift gears and fast-forward through all the positive changes that you initiated as you followed the advice in this book and worked through your situation. Consider, for example, your health and other habits and how, over time, you changed them for the better. Maybe your communication skills have improved — perhaps you're able to ask for help — and this left you in a better place with your supports, and best of all, with yourself.

At first, you may have thought that PPD was your fault or that it was a weakness. But now you know the truth — and not just intellectually, but down to your core. You now know that you didn't cause your PPD. With your newfound perspective, affirm in your deepest heart of hearts that you did not bring PPD on yourself, and that you have no need to hold onto any guilt or shame. You may have had certain traits — such as preexisting tendencies toward depression or perfectionism — that made things more difficult for you, but those weren't your fault either. You're completely blameless in what happened to you.

You took on your PPD and triumphed over it. With help, you did what it took to create and implement a recovery plan, and now you rightfully and deservedly should feel good about yourself. Allow yourself to celebrate exactly who you are, just the way you are, right this very instant. You did it! Yes, there's still more work to be done, and yes, you may still have some challenges, but you did it! Congratulations!

Completing and "anchoring in" the healing process

You may be so relieved, grateful, and happy that you're feeling better — a lot better — that you tend to forget that there's more healing to be done and more work ahead of you. You may still run across some dips, whether physically, emotionally, or otherwise. As is detailed later in this chapter, not only have you been given the opportunity to heal yourself vis-à-vis your PPD, but a silver lining may also be peeking through at this point: You have the opportunity to recreate yourself and put yourself back together even better than you were in the first place. It often takes hitting a crisis before healthful and necessary changes are finally made.

ANECDOTE

A mommy's miracle, from yours truly

As the president of Postpartum Support International, I attended the annual conference during the process of writing this book. My term was up, and I passed the torch to the incoming president. My daughter's graduation from college was scheduled for the very next morning, so I flew all night to arrive a few hours before she crossed the stage. Elana's birth and my subsequent postpartum illness had launched the beginning of my new career and mission in life. I had completed the journey, and I experienced a poetic feeling that I'm still having a hard time putting into words. From depressed special education teacher to president of our international organization to a mother watching her baby — the one who suffered through my PPD — graduate with honors. This girl was one who, due to my untreated PPD and inability to even give her eye contact, developed an attachment disorder that led to life-threatening self-destructive activities and no desire to go to college, which in turn almost led to the failing of high school. With great strength she pulled herself together,

physically and emotionally, and did what she had to do to survive and finally feel good about herself.

As I watched her at the ceremony, both of us glowing with joy, an unexplainable miracle occurred. My mind filled with visions of tenderly holding my newborn daughter, gazing at her with tremendous love, bonding with her like normal mommies do — something I had never experienced, until that moment. I welled up with tears, realizing that I was *finally* getting to experience what I thought was a long-lost opportunity!

I'm here to tell you that it's never too late. My baby girl finally knows her mommy loves her, and I'm feeling closer to her than I ever thought possible. We've been enjoying this newfound relationship for a few years now, but that graduation ceremony was my private miracle. I'm writing this book to help you from the very beginning, so you and your child can be spared what Elana and I went through. There's always hope. Never, ever give up.

REMEMBER

The point is that you need to stay present and motivated with respect to your healing process. By doing so, you can anchor in the new, healthy ways and make sure that all your new good habits, ways of thinking, and ways of relating to yourself and others really stick. Having come this far, why not make sure that you hold on to all the positive changes that you've made? And why not continue to set the stage for creating a better-than-ever you?

Some women rely on affirmations to keep themselves motivated, as I discuss in Chapter 20. Feel free to come up with an affirmation that works for you — and give it some rhythm to help you remember it. After you choose an appropriately uplifting affirmation, remember to say it to yourself (with purpose and meaning) a couple of times a day, ideally upon awakening and going to sleep. Your subconscious mind takes seriously what you say to yourself consciously.

Continuing with therapy and support groups (online or in the real world) is another useful possibility for some women. You've been through a really difficult time, so don't be too quick to cut off the support mechanisms that really made a difference to you. Slow and steady wins that race here, and if you happen to dip, you'll be glad that you still have some of your support mechanisms in place.

If and when you joined your first support group, there may have been one or two women who were then where you are now — well on their way to health. It probably felt great to have them there to give you hope. What you may not have realized is that you were giving them a gift as well. Part of recovery is seeing how far you've come. There's nothing like being the one in the group who's now saying to the newcomers, "I felt just like you do when I first started. Hang in there. You'll get through it." You'll derive great satisfaction and therapeutic benefit from doing this for others.

Taking Back the Reigns

You've probably already found that you've begun to feel more and more like your old self, and your activity level has probably picked up quite a bit. Still, it's important that you take a moderate pace after you take back the reigns and regain full control over the direction of your life. After all, you did go through an ordeal, and some of its aftereffects (including, perhaps, a wee bit of self-doubt) may potentially be lingering. Just take it one step at a time and you'll be surprised or even delighted at just how well you're able to handle things that not long ago would have overwhelmed you.

There are good, solid ways to move forward as you take back your life (and adjust to the new parts about having a baby), and I offer them to you in the following sections.

Setting realistic goals

An important task that you want to undertake as you feel better and better is setting goals for yourself. When you set goals, you give yourself something to shoot for, and as you feel good about achieving your goals, you gain even more energy and feel even better about yourself, which enables you to set and achieve additional goals.

As you start setting goals for yourself, it's critical that you set yourself up for success by setting realistic goals. After you start feeling like your old self again, it's tempting to want to bite off more than you can actually chew. You may find that you're saying to yourself something like, "Great! I'm finally coming back! Now I'm going to do all of those things that I haven't been able to do for so long. Look at that messy closet, untended garden, and all those loose pictures. I want to take care of all these chores right away!" You'll often have this sense of urgency because you're so used to these good times being suddenly ripped away again. It's difficult to trust that those times are lasting longer and longer. But, in reality, you don't have to rush and do everything to take advantage of those times. You can actually start trusting that the good times will last and eventually be here to stay.

Luckily, you have an accurate built-in feedback device — your body. If you're attempting to do too much, your body will quickly let you know, and you may find yourself dipping in mood. A better plan is to try and protect yourself from getting to this point. Instead, scale back your ambitious goals from the start. You can break down projects into manageable chunks, which allows you to feel good if you get to one or two of them.

Similarly, you can look at the calendar and say to yourself "Even though I'd love to attend all three of the local events I've been invited to — the baby shower, the neighbor's birthday party, and the community barbeque — it's probably not a good idea to commit to all three." Pick one, or maybe two of them, and that's it.

The wonderful news, of course, is that overall you feel like you can do more, and, in fact, you are doing more. Just don't do too much too soon. Life, especially life with a child or children, is like a long race, and you're much more likely to get across the finish line with poise and confidence if you pace yourself. (Even Lance Armstrong didn't ride as hard as he could on every leg of the Tour de France.) Be realistic with yourself about how you feel and about your overall energy level, and enjoy the fact that even though you may not be fully recovered yet, you're clearly doing much better than you previously were.

Making decisions again

As you feel better, you'll find that there are so many types of decisions that you're now ready and able to make — decisions that may have once overwhelmed you. As part of your healing process, you were probably deferring a great deal of the decision making in your life to your partner, if you have one, or to the other professionals or support people who you were relying on. In addition, at the beginning of this book, I specifically suggested that you not make any major life decisions (for example moving, marrying, or returning to your old job outside the house).

Depression can make any kind of decision extremely difficult, so as you're feeling better and better, take back the decision-making reigns on everything from small decisions to large ones (no need to get controlling, though!). In some cases you'll be the sole decision maker, just like you once were, and in others you'll return to the status of co-decision maker with your partner. And as you fully recover, you may just find yourself taking over the decision making in areas that you once had no interest in or were excluded from. You can continue to make changes and renegotiate these as well. In any case, you can enjoy the fact that you're once again an active participant in the many decisions that are part and parcel of your life.

If you haven't already done so, start with everyday decisions that you may have let go of. Now that you're mostly or completely through the PPD tunnel and into the light, it probably won't prove very difficult for you to decide what's for dinner, if you want to join your co-workers for an evening out, or whether to schedule an appointment. If you can, decide to take some pleasure in the sheer fact that you're once again making decisions.

Ultimately, there aren't any mistakes, just opportunities for further learning. Take, for example, the decision about using a pacifier with your baby. Well, there are as many opinions about this issue as there are "experts," and no one knows what the "right" answer is for your family. So, the best you can do is review the information that you have, make your decision, and see how things go.

If you have a tendency to put yourself down when things don't go exactly the way you planned, try to remember that beating yourself up is useless (and is an aspect of PPD that you've mostly or completely recovered from and don't want to return to). Instead, congratulate yourself for having felt well enough to make a decision in the first place, regardless of how things turned out. Think back to when you could barely make any decisions at all, take a deep breath, and then move on to the next decision.

Taking over tasks

One type of decision you want to make is whether or not you're ready to take over household chores and day-to-day tasks. Presumably you and your partner reached an understanding about your previously diminished capacities, thereby letting you out of some or all of the ongoing chores necessary to keep life going, such as cooking, shopping, cleaning, laundry, yard work, childcare, bill paying, and so on. Perhaps your partner took over most of this, or perhaps you received other outside assistance. Now that you're feeling better, it's time to get reacquainted with the day-to-day tasks of your daily life.

You don't have to suddenly start doing 100 percent (or more) of everything that you used to do all at once. Communicate with your partner or other support people about how much you feel you're ready for. Set a reasonable schedule for yourself, and check in often about whether you're able to keep that schedule. You may surprise yourself and find that you're ready for more than you think, or you may be a little disappointed when it turns out that you bit off more than you could chew. But even then, acknowledge that simply recognizing that you may have tried to do too much too soon indicates that overall you're vastly improved compared to where you once were. The point here is that if you go slowly and consciously, you can't but help come out a winner as you pick up the tasks that you once had to let go.

Some of the changes you'll want to keep, such as having your partner continue to be fully involved with taking care of the baby. (It would be sad for all of you if your recovery meant that the baby and his daddy didn't spend as much time together.) This example is another silver lining — and there are tons more. What began as a necessity due to a crisis, you and your partner may want to keep as your new, healthy way. On this note, be sensitive to your partner, because he may suddenly feel as if he's being pushed aside as the recovered you emerges. Even though he'll undoubtedly feel relief on some level and happiness for you, he can also start feeling useless or unappreciated because of all he's been doing and is no longer overseeing. Of course, don't assume that completely taking over the house or baby care is what he wants. The point is, as you recover, you can redo your expectations not only for yourself but also for your partnership and family.

Feeling Like Yourself . . . Or Even Better

You're probably wondering how you know if you're all the way back to your old self when, in reality, you're now a new self with a new child? Most of what you'll feel is the familiar "you" before pregnancy. You'll recognize her — she's the one you've been missing. Of course, the exact moment that you're back — if there is an exact moment — will be different for every woman. And then you have the adjustment to new motherhood on top — that's the new part that you'll be incorporating into your life and that will take time.

One woman I know realized she was back when she found herself singing in the shower again. (Actually, it was her husband who let her know — she wasn't even aware until he told her that she had resumed this joyful lifetime habit!) Some women have a moment when they notice that they enjoy things from the past again, such as reading mystery novels, watching movies, or even going grocery shopping. Another woman I know became aware that she had fully returned to her old self when her husband light-heartedly mentioned that she was getting ornery again.

Whenever you notice those moments that your old self is back, take time out to congratulate yourself (see the section "Congratulating yourself for pressing on the journey of healing" earlier in the chapter for tips). And while you're at it, take a quick inventory of the ways in which you're not only back to who you were, but perhaps are even a bit *better* than you were before. For example:

✔ Maybe you didn't have good communication about certain issues with your partner during your marriage and when the PPD first overtook you, but the PPD forced you to communicate with him and work things out.

✔ Maybe you weren't good at saying no to people in general or at asking for help. Or maybe you weren't particularly good at setting realistic goals and not being hard on yourself when you didn't reach them all. If any of these were the case for you, in order to emerge on the other side of that dark tunnel, you probably uncovered existing strengths and developed new ones entirely.

When you emerge from PPD, you may be aware that other moms, those who didn't go through PPD, seem a bit ahead of you regarding knowledge about everyday baby things. This is normal, so don't worry — you'll catch up quickly. You see, they jumped right into new motherhood and started adapting to their new role, doing the normal new mom things earlier than you did. It's not a judgment, just a fact. Now you'll be learning and feeling what the other moms have been doing for a while now. If you haven't already, now it would be appropriate, if you so desire, to join a regular new mother's group.

You truly are better than ever, and the coping skills and inner strength that you uncovered and learned how to use will continue to serve you as you move forward and help you create the life that you always wanted (or better!).

Chapter 18

Deciding Whether to Have Another Baby

*D*eciding whether to have another baby is a big decision for any woman. On the one hand, giving birth to new life is, in and of itself, a miraculous process, and for many women (and their partners) the excitement of expanding their family is incalculably great. On the other hand, having another baby is an all-encompassing event that has many physical, emotional, and financial implications and possible downsides. In short, even for a woman who hasn't experienced postpartum depression (PPD), the decision to bring another child into the home, whether by birth or adoption, is a breathtakingly huge one that demands careful consideration, contemplation, and planning.

Now consider the woman who has previously been afflicted by PPD. As I discuss in this chapter, her fear that she may experience PPD again — and that she's at an even higher risk of getting it than someone who has never had PPD — is a real and justifiable fear. So, the woman who previously had PPD and who's contemplating another pregnancy (or who is already pregnant) is well-advised to seek professional consultation so she can prepare herself properly. In other words, she should first make sure to carefully examine her situation, including her risk of another round of PPD, and then do whatever is possible to lessen the effects of that potential bout with PPD (or to avoid it entirely).

This chapter discusses some of the considerations of having another baby when you're at high risk for PPD and other postpartum mood disorders. I also discuss the best ways to set up your pre-pregnancy, pregnancy, and postpartum plans to help ensure the best outcome if you choose to move forward with the baby-making. Just remember: Being high risk doesn't need to scare you away from having another baby if you want one.

First Things First: Assessing Your Intentions

The decision to have another baby (whether or not you've had PPD) should be made for the right reasons — you want to expand your family and you're looking forward to having another child to love, for example — not the wrong ones. If, for example, you're saying to yourself, "This time I'll get it right and won't get depressed," or, "This time I know I'll be able to breastfeed," you may very well be setting yourself up for failure.

This kind of thinking implies that you did it "wrong" the first time, which obviously isn't true. As I point out many times in this book, you should never feel any guilt or shame if you had PPD. Yes, it's something that happened to you, but no, it's not something you were responsible for, something you caused, or something that reflects your ultimate self-worth or value. Also, thinking that having another baby will somehow "fix" things puts way too much pressure on you, your new baby, your other children, and your partner. If you do happen to encounter PPD again, you may end up blaming yourself and your new baby, which will only make things worse.

The bottom line is that having another baby won't change the past, won't prove anything to anyone, and won't heal you deep down in those places that only a competent therapist is likely to help you reach. So, just forget the idea that having another baby will make everything about your life better. If you're going to decide to have another baby, do it because you and your partner really *want* to have another baby, really *want* to bring new life into this world, and really *want* to expand your family in a way that's in alignment with your deepest beliefs and visions of a good life.

In fact, you should *want* to have another baby so badly that even if you do get PPD again, not only will you be expecting this possibility and be prepared for it, but you'll, in some fundamental sense, be okay with the PPD if it should actually hit. In other words, if you're having another baby for the right reasons — and if you have thought things through and have prepared as best you can — the possibility that you may have PPD again is something that you will have already accepted and prepared for. You'll be able to accept the possibility of going through another round of PPD as one more "cost" of having the baby, which, in the grand scheme of things, is something you'll be willing to bear.

Making an Informed Decision, Sans Fear

Ideally, the decision to have another baby is one that's made only after careful thought and consideration. Please understand that if you decide not to have another baby based on the fact that you're high risk, that's fine. Likewise, it's also fine if you decide to go ahead with plans to have another. This decision is personal, and no one but you knows what the best decision for you and your family is. About one-third of women who previously experienced PPD don't want to ever get pregnant again, and many of these women, depending on their circumstances, choose adoption, abortion (if already pregnant), or sterilization (to make certain that they never run the risk of experiencing PPD again).

Such choices — adoption, abortion, sterilization — are based on the intense and understandable fear that PPD may strike again. Depending on your specific situation and ethical values, these may be valid choices. But the fear of another bout of PPD can usually be addressed so that you don't make any of those choices out of fear. I've been working with high-risk women long enough to see them through another one, two, three (and sometimes more) pregnancies and deliveries. These subsequent pregnancies and postpartum times are much more positive. After a woman has a solid, comprehensive plan of action with physical and emotional support, medication (if needed), excellent nutrition, sleep, exercise, breaks, and whatever else she specifically needs (all of which I discuss throughout this book), PPD (or another mood disorder) doesn't have a chance to take hold. I believe in aggressive prevention, and the results I've seen have been excellent.

The only way to ensure that you're making an informed decision about whether to have another baby or how to proceed with the plan of doing so is to collect the facts. In the following sections, I present — in as condensed a form as possible (which wasn't easy!) — the relevant points that can help you make those decisions.

Sizing up your risk of getting PPD again

Whether or not you get PPD again depends on many factors, including the various reasons and predisposing factors that may explain why you got it the first time. Even though you're automatically at high risk for getting it again, it's unlikely that you (or anyone else, for that matter, including medical professionals) will be able to determine exactly how likely you are to be afflicted following a subsequent delivery. Some women with no identifiable risk factors get hit hard with PPD, and then others with many risk factors escape entirely.

Sometimes (especially in retrospect) it's obvious why a woman gets PPD after one delivery and not after another, and sometimes it seems completely random. For example, if a woman abruptly dropped her antidepressant before she delivered (never a good idea) because she heard from an untrustworthy source that it wasn't good with breastfeeding, it makes sense that she was hit hard with PPD. Or, when listing the high stress factors in a woman's life after her last round of PPD and recognizing that she had just moved away from her wonderful family, her partner was completely unsupportive and having an affair, her baby had colic, and her hypothyroid condition hadn't been diagnosed yet, it's pretty clear why she had PPD. However, even though all your ducks may be in a row and the planets are aligned just right, it's still possible that you suddenly find yourself in the pit of postpartum depression.

The key point here is that if you've had PPD once before, you're indeed more likely to be affected by it again. In any case, if you've already had PPD, it would be foolhardy to assume that you won't get it again (and to therefore not plan for it). Whether you know you're at high risk or not, you should always have a postpartum plan because you never know — no one's immune to PPD's grip.

Women who have had PPD previously have at least a 50 percent chance of having their PPD reoccur with a subsequent baby. Some women who have had PPD have the mistaken idea that, "Because I was depressed the first time, and I now understand what it's all about, having a baby won't hit me so hard this time." I have even had reports of healthcare professionals telling high-risk women that they wouldn't have PPD again. Unfortunately, this isn't the way it works, and the new mom who has experience with PPD is much better off not sticking her head in the sand and just hoping that her PPD won't come back. It's better to be prepared even though it may not happen than to be in denial of its likelihood and then go through unnecessary suffering.

Through the years I've heard couples (in which the woman is often already pregnant) squabble about whether they should "go there" and even talk about the possibility of another round of PPD. One is saying, "Let's just talk about a plan just in case it happens again — it will give me peace of mind" and the other one is saying, "Why talk about it? How could it help to think negatively?"

The person who wants to ignore the issue, whether it's the woman or her partner, is operating with the misconception that if you talk about PPD, it will happen. Not true at all. As a matter of fact, when a plan of action is in place — including a discussion about who will be on duty at night, when breaks will be, who will take care of meals, and so on — the chance of PPD happening is reduced. If the PPD still occurs, at the very least, the severity will likely be reduced). So, it's always a good idea, whether you're at high risk or not, to have a postpartum plan in place.

I've given you this realistic assessment of your odds of getting PPD again not to scare you, but so that you know the risks and can be smart about preparation. The bulk of this chapter shows you the kind of plan that you should come up with to either avoid PPD or decrease its effects. At the very first signs of depression after delivery — or depression during pregnancy (which makes PPD itself much more likely) — you should start taking active steps to implement your plan (or to come up with your plan if you don't already have one). Most of the plan to cure PPD is the same plan to help prevent it, so if you've been taking care of yourself in the best ways, chances are most of the plan is already in place.

Knowing the truth about PPD and postpartum psychosis

Even though postpartum psychosis (PPP) is fairly rare (around 2 of every 1,000 women get it), the question nonetheless may arise in the mind of a mom who has already had PPD whether having another baby may lead not just to PPD, but to PPP. After all, earlier in this chapter, I stated that having had PPD once can make a woman more likely to experience it again if she has another baby. So you may be thinking "If PPD is more likely, is it possible that PPP becomes more likely as well? Can PPD serve as a kind of gateway disorder that leads to PPP?" The answer is a resounding no.

It's important to keep the following facts about PPD, PPP, and their relationship in mind:

✔ Postpartum psychosis is *not* just a really bad case of PPD, but rather, is a very different disorder.

✔ Untreated PPD can easily become a worse case of PPD, but it does *not* turn into PPP.

✔ PPP involves a complete break with reality, and no such break with reality is experienced or observed in cases of PPD (yes, the woman with PPD may want to hide from everyone and everything or disengage from her world, but that's different from completely losing her grip on what actually constitutes her reality).

✔ Having PPD does *not* make a woman more vulnerable to, nor in any way increase the odds of her being struck with, PPP.

To read more about PPP, flip to Chapter 3, where I go over the symptoms and generalities of this and other postpartum disorders.

Andrea Yates and the risks of postpartum psychosis

In June of 2001, Andrea Yates achieved infamy by methodically drowning all five of her children (ages 7, 5, 3, 2, and 6 months) in her bathtub. She called 9-1-1 and was arrested soon after. Later, she claimed that she was suffering from a severe case of postpartum psychosis, or PPP. Her PPP was recurrent, and she had her first episode of PPP after the delivery of her fourth child. Yates may have also been suffering from other types of mental illness, which apparently run in her family.

Yates's legal defense rested on a claim of insanity because of the PPP. In March of 2002, a Texas jury rejected her insanity defense, found her guilty, and she was sentenced to life in prison with no possibility of parole for 40 years. Some four years later, in January of 2005, the Texas Court of Appeals reversed her conviction in part because a psychiatrist who had given evidence against her had given false testimony during the trial (concerning whether similar events, including a successful plea of insanity, had been televised on the show Law & Order shortly before Yates drowned her children). Most recently, in July of 2006, after deliberating for three days, a jury thankfully found Yates not guilty by reason of insanity according to the laws of Texas. At the time of this writing, Yates was committed to a state mental hospital.

Yates had previously been urged by a psychiatrist not to have more children because the psychiatrist felt that to do so would guarantee a future psychosis in her. Yates had also been on a heavy dose of anti-psychotic medication, but was taken off of all of her medications only two weeks prior to the drownings. Lastly, the family pattern was to *not* leave Yates alone with the children, because her mental state and behavior had been questionable. Unfortunately, the weekend before the drownings, Yates's husband had announced at a family gathering that he thought it would be best for her to be left alone one hour in the morning and evening so not to become overly dependent on others. Pretty outrageous.

Because the Yates case has received so much attention, it's important to bring it out in the open and discuss PPP's relationship to PPD.

Planning Ahead if You Decide to Pass Go

As the Beatles once said, "You say you got a real solution, well you know, we'd all love to see the plan." If you've already suffered from PPD and have decided to have another child, it would be simply foolish to not prepare for the possibility of another round of PPD. By putting together a comprehensive plan ahead of time, you'll be ready to deal with the illness should it arise again, and you may even be able to play a role in entirely preventing its reoccurrence. If you're ready to put together a plan, read on, because the following sections give you tips on how to be successful in your preparations.

Arming yourself early on

From telling joke punch lines to safely driving through traffic, timing is everything. In the case of your PPD plan, the right time to start putting it together is as soon as you've decided to have another baby. Even if you haven't actually started trying to get pregnant yet, it's not too early to begin putting your plan in place. In fact, the earlier you plan, the better, because by becoming the kind of "new you" capable of proactive planning, you'll decrease the chances that PPD will sneak up and surprise you. If you're a bit of a procrastinator, just remember this: To be most effective, you need to have a plan in place no later than your second trimester.

I love when women and their partners (and sometimes their whole support team) call me before the pregnancy or during early pregnancy to start discussing the plan. I know that this woman will be in good shape if PPD should surface.

If you spend the time you need to get going on your PPD plan, when you do get pregnant you'll already feel somewhat relieved and well ahead of the game. Some components of the plan will take time to put together, which is another reason to start early. For example, you'll need to spend some time talking to doctors and therapists about your history and medications. If you're taking medication for depression, anxiety, bipolar disorder, or another mood disorder, talk to a psychiatrist who specializes in medication in pregnancy. It's important to know which medications you should stay on, and which you may need to try weaning off.

Don't be surprised if certain well-meaning people in your life — whether professionals, partners, or friends — try to discourage you from putting together a PPD plan. They may try to dismiss your worry that PPD may happen again, and some people may even tell you that by thinking about it, you're making it more likely to happen. People who discourage you from putting together a plan may have a lack of information, may be in denial, or may simply be trying to help you not think about it (as if your ignorance will make it not happen). But keep in mind that not thinking about this possibility means that, like your well-meaning friends and family, you're in denial, you lack proper information that you're at high risk, or you believe that by avoiding the topic, you'll avoid the PPD. But as everyone knows deep down, sticking your head in the sand just doesn't pan out in the long run.

The good news — no, the *great* news — is that as long as you have a thorough and well-thought out plan in place, even if the PPD does surface, it won't be as bad as it was the last time around. For one thing, you know much more now. If you received proper help during your last bout with PPD, or if you're receiving good information (for example, from this book) and assistance right now, you're in good shape.

Surveying the elements of a postpartum plan

When you're in the process of creating a postpartum plan, keep in mind that the more thorough the plan, the better. A thorough plan should include at least all of the following elements:

- A list of your concerns and fears (and the concerns and fears of your partner)
- A list of professionals you want to consult. For example, you may want to contact the following:
    - Medical professionals (including a psychiatrist, if medication is in the picture)
    - Mental health professionals
    - Alternative medicine professionals, such as acupuncturists
- A list of warning behaviors that may indicate that PPD has hit you again and isn't under control or being treated effectively
- A review of what worked and what didn't work during your previous struggle with PPD, and any recommendations that may follow from this historical review
- A list of support people and support activities that you want to have in place (along with a built-in follow-up mechanism)
- A schedule of who's on duty and when during the day and night

Putting your plan on paper

Assuming that you'll remember all the details of your postpartum plan after your baby arrives is, at best, wishful thinking. Even if you can, it's better that you don't. For one, if you try to remember it, you have to continually remind and instruct all the key players. Also, the chances of misunderstandings or arguments arising are great — when a plan is written, it's more objective — not to mention the fact that your memory can be fuzzy with sleep deprivation and stress.

Identifying your concerns and fears

When people are reading self-help books of any kind and they come across an exercise involving writing something down, they often think it through but don't actually do the writing. In this case, I urge you, the mom who has already had PPD once (or more than once) and who's thinking of having another baby, to actually write down your concerns and fears. There's great power in the simple act of taking the time to actually write (or type) out what you're thinking and feeling. Writing your fears

✔ Causes you to face them head-on and puts everyone on notice — including you — that you're serious about having a much better time of things this time around.

✔ Helps you clarify what these worries actually are so you can effectively address them. (Otherwise, the worry can feel like free-floating anxiety about nothing in particular, which makes it difficult, if not impossible, to quell.)

Now is the time to get your feelings out on the table — good ones and bad ones — in order to help avoid unpleasant surprises later on and to help make this exciting next step in your journey seamless. The following suggestions may seem unimportant, and you may get the urge to skip this section. But, don't. If they make you uncomfortable, you have all the more reason to confront them. What's waiting for you (and your partner, if you have one) on the other side of these exercises is greater understanding about yourself, your partner, how to communicate honestly with each other, and what you want to create this time around as opposed to the previous one(s). It will be well worth your time.

✔ **Be completely honest as you write down your concerns, worries, and fears, even if they're pretty scary or terrible.** You may as well find out or own up to what it is you're really most afraid of with respect to PPD and having another baby. Usually your scariest worries aren't at all probable, so in the end you can let go of some unnecessary worry.

✔ **Ask your partner, if you have one, to write down his or her fears and concerns.** Having your partner do this is important for the following reasons:

• You may not know what his or her feelings are, and by having your partner write them down (or tell you so you can write them down) you'll gain the clarity needed to better understand your partner, to explain something to your partner that may shed light and resolve these worries, and to get the answers that your partner needs from the appropriate professionals.

• When you know your partner's fears and concerns, you can use the plan to address them.

• By inviting your partner into the process, you'll gain your partner's support early on.

Your partner will likely already be thinking about the possibility of PPD striking you again, so you may as well bring it out in the open (if you haven't already) and take advantage of your partner's ideas and thoughts. In this case, two heads really are better than one.

Laying out your hopes

After you've collected (in writing) your own thoughts and fears as well as your partner's, it's time to flip your thinking around. Start a new plan section in which you list how you hope this next experience will go and why you feel it will go this new, positive way.

For instance, you may want to write, "I won't have the same negative experience because I will contact professionals ahead of time and have a solid plan of action if PPD starts to occur. I will remind myself that, if I do need to deal with PPD, it isn't my fault and I'm doing a great job in taking care of it."

Create a positive scenario in a few lines or a few paragraphs, and include the fact that you've taken the time to prepare a plan that, even under the worst circumstances, will greatly help you in getting through any PPD.

Making a list of professionals to consult during pregnancy

Before you get too far in your pregnancy, you want to make sure that you're physically and mentally healthy. So, you need to consult with the right people. Trust only the professionals who have the expertise. Otherwise, ignore opinions. Here are a few suggestions:

- ✔ **Therapists, such clinical psychologists:** It's of great importance that you're working with a therapist with specialized expertise with PPD. Chapter 6 has a thorough list of types of therapists and ways to tell whether he or she has the right training.

- ✔ **Psychiatrists:** A psychiatrist is most desirable if medication has been helpful in the past because a psychiatrist can prescribe medication during your pregnancy if you need it.

- ✔ **Alternative practitioners, such as acupuncturists:** A wide variety of potential therapies can help you guard against depression and anxiety during pregnancy and postpartum. Chapter 9 may be of particular interest to you.

Creating a list of warning behaviors

If you remind yourself ahead of time of the symptoms you experienced during your first bout (or other previous experiences) with PPD, you can react to them more quickly and powerfully if you experience them this time around, which can help your situation from getting even worse.

What you want, then, is to include a list of tripwires or warning signals in your PPD plan. Just remember that this list will be specific to you. Your neighbor, who also had PPD, may have a different list of warning signs. Here are some examples of warnings to get you started on your own list:

✔ You stop enjoying things that you've always enjoyed.

✔ You start acting short with your partner, friends, or family members.

✔ You find yourself unable to sleep well at night.

If you need some more examples to jog your mind, check out Chapter 4 for an entire list of physical symptoms that accompany PPD.

Spelling out what worked and didn't work last time

Chances are that during your previous experience with PPD, some treatments didn't work for you, and other treatments didn't work at first but did as you adapted them over time. The treatments you tried may have involved meeting or working with various types of medical professionals (including alternative practitioners), interacting with your partner, children, or family members, or invoking your personal support network. As you recall your past experiences of what worked and what didn't, be ruthlessly honest with yourself, and write out a detailed list of everything relevant that you can remember. By scoping out your past successes and disappointments, you're far more likely to have only successes this time around.

Naming your support people and the activities you enjoy

PPD is never easy, but having support people and activities you enjoy — as much as enjoyment is possible for you at the time — is an invaluable piece of the plan. Hopefully, the last time around, you were able to get support from your family members, friends, and even neighbors. If, unfortunately, you didn't have this support, you probably felt isolated and overwhelmed and wished you had more support from those who you know care about you.

When you're feeling depressed and overwhelmed, nothing is quite as helpful as someone who cares. So, you want to set up a strong system of support people ahead of time, just in case PPD rears its ugly head again (see Chapter 14 for more on putting together a support team). Every new mother should have a strong support system with or without PPD, but these special people will be specifically tuned in and ready to take action if necessary. When setting up your support system, follow these steps:

1. **Let your friends and family members know that you're pregnant again and that you have a fairly high chance of getting PPD again.**

2. **Give them the list of warning signs you've prepared (see the section "Creating a list of warning behaviors" earlier in this chapter).**

   Your closest support people need to have that list of warning signs to watch out for so they can intervene on your behalf if necessary. Give them permission to act without being asked if they see it's necessary. For instance, give them permission to talk to you about what they're observing to get your feedback or insight or to call your therapist or doctor to ask for guidance.

3. **Ask (today) for their support in the future, even though you don't necessarily need their help right now.**

   If PPD does strike again, you won't have to ask for their help out of the blue when you're already feeling badly.

To make this preparation even more effective, ask them now for *specific* help in the future. For example, ask your support people for help with babysitting, preparing meals, doing the laundry for you once a week, and so on. Keep this list of people on your fridge or by your phone for easy reference. This part of the plan can be put into action with or without PPD.

Ignore the support people "shoulds." For example, ignore those people who want to be invited to your home (Aunt Betty who can't wait to nitpick at your parenting style) or those other people who are pressuring you to include (your Aunt Betty's friend who's sister's daughter had a particularly stressful week of the baby blues). Your gut knows that these people aren't really good for you. Use what you learned during your last bout of PPD, because some factors you aren't in control of, but, fortunately, this one you are.

In addition to putting together a list of prepared ("pre-asked") support people, it can also be helpful to put together a list of activities that you previously found helpful (or would have found helpful) when battling PPD. Walking in the park, going to the movies, swimming at a local pool in the summer — whatever it is, if you think it will help or at least distract you, you'll be far more likely to actually do it if it's already in your plan before PPD shows up. (Check out Chapter 12 for more ideas of how to take care of yourself.)

Undergoing professional consultations

Here are some of the main consultations that you should receive after you've decided to have another baby:

- ✔ **A thorough physical evaluation:** This evaluation should take place before you get pregnant or early during your pregnancy, both for your sake and the baby's sake — this is a good idea for any woman, not just one who's at high risk for PPD. If any health issue needs to be addressed, you can take care of it (depending on what it is, of course) before you get pregnant. Many health issues can be treated during pregnancy as well, so the sooner they're handled, the better it is for all concerned. Your thyroid should be checked as part of this evaluation, too, because a dysfunctioning thyroid can cause physical and mental health problems. Refer to Chapter 2, which tells you specifically what the doctor should be looking for.

> ✔ **A PPD screening:** Your OB's office should give you this screening every trimester to make sure no signs of depression are rearing their ugly heads.
>
> ✔ **A complete psychiatric evaluation:** If you've previously suffered from PPD, make sure you receive this evaluation from a therapist who's qualified with specialized expertise to check out your mental health (see Chapter 6 on how to find one).

Considering an antidepressant as a preventive means

Taking medication (antidepressants) during pregnancy as a prevention of PPD is an area of controversy within the medical community — even among those specializing in treating PPD. Most believe that the benefit of preventing a probable and potentially serious illness (or at least lessening its effects) is worth the possible unknown risk to the baby. The reasoning is that because an antidepressant can take a few weeks to start working, it makes sense to start the medication in the third trimester to give the medication time. If she starts medication only after the PPD hits, during the weeks that she's waiting for the medication to start working, mom spends her precious time being depressed instead of enjoying her baby.

For the purposes of writing this section, please note that I am using the word "medication" to mean antidepressant medication. There are other types of medication that you shouldn't use during pregnancy. This is another reason why you need to work with a psychiatrist or other MD who has specialized training in this area.

Many people (including doctors without specialized training) believe that a depressed pregnant women should take the lowest dose of medication possible —just enough to take the edge off. This theory isn't true. The goal is to take the lowest *effective* dose possible, which is a very different idea. The woman should be treated to 100 percent wellness. It's important not to be undertreated, because that situation can lead to chronic depression.

Ultimately, of course, the decision to take (or not take) medications during pregnancy and breastfeeding (if you choose to breastfeed) is yours and yours alone because only you know how you really feel. Still, if you have a partner, it's a big help if he is on board with you. So, when you're collecting information, have him accompany you to your doctor or psychiatrist appointments so he can ask questions and voice possible concerns as you're making your decision.

Understanding the effects of depression and meds on fetuses

Until a few years ago, most of the focus with respect to taking medications while pregnant was on the possibility of harming the fetus. Today, the focus has shifted to the possible harm to the fetus from *not* taking medications if the pregnant woman needs them to relieve ongoing depression.

Women sometimes abruptly take themselves off their antidepressants or are told by misinformed doctors to abruptly stop when the women find out they're pregnant. Fifty to 75 percent of women relapse after discontinuing medication abruptly, and over 40 percent resume medication during the pregnancy, which is thought to be even riskier for the fetus. First, before the woman knows she's pregnant, the baby is exposed to the medication. Then, the mother quickly stops the medication, so it leaves the baby's system abruptly too. Then the mom becomes ill so the baby is now exposed to both the chemicals involved in depression as well as the possible negative behavior changes (poor prenatal care, not eating well, and so on) of the mother, and then the mother resumes medication, reintroducing it into the baby's system. This scenario, which unfortunately happens way too often, is definitely not good for the baby.

On the same note, 50 percent of the women who have bipolar illness and who stop their medication when they find out they're pregnant relapse (have a manic episode, which can be dangerous) within the first three months of pregnancy. Seventy percent relapse within the first six months. These facts hopefully make the point stronger that preconception counseling, putting a plan together before the pregnancy, is critical.

Understanding the effects of depression and meds on breastfeeding babies

Even though virtually undetectable traces of certain medications have shown up in the blood of breastfeeding babies who have been tested, no serious adverse effects on these babies have ever been noted; no increased risk of malformation, miscarriage, neonatal complications or developmental problems of any kind. So, if you think you're doing your baby a favor by sacrificing your mental health by not taking an antidepressant if you need one, think again. If you're depressed or anxious, enjoying your new baby will be difficult, and this will undoubtedly do far more harm to your baby than any medication traces that may make their way to him or her. In fact, it's clear that depression and anxiety in pregnancy can chemically hurt growing babies. Depression during pregnancy can cause low birth weight and preterm delivery, and anxiety may cause harm by constricting the placental blood vessels and raising cortisol.

If for any reason you find that you're completely opposed to being on medication while you're breastfeeding, and you clearly need medication, the better choice is to take the medication and forego breastfeeding. It's far better to choose to be mentally and emotionally stable than to breastfeed your baby. Your child will benefit much more from having a comfortable, happy, and emotionally grounded mom who's present than he or she would lose from being bottle-fed with formula. And it goes without saying that if your symptoms are severe enough to impair your daily life or your ability to bond with your baby, you really have no choice but to go with medication. While there's no perfect decision without any risk (many factors have to be taken into account, including the severity of your symptoms, your comfort level with a given treatment, and how strong your support system is) not taking medication when you really need it simply isn't a viable option.

 If you aren't experiencing depression in pregnancy but want to be aggressive in trying to avert another episode of PPD, you can speak with your doctor about taking your first dose of an antidepressant right there on the delivery table and not wait and see if PPD will surface. Many women don't want to give it a chance — and who could blame them?

Trusting Your Decisions

Seeking advice from other people you trust can be useful and helpful when making the decision to have another baby. But, be careful not to ask too many people as to what they would do. Resist the temptation to ask just one more person what *she* would do (this also applies to decisions about taking medication during pregnancy or breastfeeding). Requesting advice from one person too many, especially if that person replies differently from the way others have or the way you're already leaning, may throw you into severe doubt and can turn your days into a never-ending, spinning whirlpool of worry. Usually, you'll be tempted to ask "just one more person" for advice because you want reassurance and validation that your choice is the right one.

Here are a couple of hints that can save you lots of wasted, anxious time:

✔ **The validation you're seeking can never be found outside of yourself.** Only you can be the one to reassure yourself that you made an excellent decision (of course it's nice to hear it from others, but you shouldn't *need* it). Every time you feel an urge to ask another person if you were right or what she would've done (you may get an uncomfortable anxious feeling in your stomach), don't do it. Literally stop and repeat with strength to yourself, "I made the right decision with all the information I needed." Then distract yourself if necessary.

✔ **Don't confuse feeling worried about the outcome of your decision with having made the wrong one.** If, for example, you decide to take medication for depression in pregnancy, and then you start obsessing about whether this was the right choice, don't assume that your worry means you should necessarily change your mind. If you do switch your decision, you'll inevitably find yourself doing the exact same thing with the other choice.

✔ **The quicker you can go from worrying to reassuring yourself, the better your mental health will be.** And, when you're feeling better with yourself, your relationships with your friends and family will be healthier, too.

You can't make a perfect decision, because each decision has some kind of risk. For example, taking a medication during pregnancy may have a potential risk, and not taking a medication may also have a risk. So, whatever decisions you make — whether to have another baby or whether to take medication (and when) — feel good about them. Because second-guessing is never helpful, every time one of those I-should-have-chosen-the-other-way thoughts pops into your head, say "I made my decision with good, solid, information."

Part VI
The Part of Tens

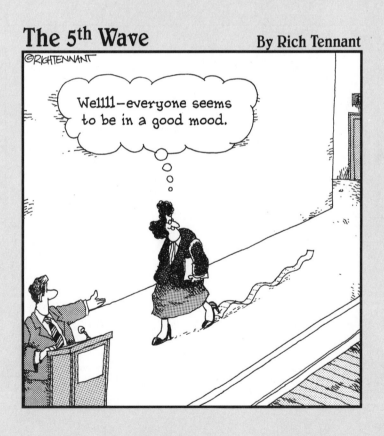

In this part . . .

When you're suffering from postpartum depression, the only thing you want to do is feel better — and you want it to be quick. Unfortunately, recovery takes time, but, in this part, I include two top-ten lists to get you the information that you need fast, including the ten most common fantasies (or myths) about motherhood and ten thoughts for you to focus on to help you get through the day.

Chapter 19

Ten Common Fantasies about Motherhood

● ●

In This Chapter

▶ Recognizing the damaging misperceptions of motherhood

▶ Doing what's right for you and your family no matter what society says

● ●

*I*n this tens chapter, I give you some of the most common myths that mothers have about motherhood. You can find plenty of mothers who actually believe that these fantasies are true. It's wonderful for them if one or more of these fantasies do come true, but the danger is when women *expect* these fantasies to happen. When women expect motherhood to be one way and it turns out the exact opposite, they feel inadequate and as if they've failed.

So, it's important not to begrudge a woman for having had one or more of these fantasies come true in her life — it's nice for her. But, at the same time, remember that just because she ran across some luck doesn't mean you've failed.

The following are ideas that many mothers, with or without depression, tend to believe. When PPD is present, however, believing these fantasies becomes even more painful because the feelings of self-worth and inadequacy are even more pronounced. In this chapter, I aim to help you blow these myths to smithereens so you can more comfortably embrace what's true and real.

This Should Be the Happiest Time in My Life

"If this is supposed to be the happiest time in my life," you may be saying, "then I'm really doomed." The truth is, when a baby first joins your family, it's more like boot camp. So don't worry if your days aren't all filled with laughs, giggles, and smiles — this is hardly the happiest time in your life! Between recovering from stitches, aching in places you didn't know existed, fatigue, hormonal sweats, mood changes, and a small but loud stranger demanding full-time care with no manual of directions, it's no wonder that you shouldn't expect this to be the happiest time in your life. You can certainly have joyful times during this period (finding these times is easier if you have only a mild case of PPD), but most of the happy times come later.

1 Should Be Able to Do Everything Myself

Today's society values self-reliance to the point that people are often embarrassed to ask for help. They're embarrassed because dependence, unfortunately, is often still equated with weakness. So, the faster you can free yourself from that unenlightened point of view, the better. Just remember that emotional, social, and physical support is necessary for everyone — even when there's no baby and no depression.

As an example of society's love of self-reliance, consider how many mothers (with partners to share the duties!) work full time outside the home and still expect themselves to have dinner ready immediately after work. Who made that rule? More importantly, why would anyone allow this rule to continue? Mothers who work inside their homes taking care of their children know very well that their efforts equate to more than a full-time job. To expect yourself to take care of a child and then have dinner made is asking a lot of yourself. If you're able to achieve this feat sometimes, kudos to you, but don't expect it. I suggest that if you have a partner or support person living with you, you share who puts dinner on the table. Or, decide that whoever makes dinner shouldn't be watching the children at the same time.

With any other new job, you'd have a mentor showing you the ropes, and the first three months would be an introductory period in which you didn't have a full workload. So, as you get used to your new job as mom, cut yourself some slack.

1 Shouldn't Need Breaks

A myth that often accompanies this damaging fantasy is, "If I love my child enough, I shouldn't need a break from her." There's also the one that says, "My child is my responsibility. I don't feel right asking other people to take care of her." But, the truth is that every mom needs a break (and she isn't a bad mom for believing so).

There are many different kinds of breaks to choose from. There's the quickie ten minutes alone to take a shower kind and the spontaneous kind you get when your baby naps (unfortunately you never know for sure how long you'll get). And then there's the really nurturing kind that I focus on here. I describe this nurturing kind as at least two hours off duty to do something pleasurable for yourself. In other words, someone else is watching the children. You can be in your home or not, and it can take place at any time of the day. It doesn't matter as long as you follow the pleasure and off-duty rules. If you're a stay-at-home mom, you should aim for at least four two-hour breaks per week (I go into detail on how you can manage this in Chapter 12).

Breaks are mandated by law for almost all jobs. These laws are in place so employers can't abuse workers by refusing to let them take care of their needs. If you're working in your home, you're your own employer. It's up to you to make sure your needs are being taken care of so you stay healthy, both physically and emotionally, and so you can be the mother and wife you truly want to be. Raising a baby is labor of love, but it's still labor. By taking breaks, you'll also be modeling healthy habits to your little ones.

My Life Won't Change That Much

A major fantasy that many pregnant women have is that they'll be able to take their babies everywhere they go. These women are in the camp that says it'll just be your life plus a baby — no big deal. They think that a baby is really portable: Just pop him into a baby carrier and off you go to that fancy restaurant. He'll sleep right through dinner and you and your partner will gaze romantically into each other's eyes, and no one in the restaurant will be disturbed. Are you laughing out loud yet?

One of the best things you (and your partner, if you have one) can do, is acknowledge the many ways your life will change — or is already changing — when a baby is present. For example, simply leaving the house with an infant in tow can take hours — even for a woman who's mentally healthy. With depression and anxiety added to the mix, even the simplest of tasks are over-whelming and worrisome. What you'll be able to do with your baby depends on many factors, two of which are the temperament of your child and your mental health. So, no matter what anyone else tells you, it's okay if the family camping trip with your baby has to wait.

My Needs Shouldn't Matter

If one person in the family unit is continually sacrificing his or her needs, the family unit can't be healthy. On the other hand, however, I don't mean that everyone's needs will be fulfilled at all times — that just isn't realistic, especially with children. It isn't always going to be exactly even every day, but the main point here is that, in order to have a happy and healthy family, each member of the family — young and old — needs to experience a family life in which all members "count." A child can't easily grow up to feel that she's important and that her needs matter if she sees her dad constantly squashing his own needs. And, if the child is the only one who's nurtured for years, her parents will burn out and it won't be a happy home. So, it's good for each member, including young ones, to learn to wait their turn and consider other people's needs and wants.

The bottom line is that the days of the self-sacrificing woman who buries herself under loads of laundry and says, "That's okay, in a few years I'll be able to see my friends again" are over. It's not selfish to take care of yourself emotionally, spiritually, and physically. Rather, your family benefits tremendously when you take care of yourself in these ways on a regular basis.

Bonding Happens Immediately at Birth

With certain species, bonding is fairly immediate after birth (for example, geese). But for humans, bonding is a gradual process in which the mom and baby learn how to communicate with each other. The mom is taught, so to speak, by her baby what his signals mean, which allows her to learn how to respond to him. So, as you get to know your baby and spend time with him, bonding will happen more and more. Unfortunately, the depression and anxiety caused by your PPD can often interfere with the bonding feelings for your new baby.

Your baby is still bonding with you, even if you aren't feeling much for him. He knows you're mom — he's quite familiar with your smell, heartbeat, and voice. When the PPD and anxiety lift, though, all those feelings that you were looking forward to feeling for your baby will be there — they aren't gone forever as so many moms seem to believe.

For example, there's so much unnecessary worry from moms who are separated from their infants at birth (due to health complications of either mom or baby). They're anxious that the so-called "magic moment" is forever lost and that bonding won't ever happen. Just remember, even infants who need to stay in the hospital for days, weeks, or months still bond fine with their moms. And rest assured that even though your baby will feel comforted and safe with the nurses at the hospital, no one will ever be able to replace you. If bonding only occurred immediately after birth, many adopted babies couldn't bond with their adoptive moms — and you know that doesn't make sense.

Breastfeeding Is Natural, So It Should Come Easily

Stress is suddenly having two watermelons hanging from your chest and thinking you should automatically know what to do with them. After all, women have been breastfeeding for thousands of years — how difficult could it be? No matter how many classes you've taken with a doll positioned at your breast, having a real, squirming, chomping, fussing newborn is a whole different experience.

Even when you figure out how to position yourself and the baby just right, more challenges can arise if your baby refuses to nurse or has a difficult time latching on. When this happens, some moms will say "My baby doesn't like me." (I tell nurses in the postpartum unit that this type of statement is a warning sign of a depressed mom.) So, just remember that when a baby has difficulty or doesn't want to nurse, which is extremely common, this has nothing to do with you — it's not personal.

Mothering Is Instinctual

Parenting, like many things, is learned by trial and error — it isn't at all instinctual. After all, there's a reason why so many parenting books are on the market — every parent is searching frantically for the answers. If mothering came naturally, none of these books would be sold. To make things even more complicated, one method of sleep-training, for instance, may work for your first child but not at all for your second. So, as a parent, it's back to the drawing board.

During my first bout with PPD, I remember thinking "The next person who tells me that I should just 'know' what my baby's cries mean will get a pie in the face." Either that or I'd start crying because I felt so inadequate. All my daughter's cries sounded identical. If you feel the same, it doesn't mean you're a bad mom. And it doesn't mean you aren't "in tune" enough with your child. Some babies are just more difficult to read both visually and audibly. Just don't take it personally. In fact, if you ask your partner or a support person if he or she can tell the difference between your baby's cries, chances are you'll see you're not the only one.

I Should Feel Satisfied Being a Stay-at-Home Mom

Some women, even if they held high-powered positions in the workplace before parenthood, feel satisfied working full time at home with their children. If this is you, it may have taken you by surprise. If you're pleased with your reaction, great. If you're embarrassed and think, "This shouldn't be enough to fulfill me," remember that the most liberated attitude you can have is total acceptance for whatever it is you feel. Discard the "shoulds."

On the other hand, some women, in order to be the best moms they can be, need to have their intellect stimulated and need to have interesting adult interaction at work outside the home. This is totally normal and it doesn't make you a bad mom. Remember: To each her own.

Even when you think that you'll love staying home, you can never tell until you're there. Most importantly, remember that no one has the "right" answer. Whatever works the best for you and your family is the right answer for you.

My Baby Will Be My Companion

You can and will, I'm sure, have lots of fun mother-child time together, especially as your PPD lifts. Enjoying each other's company is special and is something to treasure. Be careful with this fantasy, though, because it's one that places unfair expectations onto your child. If you need your child to keep you company, you may end up running into problems, especially as she gets older and would, for example, rather play with a friend instead of you (which is normal).

If you're having (or have had) a baby to, say, take care of your own loneliness or another need of yours, I suggest you find a therapist right away. Expecting a child to fill your void is inappropriate at best, and is a set-up for you both. Especially as your child grows up, becomes more independent, and starts voicing her opinions, it will be extra challenging for both of you if you're expecting your child to take care of your needs. She has her own, and they need to be respected. And she needs a mom who will take care of her own needs as well.

Chapter 20

Ten Thoughts to Focus on Throughout the Day

*R*epeating truths to yourself is quite powerful and can advance your postpartum depression (PPD) recovery in a huge way (and likewise, repeating falsehoods can greatly slow it down). So, in this chapter, I give you ten positive thoughts to focus on. You may have a difficult time feeling the truth of these statements at first because the PPD makes you doubt your worth. But, this difficult and doubtful time is when you need to focus on these statements the most.

PPD Is an Illness, Not a Weakness

No matter what you think or what you may hear from others who don't have experience or training in dealing with PPD, postpartum depression is not a character flaw or a personality weakness. PPD is a diagnosable mood disorder with real causes, symptoms, and treatments (refer to Chapters 2 and 4 for a list of physical and emotional symptoms). And, PPD is 100 percent treatable when the right kind of help is received.

Just as you wouldn't put someone down for getting cancer, it makes no sense to blame yourself for being hit with postpartum depression.

Seeking Help is Courageous

Courage is when you feel scared or otherwise uncomfortable, but you *do what it takes anyway*. Seeking and receiving help when you need it is smart and strong (and, well, courageous!). The great news is that, unlike when I went through my bouts of PPD in the 80s, excellent help is available for you now. I remember how just moving from one room to another was an effort, which meant that making a phone call to get help (or buying a book on the topic) was out of the question. Even if you've done nothing else yet, you're reading this book, and that's worth an acknowledgment. Whatever you're doing to move forward toward full recovery, no matter how miniscule those steps may seem, congratulate yourself and consider these baby steps excellent progress.

I'm a Good Mom

Before you write me off for good, hear me out: You truly are a good mom. Good moms want to do whatever they can to recover, because they know that their children will reap the benefits too (and you obviously fall into this camp or you wouldn't have bought this book). If you had PPD before, and you were unable to reach out for help that time, please don't feel bad. I'm just glad that you now feel ready to get help.

By reading this book, you're taking action to help yourself and your family, and therefore, you're clearly a good mom. Even if you're raising your voice at those you love, and sometimes think, "I don't want to be a mom," or "I want to give my baby away," or if you have scary thoughts about your baby, don't worry, you're still a good mom. You're a good mom who just needs help. Even if you're in the hospital or otherwise unable to care for your baby in person, you're still a good mom. A good mom makes sure that even if she can't care for her children physically or emotionally, someone else is.

PPD is Temporary — I Will Recover

Out of the 15,000 women who I've counseled individually and in groups, I have yet to meet anyone who doesn't fully recover from postpartum depression when given proper care. But these women all have another thing in common: At one time or another during their illnesses, each one of them doubted that she'd ever be well again. The nature of depression makes it difficult to see a future at all, let alone a positive one. Each mom thinks that she's the only one who has ever felt this bad, and that she'll be the first one who's unable to come through the tunnel. Remind yourself frequently that "this too shall pass."

It's Important That I Take Care of Myself

Taking care of yourself isn't a luxury — it's an absolute necessity (see Chapter 12). Your health (and your family's health) depends on it. You, along with many other women, may have been socialized to believe that when you become a mother your needs — even basic ones such as sleeping and eating — shouldn't matter any more. But, if you take a good look at the healthiest, happiest, and most fulfilled mothers around you, they're probably making sure that they're caring for themselves too.

Now, take a look at your own life: What are those things that you know you need to do to take care of yourself? Why are these important for you to do? What will happen to you and those around you if you don't do these things? If nothing else inspires you to take care of yourself, think of it this way: By doing so, you'll be modeling healthful behavior for your children — when your kids are older, they will do exactly what they saw you do as they grew up.

I'm Doing the Best I Can

So maybe you aren't functioning the way you want to or maybe you aren't reacting with the patience you think you ought to these days. Don't worry. Just remember that you're doing the best you can. Your "best" will get better as you recover, but at any given time, you're doing what you can with what's available.

If you tend to be a perfectionist, you may argue that you aren't doing your best. If this is the case, be careful not to define *best* as *perfect*. Accept your progress and give yourself credit for what you're doing well, instead of focusing on what you're unable to do right now.

To keep your perspective in the positive, contemplate how you're doing your best in at least five ways (trying to smile at your baby, getting out of bed in the morning, preparing breakfast for yourself, and so on).

I'm Practicing Love toward Myself

It's normal to feel frustrated when you've been feeling pretty good for a week or two, and then you suddenly dip (check out Chapter 11 for more on handling PPD dips). However, it's important not to blame yourself or yell at yourself for the dip. Instead, have patience and say, "Like it or not, this is the nature of the illness, and it's not my fault."

You're allowed to not enjoy the fact that you're still dealing with this illness, and you're allowed to look forward to being totally well, you just have to be kind to yourself. So, you need to speak to yourself the same way you'd speak to a friend who was handling a stubborn illness — with compassion. You wouldn't say to your friend, "What's wrong with you? Why can't you get rid of your cancer sooner — what's taking you so long?" Instead, you'd say, "Wow, this illness must be difficult for you. Hang in there — you're getting better, and you're doing a great job."

I'm Surrounding Myself with Positives

Support should feel good and should be positive, so right now, you want to be around only positive people and things. Positive people will be encouraging, helpful, and reassuring — not judgmental, demanding, or critical. As far as positive *things* go, you should stick to positive books, movies, and TV shows that make you feel good (preferably comedies). Listen to happy music, such as upbeat Broadway tunes, the Beatles (I'm dating myself), or soothing and relaxing melodies like those you'd hear during a massage. Avoid the news shows at all costs! They're filled with fear-producing negativity of all types, none of which will help you recover. Stay away from the Internet unless you're visiting a trusted site with a positive influence, such as www.postpartumdepressionhelp.com and www.postpartum.net.

PPD Isn't My Fault

You didn't cause your PPD, so don't blame yourself. Women (especially depressed women who have low self-esteem) are always ready to blame themselves for anything and everything — even their own illnesses. PPD happens to women of all personalities, ethnicities, backgrounds, and habits. I once had a client who was convinced that if she had eaten more broccoli after her baby was born, she wouldn't have suffered from PPD — and she now knows that idea was a bunch of bologna.

I'm Not Alone

Because of your PPD, you may feel like you're all alone. And even worse is that symptom that makes you feel alone even when you're surrounded by people who love you. I painfully remember being at a family party when I was suffering from PPD. I knew rationally that many of the people there cared about me, but I still felt like I was in a dark, isolated box where no one could reach me. Just remember that you're in good company: About one in five mothers are feeling what you're feeling right now.

Appendix

Resources

• •

A s you probably know, it's easy to get lost in a maze of resources on the Internet, in the bookstore, and in the phonebook when you start searching. And, unfortunately, many of those resources may not be as helpful as they claim. So, here I provide you those that I think may offer you the most help.

Web Sites

This section lists just a few of the excellent Web sites that may be of use to you. Some are clinical and research-oriented for those of you who want to study the latest data, while others are more for locating support and helping you on a practical level.

As always, if you're obsessive or anxious, stay off the Internet until you're better because browsing can make you even more anxious. If you want to ask a support person to search for you, however, go right ahead. Either way, to make it easier, I have listed specific sites that have reliable information. This way, you or your support person won't have to start from scratch and screen the sites yourselves.

Information

The following sites all provide you with accurate and reliable information about postpartum depression — from professional journal articles to those for the general public:

- **Pregnancyanddepression.com:** At this site, you can find professional medical articles on the treatment of depression during pregnancy.

- **Depression Central** (`www.psycom.net/depression.central.post-partum.html`): This site has information regarding the many depressive disorders. You can also find helpful links to specific information and materials regarding postpartum depression.

- **Womensmentalhealth.org:** Here you have access to the latest research regarding mood disorders during pregnancy and postpartum.

- **U.S. Department of Health and Human Services:** (`www.4woman.gov/faq/postpartum.htm`): This is a site sponsored by the federal government that gives solid information about depression during and after pregnancy.

Support resources

If you're in need of some support, take a look at the following organizations' Web sites, which are specifically set up to provide support to you when you contact them:

- **Postpartum Assistance for Mothers** (`www.postpartumdepressionhelp.com`): I founded Postpartum Assistance for Mothers in 1988 as I was recovering from my second serious, undiagnosed bout with postpartum depression. This organization provides individual assessments and consultation by phone or Webcam to women nationally and internationally. My organization also provides training for support group leaders, hospital staff, and all the various medical and mental health professionals who are working with pregnant and postpartum women. A free e-zine informs readers about upcoming postpartum trainings.

  The best way to reach me is through my Web Site, but feel free to write me at Dr. Shoshana Bennett, 342 South Overlook Drive, San Ramon, CA 94582; phone 925-735-3099.

- **PostpartumDads** (`www.postpartumdads.org`): This volunteer outreach project (in association with Postpartum Support International) gives new dads information on how to deal with a partner who has postpartum depression. They can also read stories from other dads about their experiences with PPD. Dads who feel as if they're being rejected by their partners due to PPD can also get advice here.

- **The Online PPD Support Group** (`www.ppdsupportpage.com`): At this site, women and their friends and families can get information, support, and assistance in dealing with postpartum disorders. This site has real-time chats, discussion forums, and other downloads and resources.

  You can contact the group at 821 S. Avenida Del Oro E, Pueblo West, CO 81007.

- **www.postpartumexperience.com:** This is a site full of resources for women suffering from postpartum depression.

- **The Pacific Post Partum Support Society** (`www.postpartum.org`): This is a nonprofit society that provides support to women and families experiencing depression or anxiety related to the birth or adoption of a baby.

You can contact the society at #104-1416 Commercial Dr., Vancouver, BC (Canada) V5L 3X9; phone 604-255-7999.

✔ **The Ruth Rhoden Craven Foundation, Inc., for Postpartum Depression Awareness** (`www.ppdsupport.org`): This foundation is a nonprofit organization providing information and support to women suffering from postpartum depression and their families. The foundation also aims to serve as a resource to those in the medical community.

You can contact the foundation at 1339 Outreach Ln., Mt. Pleasant, SC 29464; phone 843-881-2047.

Support Numbers

You can call the numbers in this section for information and support. The first number listed (Motherisk) is for information only. However, the last three toll-free numbers provide support to the suffering mom through trained volunteers. Keep these numbers handy as you go through the PPD recovery process because it's always good to be within arm's reach of someone who understands and who can lend a compassionate ear.

✔ **Motherisk (416-813-6780):** This hotline is an excellent resource for pregnant and breastfeeding women. When you call, you can receive answers to questions about the risk or safety of medications, herbs, diseases, or chemical exposure.

✔ **Postpartum Stressline (888-678-2669):** All of the trained volunteers at this stressline are survivors of postpartum depression, and they're hoping to help others (you) who are now going through what they did.

✔ **Postpartum Support International (800-944-4773):** This postpartum hotline has well-trained volunteers waiting to answer your questions.

✔ **National Hopeline Network (800-773-6667)**

International Organizations

A few excellent international organizations are devoted specifically to maternal mental health. Any therapist or MD who claims to be a specialist in this field should be a member of at least one of these organizations. Although any individual will gain a plethora of knowledge by joining one or more of these organizations, I indicate in my description of each organization whether it's mainly geared toward professionals or the public.

Postpartum Support International

Postpartum Support International (PSI) is an international network that focuses on postpartum mental health and social support. It was formed on June 26, 1987, in Santa Barbara, California, by Jane Honikman who's the founding director. The purpose of the organization is to increase awareness among public and professional communities about the emotional changes that women often experience during pregnancy and after the birth of their babies. PSI holds an annual conference and mails a quarterly newsletter to members. This organization is primarily geared toward the public, but an increasing number of professionals are joining. You can find out more about PSI at www.postpartum.net.

You can contact Postpartum Support International at 927 N. Kellogg Ave., Santa Barbara, CA 93111; phone 805-967-7636; support line 800-944-4773.

Marcé Society

The Marcé society (www.marcesociety.com) was formed at an International Conference in 1980. The purpose of that conference was to bring together different strands of research in postpartum mental disorders. The society was named after Louis Victor Marcé, a French psychiatrist who wrote the first treatise entirely devoted to postpartum mental illness, published in 1858. This organization is mainly geared for professionals, and members receive an annual newsletter.

The principal aim of the society is to promote, facilitate and communicate about research into all aspects of the mental health of women, their infants and partners around the time of childbirth. This involves a broad range of research activities ranging from basic science through to health services research.

The Society encourages involvement from all disciplines, as well as consumer and self-help groups. It also holds an international meeting every two years that brings together researchers, clinicians and consumers from around the world.

You can contact the president of the Marcé Society, Dr. Carol Henshaw MD FRCPsych, via e-mail at chenshaw@doctors.org.uk.

North American Society for Psychosocial Obstetrics and Gynecology (NASPOG)

The aim of NASPOG is to foster scholarly, scientific, and clinical study of the biopsychosocial aspects of obstetric and gynecologic medicine. This organization was formed in 1971. It had been a special interest group of the

American College of Obstetricians and Gynecologists and remains an affiliate. There's an annual conference presenting the latest research, which serves as a forum for scientific and clinical discussions. NASPOG is mainly geared to researchers and practitioners. Members will receive an annual journal called *Archives of Women's Mental Health,* which contains the latest research.

You can contact NASPOG at 409 12th Street, S.W., Washington, D.C. 20024; phone 202-863-1628; Web site www.naspog.org.

Further Reading

For those of you who are thirsty for more, you may enjoy reading the following books. They're filled with the real scoop (and sprinkled with humor) about the joys and challenges of motherhood:

- ✔ *Beyond the Blues: A Guide to Understanding and Treating Prenatal and Postpartum Depression:* Written by Shoshana S. Bennett, PhD, and Pec Indman, EdD, MFT, and published in both English and Spanish, this concise guide describes mood disorders in pregnancy and postpartum, and gives you information on what to do about them (Moodswings Press, 2006).

- ✔ *Why Didn't Anyone Tell Me? True Stories of New Motherhood:* In this book, which is compiled by Melanie Bowden, first-time moms tell what worked and what didn't as they adjusted to parenting, including info on conflicts with relatives, colic, single-parenting, C-sections, and babies who are ill (Booklocker.com, Inc, 2006).

- ✔ *Mother Shock: Tales from the First Year and Beyond, Loving Every (Other) Minute of It:* Written by Andrea Buchanan, this personal account of the challenges of new motherhood is at times humorous. It provides an honest look at many things, including ambivalent feelings about motherhood (Seal Press, 2003).

- ✔ *The Birth of a Mother: How the Motherhood Experience Changes You Forever:* This book, written by Daniel Stern and Nadia Bruschweiler-Stern, approaches the psychological and emotional changes and experiences associated with becoming a mother (Basic Books, 1998).

Index

BUSINESS, CAREERS & PERSONAL FINANCE

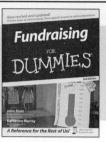

0-7645-9847-3

0-7645-2431-3

Also available:
- Business Plans Kit For Dummies
  0-7645-9794-9
- Economics For Dummies
  0-7645-5726-2
- Grant Writing For Dummies
  0-7645-8416-2
- Home Buying For Dummies
  0-7645-5331-3
- Managing For Dummies
  0-7645-1771-6
- Marketing For Dummies
  0-7645-5600-2

- Personal Finance For Dummies
  0-7645-2590-5*
- Resumes For Dummies
  0-7645-5471-9
- Selling For Dummies
  0-7645-5363-1
- Six Sigma For Dummies
  0-7645-6798-5
- Small Business Kit For Dummies
  0-7645-5984-2
- Starting an eBay Business For Dummies
  0-7645-6924-4
- Your Dream Career For Dummies
  0-7645-9795-7

HOME & BUSINESS COMPUTER BASICS

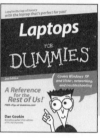

0-470-05432-8

0-471-75421-8

Also available:
- Cleaning Windows Vista For Dummies
  0-471-78293-9
- Excel 2007 For Dummies
  0-470-03737-7
- Mac OS X Tiger For Dummies
  0-7645-7675-5
- MacBook For Dummies
  0-470-04859-X
- Macs For Dummies
  0-470-04849-2
- Office 2007 For Dummies
  0-470-00923-3

- Outlook 2007 For Dummies
  0-470-03830-6
- PCs For Dummies
  0-7645-8958-X
- Salesforce.com For Dummies
  0-470-04893-X
- Upgrading & Fixing Laptops For Dummies
  0-7645-8959-8
- Word 2007 For Dummies
  0-470-03658-3
- Quicken 2007 For Dummies
  0-470-04600-7

FOOD, HOME, GARDEN, HOBBIES, MUSIC & PETS

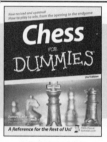

0-7645-8404-9

0-7645-9904-6

Also available:
- Candy Making For Dummies
  0-7645-9734-5
- Card Games For Dummies
  0-7645-9910-0
- Crocheting For Dummies
  0-7645-4151-X
- Dog Training For Dummies
  0-7645-8418-9
- Healthy Carb Cookbook For Dummies
  0-7645-8476-6
- Home Maintenance For Dummies
  0-7645-5215-5

- Horses For Dummies
  0-7645-9797-3
- Jewelry Making & Beading For Dummies
  0-7645-2571-9
- Orchids For Dummies
  0-7645-6759-4
- Puppies For Dummies
  0-7645-5255-4
- Rock Guitar For Dummies
  0-7645-5356-9
- Sewing For Dummies
  0-7645-6847-7
- Singing For Dummies
  0-7645-2475-5

INTERNET & DIGITAL MEDIA

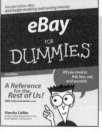

0-470-04529-9

0-470-04894-8

Also available:
- Blogging For Dummies
  0-471-77084-1
- Digital Photography For Dummies
  0-7645-9802-3
- Digital Photography All-in-One Desk Reference For Dummies
  0-470-03743-1
- Digital SLR Cameras and Photography For Dummies
  0-7645-9803-1
- eBay Business All-in-One Desk Reference For Dummies
  0-7645-8438-3
- HDTV For Dummies
  0-470-09673-X

- Home Entertainment PCs For Dummies
  0-470-05523-5
- MySpace For Dummies
  0-470-09529-6
- Search Engine Optimization For Dummies
  0-471-97998-8
- Skype For Dummies
  0-470-04891-3
- The Internet For Dummies
  0-7645-8996-2
- Wiring Your Digital Home For Dummies
  0-471-91830-X

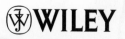

SPORTS, FITNESS, PARENTING, RELIGION & SPIRITUALITY

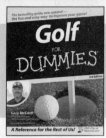

0-471-76871-5

0-7645-7841-3

Also available:
- Catholicism For Dummies
  0-7645-5391-7
- Exercise Balls For Dummies
  0-7645-5623-1
- Fitness For Dummies
  0-7645-7851-0
- Football For Dummies
  0-7645-3936-1
- Judaism For Dummies
  0-7645-5299-6
- Potty Training For Dummies
  0-7645-5417-4
- Buddhism For Dummies
  0-7645-5359-3

- Pregnancy For Dummies
  0-7645-4483-7 †
- Ten Minute Tone-Ups For Dummies
  0-7645-7207-5
- NASCAR For Dummies
  0-7645-7681-X
- Religion For Dummies
  0-7645-5264-3
- Soccer For Dummies
  0-7645-5229-5
- Women in the Bible For Dummies
  0-7645-8475-8

TRAVEL

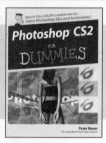

0-7645-7749-2

0-7645-6945-7

Also available:
- Alaska For Dummies
  0-7645-7746-8
- Cruise Vacations For Dummies
  0-7645-6941-4
- England For Dummies
  0-7645-4276-1
- Europe For Dummies
  0-7645-7529-5
- Germany For Dummies
  0-7645-7823-5
- Hawaii For Dummies
  0-7645-7402-7

- Italy For Dummies
  0-7645-7386-1
- Las Vegas For Dummies
  0-7645-7382-9
- London For Dummies
  0-7645-4277-X
- Paris For Dummies
  0-7645-7630-5
- RV Vacations For Dummies
  0-7645-4442-X
- Walt Disney World & Orlando
  For Dummies
  0-7645-9660-8

GRAPHICS, DESIGN & WEB DEVELOPMENT

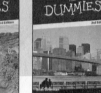

0-7645-8815-X

0-7645-9571-7

Also available:
- 3D Game Animation For Dummies
  0-7645-8789-7
- AutoCAD 2006 For Dummies
  0-7645-8925-3
- Building a Web Site For Dummies
  0-7645-7144-3
- Creating Web Pages For Dummies
  0-470-08030-2
- Creating Web Pages All-in-One Desk
  Reference For Dummies
  0-7645-4345-8
- Dreamweaver 8 For Dummies
  0-7645-9649-7

- InDesign CS2 For Dummies
  0-7645-9572-5
- Macromedia Flash 8 For Dummies
  0-7645-9691-8
- Photoshop CS2 and Digital
  Photography For Dummies
  0-7645-9580-6
- Photoshop Elements 4 For Dummies
  0-471-77483-9
- Syndicating Web Sites with RSS Feeds
  For Dummies
  0-7645-8848-6
- Yahoo! SiteBuilder For Dummies
  0-7645-9800-7

NETWORKING, SECURITY, PROGRAMMING & DATABASES

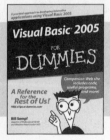

0-7645-7728-X

0-471-74940-0

Also available:
- Access 2007 For Dummies
  0-470-04612-0
- ASP.NET 2 For Dummies
  0-7645-7907-X
- C# 2005 For Dummies
  0-7645-9704-3
- Hacking For Dummies
  0-470-05235-X
- Hacking Wireless Networks
  For Dummies
  0-7645-9730-2
- Java For Dummies
  0-470-08716-1

- Microsoft SQL Server 2005 For Dummies
  0-7645-7755-7
- Networking All-in-One Desk Reference
  For Dummies
  0-7645-9939-9
- Preventing Identity Theft For Dummies
  0-7645-7336-5
- Telecom For Dummies
  0-471-77085-X
- Visual Studio 2005 All-in-One Desk
  Reference For Dummies
  0-7645-9775-2
- XML For Dummies
  0-7645-8845-1